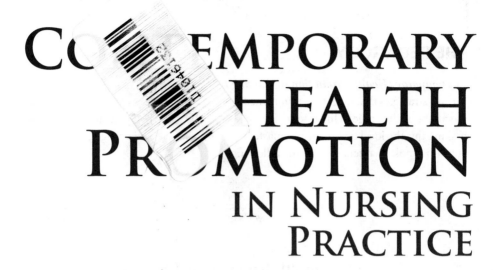

CONTEMPORARY HEALTH PROMOTION
IN NURSING PRACTICE

THE PEDAGOGY

Contemporary Health Promotion in Nursing Practice drives comprehension through various strategies that meet the learning needs of students, while also generating enthusiasm about the topic. This interactive approach addresses different learning styles, making this the ideal text to ensure mastery of key concepts. The pedagogical aids that appear in most chapters include the following:

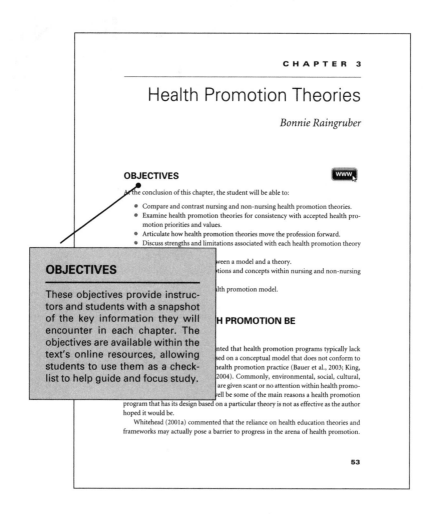

CHAPTER 3

Health Promotion Theories

Bonnie Raingruber

OBJECTIVES

At the conclusion of this chapter, the student will be able to:

- Compare and contrast nursing and non-nursing health promotion theories.
- Examine health promotion theories for consistency with accepted health promotion priorities and values.
- Articulate how health promotion theories move the profession forward.
- Discuss strengths and limitations associated with each health promotion theory

between a model and a theory.

tions and concepts within nursing and non-nursing

health promotion model.

OBJECTIVES

These objectives provide instructors and students with a snapshot of the key information they will encounter in each chapter. The objectives are available within the text's online resources, allowing students to use them as a checklist to help guide and focus study.

H PROMOTION BE

nted that health promotion programs typically lack sed on a conceptual model that does not conform to health promotion practice (Bauer et al., 2003; King, 2004). Commonly, environmental, social, cultural, are given scant or no attention within health promo-ell be some of the main reasons a health promotion program that has its design based on a particular theory is not as effective as the author hoped it would be.

Whitehead (2001a) commented that the reliance on health education theories and frameworks may actually pose a barrier to progress in the arena of health promotion.

healthcare redesign must involve utilizing the nursing workforce to transition the United States healthcare system to a health-promotion and disease-prevention service model. Arguably, there is no place more critically in need of the contributions of nursing health-promotion and disease-prevention services than in the underserved and often disadvantaged rural communities. The Patient Protection and Affordable Care Act of 2010 specifically recognized the importance of nursing services and community-based health centers in addressing the urgent health care needs of the American public (English, 2010). It is now up to the nursing profession to respond to the critical healthcare needs of rural America through nursing health-promotion practice, program development, nursing research and policy advocacy.

DISCUSSION QUESTIONS

1. How does the cultural climate and socioeconomic status of the rural community affect the provision of nursing health promotion services?
2. Identify three theoretical frame
   resource, that could be used in
   promotion services or a rural hea
   retical frameworks might apply
   health-promotion service or rese
3. Identify three Healthy People 20
   rural communities in America.
4. Identify three potential resourc
   health-promotion services in rel

DISCUSSION QUESTIONS

Students can work on these assignments individually or in a group after reading through the material. Students can delve deeper into concepts by completing these exercises online.

CHECK YOUR UNDERSTANDING

1. In general, how do the current and projected future demographics of the rural community differ from suburban and urban populations?
2. Identify five major health issues affecting rural populations.
3. Identify three potential influences that may increase health disparities among rural populations.
4. Identify three factors that may contribute to birth disparities among rural
   [...] immunization in the rural community.
   [...] in rural dental health affect the overall

CHECK YOUR UNDERSTANDING

Review key concepts from each chapter with these questions at the end of each chapter. The questions can also be found in the text's online resources, where students can submit their answers directly to the instructor.

7. Identify three factors that may influence the obesity health disparity in the rural community.
8. Identify three adolescent health issues of particular concern to rural residents. What are some potential barriers to care experienced by rural adolescents?
9. Identify three social determinants of mental health pertinent to the rural community.
10. Identify three occupational health issues particularly pertinent to rural residents in America.
11. Identify three health issues particularly relevant to the migrant worker population and discuss potential barriers to care for these health concerns.
12. Describe primary, secondary, and tertiary nursing services to improve outcomes in the management of cardiovascular and respiratory chronic disease among older rural residents.
13. Design a nursing health-promotion proposal for a rural health issue within a specific population and an identified rural region. The proposal should include:
    A. a discussion of the health issue as it relates to the rural community and the Healthy People 2020 objectives,
    B. an ecological community assessment,
    C. a nursing health-promotion intervention plan based in an appropriate theoretical framework and reflective of applicable cultural concerns,
    D. a consideration of available resources and interdisciplinary collaboration opportunities to support the health-promotion interventions, and
    E. an outline of the desired outcomes of the health-promotion intervention and an outcomes evaluation plan.

WHAT DO YOU THINK?

1. How would you apply the principles of patient-centered care to the provision of nursing health-promotion services in the rural community? Describe a patient-centered care approach to the provision of nursing health-promotion services in relation to a particular rural health issue.

[...] ealth policy trends in America in relation to the provision of [...] motion services for a specific rural health issue. How would [...] change in the delivery of healthcare services to reduce rural [...]

[...] problem or research question that could potentially add [...] rature to improve the provision of evidence-based nursing [...] services in the rural community. How might you design a [...] investigate the research problem?

WHAT DO YOU THINK?

These questions are designed to prompt students to expand upon the concepts in the text. These activities can also be completed and submitted online.

---

24 CHAPTER 1 Health Education, Health Promotion, and Health

Whitehead, D. (2008). Health promotion: An international Delphi study examining health promotion and health education in nursing practice, education and policy. *Journal of Clinical Nursing, 17*, 891–900.
Williamson, D. L. & Carr, J. (2009). Health as a resource for everyday life: Advancing the conceptualization. *Critical Public Health, 19*(1), 107–122.
Wilson-Barnett, J. (1993). Health promotion and nursing practice. In A. Dines and A. Cribb (Eds.), *Health promotion: Concepts and practice* (pp. 195–204). Oxford, UK: Blackwell Scientific Publications.
World Health Organization [WHO]. (1948). *Preamble to the constitution of the WHO*. Official records of the WHO (No 2, p. 100). Entered into force April 7, 1948.
World Health Organization [WHO]. (1986). *The Ottawa charter for health promotion*. Ontario, Canada: Canadian Public Health Association, Health and Welfare Canada, and the World Health Organization.

www For a full suite of assignments and additional learning activities, see the access code at the front of your book.

Redeem the access code at the front of your book at www.jblearning.com. If you do not have an access code, one can be purchased at the site.

CONTEMPORARY HEALTH PROMOTION
IN NURSING
PRACTICE

Bonnie Raingruber, PhD, CNS, RN

Professor of Nursing
California State University—Sacramento
Sacramento, California

Nurse Researcher
Center for Nursing Research
University of California—Davis Medical Center
Sacramento, California

Adjunct Professor
Department of Internal Medicine
Department of Hematology and Oncology
University of California—Davis
Sacramento, California

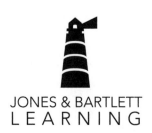

JONES & BARTLETT
LEARNING

World Headquarters
Jones & Bartlett Learning
5 Wall Street
Burlington, MA 01803
978-443-5000
info@jblearning.com
www.jblearning.com

Jones & Bartlett Learning books and products are available through most bookstores and online booksellers. To contact Jones & Bartlett Learning directly, call 800-832-0034, fax 978-443-8000, or visit our website, www.jblearning.com.

Production Credits

Executive Publisher: Kevin Sullivan
Acquisitions Editor: Amanda Harvey
Editorial Assistant: Rebecca Myrick
Production Editor: Cindie Bryan
Marketing Communications Manager:
    Katie Hennessy
V.P., Manufacturing and Inventory Control:
    Therese Connell
Composition: Paw Print Media
Cover Design: Scott Moden

Rights & Photo Research Assistant: Joseph Veiga
Front Cover Images: Clockwise from top left:
    © Goodshoot/Thinkstock,
    © Ingrid Balabanova/ShutterStock, Inc.,
    © iStockphoto/Thinkstock,
    © iStockphoto/Thinkstock
Back Cover Image: © BananaStock/Thinkstock
Printing and Binding: Edwards Brothers Malloy
Cover Printing: Edwards Brothers Malloy

To order this product, use ISBN: 1-978-1-4496-9721-1

Library of Congress Cataloging-in-Publication Data
Raingruber, Bonnie.
  Contemporary health promotion in nursing practice / Bonnie Raingruber.
     p. ; cm.
  Includes bibliographical references and index.
  ISBN 978-1-4496-2812-3 (pbk.) -- ISBN 1-4496-2812-5 (pbk.)
  I. Title.
  [DNLM: 1. Health Promotion. 2. Nurse's Role. WA 590]
  613--dc23
                                                2012031086

6048

Printed in the United States of America
17 16 15 14 13   10 9 8 7 6 5 4 3 2

Contents

CHAPTER 3

Health Promotion Theories   **53**

Bonnie Raingruber

CHAPTER 10

**Evaluation, Research, and Measurement in Health
Promotion Practice**   **323**

Bonnie Raingruber

CHAPTER 11

Entrepreneurship and Health Promotion 375

Bonnie Raingruber

Preface

WHY I WROTE THIS BOOK

Recent years have brought with them an amazing amount of new knowledge related to health promotion. An astounding number of innovative policies, emerging priorities, newfound disciplines, evolving research methods, and challenging settings confront the nurse engaged in health promotion practice. These innovations and challenges demand that nurses develop familiarity and expertise with a large amount of new content. This book was developed to address these newly emerging fields, content, methods, and settings, as well as the multitude of challenges confronting students and nurses engaged in health promotion practice. The book includes a chapter on the history of health promotion including recent critical developments; a chapter on social determinants of health, genomics, epigenetics, and plasticity; a chapter on health literacy; a chapter on health disparities and social capital; a chapter on nursing informatics (electronic medical records, biometric screening, virtual reality, avatars, simulation, telehealth); and a chapter on recent events that will shape health policy work. The book includes content on community-based participatory research, calculating quality-adjusted life years, common health screening tools, logic models, outcome evaluation, neighborhood mapping, and cost–utility and cost–benefit analysis. Also included is content on entrepreneurship and aesthetic/creative approaches to health promotion such as reminiscence therapy, mutual storytelling, street theater, photo-voice, motivational interviewing, and dance. The nurse's role in health promotion is emphasized by using a historical, theoretical, and philosophical perspective. The importance of social, linguistic, and cultural determinants of health is highlighted throughout the text. Each chapter was designed to address critical new information that shapes contemporary health promotion practice.

Health promotion has long been a central part of nursing practice, but at this juncture it is increasingly vital that nurses adopt an active role in promoting the health of individuals, families, communities, and nations. Empowering individuals and communities, facilitating public awareness of health disparities, advocating for the underserved, enhancing access to care, involving patients in their care, connecting individuals with community resources, and engaging in health policy work is critical if nurses are to have a role and a voice in the future of healthcare delivery. At no time in our history have social pressures, stresses, economic and environmental uncertainties, political forces, and a complex healthcare delivery system posed more challenges to the health of individuals and communities than currently exist. This book is written to provide current content for nurses and to encourage them to empower, advocate for, and involve clients in their care. Nursing is a trusted profession with a broad knowledge base and a history of working with the community. As such, nurses are well situated to become leaders in health promotion, disease prevention, and healthcare advocacy. We need to prepare ourselves to adopt a visible role in shaping the future of health promotion practice. This book was developed to assist nurses to take on that leadership role.

Active learning is necessary if students are going to apply what they have learned in their practice. Therefore, each chapter in this book includes an introduction and learning outcomes as well as end-of-chapter exercises that enable students to check their understanding. The end-of-chapter exercises include discussion questions that an instructor can use for essay assignments or group discussions, and students can use these discussion questions to reflect on the chapter content. The end-of-chapter exercises also include a section titled "Check Your Understanding," where students complete critical thinking activities, evidence-based applications, matching exercises, short essay questions, fill-in-the-blank activities, and compare their answers to responses offered by the authors. Finally, the end-of-chapter exercises include a section titled "What Do You Think?," in which students are encouraged to reflect on and articulate their views and consider the significance of presented content. Each of these sections as well as the case studies and clinical scenarios included in each chapter are designed to involve students in the learning process, to highlight the relevance of the material to clinical practice, and to prepare students for their health promotion role. The book contains an abundance of clinical examples, critical thinking and reflective practice activities, and application exercises.

TARGET AUDIENCE

The primary target audience is nursing students enrolled in a health promotion, community health, health assessment, or health education course. Given the rapid nature of change within health promotion practice over the last few years, the book will also be an excellent resource for all nursing students and nursing faculty who need a concise resource that outlines recent practice-based changes. Other professionals as well may benefit by using this text as a reference and as a way to discover parallels between their practice and that of nurses who are engaged in health promotion.

USING THIS BOOK

The initial chapter describes why health promotion is an integral part of nursing practice. Three subsequent chapters—the history of health promotion, health promotion theories, and genetic and social determinants of health—form the basis for the remainder of the book. Other chapters can be read or assigned in any order, as they address freestanding content. The chapters on evaluation and health promotion policy are best left for last since they summarize content that was introduced in earlier chapters. The "Discussion Questions," "Check Your Understanding" sections, and "What Do You Think?" sections can be used by both students and instructors to stimulate creative thoughts, to verify understanding, and to apply the content to practice.

Acknowledgments

I would like to thank my many clients and students, whose curiosity and input made this book possible. In particular I would like to acknowledge the case studies contributed by two students, Mary Ann Sandoval and Yuri Vorobets. I am especially grateful to Dr. Michelle Dang, Dr. Alexa Curtis, and Amy Zausch for their content-based expertise and tireless efforts in contributing to this work. In addition, I appreciate the constant efforts of Amanda Harvey, Sara Bempkins, Cindie Bryan, and Rebecca Myrick as well as the rest of the staff at Jones & Bartlett Learning who have encouraged and assisted me throughout this process. I would like to acknowledge my mentor, Dr. Patricia Benner, for the motivation and vision she embodied and shared with all her students.

About the Author

Dr. Raingruber is a mental health clinical nurse specialist who has taught nursing for 26 years in bachelor's, master's, and Doctor of Nursing Practice (DNP) programs. She has done extensive research focused on health promotion and health disparities and has been funded by the National Institutes of Health, the Substance Abuse and Mental Health Administration, the Health Resources and Services Administration, as well as private foundations. Dr. Raingruber maintains a private health promotion practice and has worked in university settings, county facilities, public and private hospitals, and community-based organizations. She is the author of over 30 peer-reviewed journal articles, 2 books, and 6 book chapters.

Contributors

Michelle Dang, PhD, APHN-BC, RN
Assistant Professor, California State University—Sacramento

Alexa Colgrove Curtis, PhD, FNP-C, RN
Associate Professor, California State University—Sacramento

Amy Zausch, MSN, RN
Clinical Nurse, University of California Davis Medical Center

Health Education, Health Promotion, and Health: What Do These Definitions Have to Do with Nursing?

Bonnie Raingruber

OBJECTIVES

At the conclusion of this chapter, the student will be able to:

- Define health education, health promotion, health, and wellness, and compare and contrast each concept.
- Discuss criticisms of the accepted definitions of health.
- Apply health promotion concepts to several case studies and identify how a nurse could work with a patient, family, or community to foster health.
- Analyze health promotion core competencies.
- Explain why health promotion is a vital part of nursing practice.

INTRODUCTION

Health promotion is a key component of nursing practice. As we will discuss, by promoting the health of individuals, families, communities, and populations, nurses help transform the health of individuals, our society, and our healthcare system. As one looks carefully at the varied definitions of nursing, it is interesting to see how often health promotion activities are highlighted as being a central nursing role.

Florence Nightingale influenced modern definitions of nursing by focusing on the triad of the person, health, and the environment while stressing the promotion of health and healing as being central to definitions of nursing (Nightingale, 1859).

The American Nurses' Association (ANA) defined nursing as "the protection, promotion and optimization of health and abilities, prevention of illness and injury, alleviation of suffering through the diagnosis and treatment of human response and advocacy in the care of individuals, families, communities and populations" (ANA, 2010, para 2). In the ANA social policy statement (1995), we see that "nursing involves policies that are restorative, supportive, and promotive in nature . . . . Promotive practices mobilize healthy patterns of living, foster personal and family development, and support self-defined goals of individuals, families, and communities (p. 11).

The International Council of Nurses (2010) defined nursing as "including the promotion of health, the prevention of illness and the care of ill, disabled and dying people" (para 1). Advocacy, promotion of a safe environment, research, participation in shaping health policy, and health systems are also described as key nursing roles (International Council of Nurses).

Irrespective of which definition of nursing is used, we see that health is the central concept and that health promotion is a key nursing activity. As Morgan and Marsh (1998) suggested, nurses promote the health of individuals, families, and communities by educating about needed lifestyle modifications and advocating for conditions that foster health.

HEALTH EDUCATION VERSUS HEALTH PROMOTION

Within the nursing literature and within practice, the terms health promotion and health education have mistakenly been used as interchangeable concepts. In reality, health education and health promotion are distinct activities. The concept of health promotion, which focuses on socioeconomic and environmental determinants of health and participatory involvement, includes the narrower concept of health education (Whitehead, 2008).

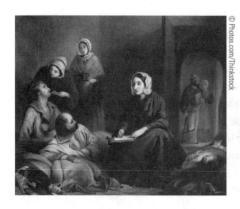
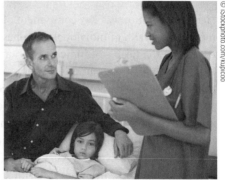

Health education involves giving information and teaching individuals and communities how to achieve better health, a common role within nursing. Health education has been defined as those "activities which raise an individual's awareness, giving the individual the health knowledge required to enable him or her to decide on a particular health action" (Mackintosh, 1996, p. 14). Whitehead (2004) defined health education as "activities that seek to inform the individual on the nature and causes of health/illness and that individual's personal level of risk associated with their lifestyle behavior. Health education seeks to motivate individuals to accept a process of behavioral change through directly influencing their values, beliefs, and attitude systems" (p. 313). In contrast, health promotion "involves social, economic, and political change to ensure the environment is conducive to health . . . it requires a nurse educate an individual about his or her health needs, but also demands that the nurse play a role in attempting to address the wider environmental and social issues that adversely affect people's health" (Mackintosh, 1996, p. 14).

For years health education was seen as synonymous with health promotion and the terms were used interchangeably. Whitehead (2003a), however, argued that there is in fact a paradigm war or tension between disease-centered health education and the larger concept of health promotion that includes a focus on environmental, educational, cultural, and sociopolitical determinates of health. Whitehead (2003b) explained that nurses working in inpatient settings are socialized to use the biomedical model, focusing to a greater extent on health education rather than health promotion. The biomedical model, according to Whitehead (2003b) is reductionistic, views the body and mind as separate, and promotes an illness perspective, not a health promotion perspective.

Although acute care nurses report that they are engaged in health promotion activities, they are often conducting behavioral, lifestyle-oriented, or risk-oriented health education (Whitehead, 2006). Whitehead (2006) suggested that nurses need to extend their activities into the realm of health promotion by becoming more involved in legislative reform, empowering communities, paying attention to ethnic/racial or economic health disparities, facilitating public consciousness-raising, adopting a role as a political advocate for underprivileged individuals who cannot lobby for themselves, and influencing health-related policy development.

Many authors (Robertson, 2001; Tones, 2000) have argued that health education is a component of health promotion. Certainly, health education, a traditional nursing role, is an integral and essential part of health promotion. However, achieving health is not just about being educated or coached to change one's behavior by a healthcare provider. Oftentimes patients have attempted to alter a health-related behavior before talking with a healthcare provider. In these situations, talking with a patient and developing a comprehensive understanding of what they want to change, what they have previously tried, and their barriers to change is vital.

Health is influenced by adaptive potential, perceptual capability, environmental stress, and coping resources (King, 1994). Therefore, health promotion includes empowering individuals and communities and implementing larger sociopolitical interventions designed to foster health (Whitehead, 2003a). These additional aspects of health promotion make it possible for nurses to play a role in reforming healthcare delivery systems, addressing the health needs of local communities, and improving the health of society overall.

Everyone's health is influenced by their family situation, their community, the environment, and the political climate in which they live. In fact, socioeconomic factors often have a larger impact on a person's health than their individual health maintenance behaviors (Williamson & Carr, 2009). For that reason, health promotion must include health education plus the related legal, economic, environmental, educational, legislative, and organizational interventions necessary to facilitate health (Tones, Tilford, & Robinson, 1990). This does not mean a nurse must be a lobbyist, a Senator or Representative, an epidemiologist, a community organizer, a community health nurse, or work at the National Institutes of Health to facilitate health promotion.

All nurses can engage in health promotion. Harm (2001) suggested that nurses who work in busy inpatient settings who wish to engage in health promotion need to integrate a holistic perspective into their practice. Health promotion requires individualizing care to match patient and family needs; assessing the economic, sociocultural, political, and organizational factors that shape health; involving patients in care planning; connecting them with community resources; serving in an advocacy role; and promoting continuity of care between inpatient and outpatient or community-based settings.

Larsson and colleagues (1991) stressed that the frequency and intensity of daily hassles in life affect health. Poverty brings with it a burden of chronic stress and predisposes people to make unhealthy lifestyle choices, including smoking; using drugs or drinking; not exercising; living in unsafe areas; and eating foods that are affordable, readily available, and typically high in calories. In addition, many individuals do not have access to regular, preventive health care or the educational background to fully understand what healthcare providers are trying to communicate. Therefore, a component of health promotion is paying attention to health literacy, issues of access to care, and poverty-related barriers that prevent individuals and communities from engaging in health-promoting activities.

Advocacy as an Aspect of Health Promotion

Cribb and Dunes (1993) stressed that empowerment and advocacy are vital aspects of health promotion that help individuals and communities make healthy choices. Maben and Macleod-Clark (1995) suggested that health promotion "is concerned with making healthier choices easier choices" (p. 1161). Health promotion involves lobbying for healthy communities, access to health care and nutritious food, safe homes, understandable healthcare information, and involvement of patients in care planning, and healthcare policy changes as needed.

Consider for a moment healthcare policies that nurses have been involved in implementing in your community. Do you know any nurses who have participated in seat belt or bicycle helmet safety campaigns, health screenings, discussions on water or air quality issues, dialogue about nurse–patient ratios, or debates about access to health care? Have you talked with any of your patients about ways to incorporate healthier lifestyle choices into their routine while assessing the barriers they have to deal with on a daily basis? Have you advocated for a patient by helping them apply for food stamps or the Women, Infants, Children (WIC) program? Have you empowered a patient to believe they could make needed lifestyle modifications irrespective of the barriers that exist in their environment? If so, you were engaged in health promotion activities as part of your nursing role.

Assessing and Building on Patient Strengths as an Aspect of Health Promotion

Health promotion requires carefully assessing your client's background, challenges, and strengths and determining what they want to change, how they plan to modify their lifestyle, how they best learn, and what help they need from you as a nurse. It is critical to identify the strengths and past successes that individuals and communities have had in improving their health. As Eldh, Ekman, and Ehnfors (2010) commented, patients need to be active participants in their care, to feel like they are knowledgeable partners whose input is respected and believed, and to share in decision making about their health.

For example, it is important to assess how a patient lost weight in the past when discussing how they will begin their current weight loss program. You need to discuss what interfered with their weight loss program and what worked for them in the past. When talking with a patient who needs to decrease the amount of salt in his or her diet, it is very helpful to assess whether there are family members or friends who will help with that lifestyle modification. Are there situations, like eating at fast food restaurants, that will make it harder to eat less salt? Do the patient and family understand why eating less salt is important? Are the patient and family committed to changing their behavior by buying foods that are low in salt? Do they have the financial resources necessary to modify their diet? Are fresh foods available in their community? Do they know which canned, frozen, and prepared foods are highest in salt? Are there any cultural preferences that influence their dietary habits?

As another example, when exploring how a patient will stop smoking it is necessary to talk about how the person tried to stop smoking in the past. What successes did they have? What challenges interfered with their success? Was it hardest not to smoke after meals or when going out on the town for the evening? Does the patient have enough money to purchase nicotine patches? Does he or she have insurance that will cover acupuncture or hypnosis for smoking cessation? Would text message reminders and motivational comments help the patient? Which smoking cessation method does the patient want to use?

At the community level, what would work when designing an HIV prevention program for young migrant farm workers age 19 to 25? Would HIV prevention information broadcast on a Spanish-speaking radio station work better than cell phone text messages sent directly to individual farm workers? Would posters placed in local health clinics be effective or are visits to health clinics too rare for young migrant workers? Should personal stories or novellas of how other migrant workers got HIV be used to motivate behavioral changes? Does the fact that a significant number of agricultural employers bring professional sex workers to the migrant camps on a weekly basis create a challenge that needs to be addressed? Do commonly held beliefs like the idea that showering in beer after having sex kills the HIV virus need to be addressed? Should health education be provided by Spanish-speaking males or females? What resources exist within the farm worker community that could be used to design an effective HIV prevention program?

DEFINITIONS OF HEALTH PROMOTION

The term health promotion has been defined in myriad ways (Maben & Macleod-Clark, 1995). Tones (1985) defined health promotion as any intervention designed to foster health. Pender and colleagues (2002) defined health promotion as "increasing the level of well-being and self-actualization of a given individual or group" (p. 34). Others have defined health promotion as lifestyle coaching designed to promote optimal health, quality of life, and well-being (Saylor, 2004). Health promotion includes health education, identification and reduction of health risks for selected individuals and populations, empowerment, advocacy, preventative health care, and health policy development.

Although television commercials, billboards, and Twitter messages have all been used to promote the health of communities, health promotion does not mean "promoting" in the sense of marketing or selling (Maben & Macleod-Clark, 1995). In fact, a danger associated with viewing health as a commodity or as capital is that health is then seen as having no inherent value unless it generates positive returns such as economic productivity. Such a stance can provide the rationale for denying health care to the disabled, unemployed, or elderly if their years of productive life do not warrant an expensive operation or treatment (Williamson & Carr, 2009).

Rather than being a commodity to be marketed, health promotion includes health education and motivating lifestyle and behavior change based on a careful understanding of the patient's situation, economic resources, educational background, social supports, cultural beliefs, and environmental factors within their community. To motivate individuals, families, and communities to make lifestyle changes, it is necessary to understand the factors that keep people from changing as well as those that prompt them to adopt new behaviors. It is vital to understand the perspective of the patient or the community with whom one is interacting.

Definitions of health promotion and health include numerous subjective components that require careful assessment (Sullivan, 2003). Health is influenced by feelings such as pain levels, energy levels, and the ability to perform one's job or social role. Some people describe their health as poor, even if they don't have a major disease, when they can no longer do what they want to do on a daily basis. Likewise, people who have some degree of disease can still consider themselves to be in good health. In addition, one's view of whether they are healthy changes depending on the culture and age of the person (Larson, 1999). A nurse must begin by understanding what a patient understands about their current health condition, what lifestyle change(s) the patient is willing to make, what barriers they will encounter, and how best to motivate the person to make those modifications. For example, does the 30-year-old patient you are working with regarding their exercise routine hope to return to being a marathon runner after his or her broken leg heals, or does the 80-year-old patient hope to be able to take a 5-minute walk without experiencing pain? The nurse should find out what activities bring satisfaction and enjoyment to the patient so that changes can be planned that build on existing health habits; incorporate social supports; substitute realistic alternatives to unhealthy behavior given the patient's preferences; and consider relevant economic, cultural, and environmental influences (Saylor, 2004).

MEDICAL MODEL AND WORLD HEALTH ORGANIZATION DEFINITIONS OF HEALTH

Health, in the medical model, has been defined primarily as an absence of physical and mental disease. The illness paradigm typically emphasizes disease rather than health and well-being (Larson, 1999).

Health has also been defined much more broadly by the World Health Organization (WHO) (1948) as a complete state of physical, mental, social, and emotional well-being, not merely the absence of disease. The Ottawa Charter of the WHO (1986) stressed that peace, shelter, education, food, income, a stable ecosystem, sustainable resources, social justice, and equity are necessary for health. Therefore, their definition of health included attention to conditions where peace is uncertain because of war, areas ravaged by natural disasters such as earthquakes and floods, countries where infectious disease abounds, situations where pollution is widespread, and locales where education is not available to everyone. Included in the WHO definition is the idea that physical, mental, and social health is a fundamental right of all people (Larson, 1999).

Since few of us are in a complete state of physical, mental, social, and emotional well-being at all times, the WHO definition gives us a goal to motivate us to grow in a multitude of ways. Consider for a moment what physical challenges, mental constructs, social obligations, or emotional feelings are keeping you from a holistic sense of well-being as you pursue your nursing studies.

This case study about Jane illustrates how nursing school affected her well-being. Jane was delighted when she was admitted to nursing school, but she had a persistent worry that someday a clinical instructor would recognize what she didn't know and she would then be abruptly removed from the program. The stress of worrying about exams and late night clinical write-ups kept Jane from sleeping as much as her body required. She was so busy with school work that she felt isolated from her family and friends. Jane gained 5 pounds in one semester just by snacking during late night study sessions in the weeks before exams. She went into each exam believing she would get the lowest grade in the class and be humiliated. What else would you want to know about Jane before you began a conversation about promoting her well-being and health? What barriers could be interfering with Jane's health promotion goals?

Additional Definitions of Health

The WHO definition of health is the most accepted definition, but numerous other definitions of health have been proposed. Authors have defined health as a capacity for living (Carlson, 2003); an optimal individualized fitness so that one lives a full, creative life (Goldsmith, 1972); as having a good quality of life (Brown et al., 1984); or as actualization of inherent and acquired human potential through goal-directed behavior, competent self-care and stratifying relationships with others . . . while maintaining harmony with relevant environments (Pender, Murdaugh, & Parsons, 2002, p. 22). Yet other definitions of health include: (1) the state of optimum capacity to perform roles and tasks one has been socialized into; (2) a joyful attitude toward life and a cheerful acceptance of one's responsibilities; and (3) the capacity to maintain balance and be free from undue pain, discomfort, disability, or limitation of action including social capacity (Goldsmith, 1972, p. 13).

Meaning and Purpose as Part of Health

The concept of health also includes a sense of meaning and purpose or knowledge that one's life makes a difference (Pender, Murdaugh, & Parsons, 2002). Nurses need to explore what brings a sense of meaning to the patients and communities they work with to effectively design health interventions that will be satisfying. Perception is a vital aspect of health that nurses must consider. Nurses should explore how a patient's lifestyle will be altered by their illness, what that change will mean to the patient, how the patient previously coped with similar challenges, and which family members/friends will be influenced by this illness.

Many authors have argued that illness can be a catalyst for health and growth. Illness often prompts individuals to reflect on their life, to consider what is most important to them, and to imagine how life will be after the acute phase of their illness is over and their health is restored (Diemert-Moch, 1998). Relationships, health behaviors, and daily routines that the individual previously took for granted are now redefined by the current threat to their health. Illness can offer individuals an opportunity to recreate and shape their health.

Likewise, health crises that affect entire communities can bring an opportunity to rebuild infrastructures, laws, and policies that support health. Consider how the people of New Orleans were affected by Hurricane Katrina, which flooded their hospitals, schools, homes, and places of employment. Have there been any improvements to that community since the hurricane? What remains to be done? Think about the economic, social, and physical devastation faced by the people of Germany in the years following World War II. Were there any economic, social or political changes that followed decades later that helped reorganize their society in a positive way?

CRITIQUES OF DEFINITIONS OF HEALTH

Each of the commonly used definitions of health, along with the WHO definition, is holistic and includes aspects of well-being. However, these definitions have been criticized for being difficult to measure, idealistic, and hard to implement in busy healthcare settings.

The RAND Health Insurance Experiment used measurement methods to assess whether the WHO definition of health was practical and measurable. Physical health was measured by a standardized functional health status tool and the ability to complete daily self-care, household work, and leisure activities. Mental health was measured using depression scales, anxiety scales, measures of positive well-being, and self-control. Social health was measured in terms of participation in social activities. Physical and mental health was found to be an independent dimension of health that could be measured. Social well-being in the RAND study was not found to be an independent dimension of health. RAND researchers summarized that although social factors affect health, they should not be used to define personal health status. It is important to remember the RAND study summarized findings from only one study (Ware, Brook, Davies, & Lohr, 1981).

Other authors have criticized the WHO definition for being too utopian and abstract, emphasizing that there is no consensus about the meaning of well-being, and commenting that meanings of health differ in different countries and cultures (Larson, 1999; Saylor, 2004). Even though different cultural views influence how health is defined and what interventions are acceptable, and in spite of the fact that well-being can be measured in multiple ways, still the WHO statement is the most accepted and comprehensive definition of health worldwide. Some have suggested that the WHO definition represents a goal more than a guideline for concrete action (Larson, 1999).

Each individual nurse must reflect on the concepts included in the WHO definition (physical, mental, social, and emotional well-being) and apply them in an individualized manner in their daily practice (Larson, 1999). Nurses also need to think about the organizational, environmental, economic, and sociocultural factors that influence the health of patients, families, communities, and populations.

Do you agree that social factors are a defining part of health for individual patients? Have you worked with a patient who struggled with social factors that influenced his or her health? Have you ever seen the discharge of a heart patient delayed or a rehabilitation facility transfer be needed because the patient's spouse had Alzheimer's disease and could not assist in the recovery? Have you worked with homeless patients who did not have anyone to help them pick up a prescription or change a dressing after they left the hospital? What other examples of social factors have you observed that have influenced the health of patients?

Organizational Factors Affecting Health

Considering which organizational factors influence health is an important aspect of what nurses do when promoting the health of their patients. Think about an organizational factor that affected the health of a patient you cared for during the last year. Did you encounter anyone who had to wait a long time for a healthcare appointment, schedule a health visit at a time that was really difficult for them, wait to get their medications refilled, or work to understand what a busy healthcare provider was actually saying?

Consider the case of Ramon, who spoke very little English. When he came to the Urgent Care Clinic he had difficulty registering because he did not feel comfortable standing at the front counter, where everyone could hear, and saying that frequent urination brought him to the clinic. Once he met with the nurse practitioner (NP) and a urine screen showed he had a urinary tract infection, he did not know how to tell the busy NP he did not have enough money to get the antibiotic prescription filled for 5 more days. Frustrated, he left the clinic and went home. Discomfort, burning, and frequency prompted him to go to the emergency room later that night, where he had to wait 12 hours before being seen. Which organizational factors interfered with Ramon getting adequate care? What could a nurse do to advocate for Ramon?

Think about the introduction of electronic medical records, the use of bar codes for dispensing medications in hospitals, and pill bottles that buzz to remind patients to take their medications at home. How have those organizational changes affected the health of patients and the workload of nurses who care for those patients? What are the advantages and challenges associated with these changes? Has the hospital where your clinical placements are scheduled incorporated nursing notes, pharmacy orders, laboratory results, pain assess-

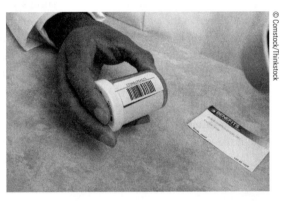

ment inventories, fall risk tools, pressure ulcer rating systems, and advance directives as part of their electronic medical record system? How has the introduc- tion of each of those compo- nents affected the health of the patients you have cared for in that hospital? Have you used bar code scanning as part of medica- tion administration? If so, what did you like about bar code scanning? What sort of errors could occur with bar code scanning for medication administration? Have you seen wristband reminders or pill bottle caps that include a microchip used to remind patients to take their medication at home? So far these devices have been used with blind, noncompliant, congestive heart failure, organ transplant, and elderly patients. Are there other populations in which talking pill bottles might be useful?

Environmental Factors Affecting Health

It is necessary for nurses to consider environmental factors that influence health before working with clients. Think about an environmental factor that affected the health of a client you cared for in the last year. The two case studies that follow illustrate environ- mental factors that impact the health of two very different 10-year-old children. What would you, as a nurse, do in each case to promote the health of the child?

Marcella was a 10-year-old girl who lived in a low-income, urban area where gang activity, prostitution, and drug abuse was rampant. Her mother would not let her go outside after 4 PM because several other children in her neighborhood had been shot while riding their bikes. Marcella lived in a small apartment with her three sisters and her mother. Due to their limited budget, her mother routinely bought foods that were high in calories because they were convenient and affordable. There was no space inside the crowded apartment to exercise. However, the school nurse kept telling Marcella that she was 25 pounds overweight, so she had to exercise and change what she ate. What else could the school nurse do to actually be helpful to Marcella? What could the school nurse learn by placing a telephone call to Marcella's mother or scheduling a home visit?

Aboyo was a 10-year-old girl who lived in a rural village outside of Kumasi, Ghana in West Africa. The power went out in her village on a regular basis, leaving the community without water when the electric pumps stopped working. To earn money for food, children in the village regularly went to the dump barefoot to collect plastic water bottles that had been discarded. The children would refill the bottles with stagnant water and superglue the lids back on the bottles before reselling them in the market. All of the bottles that were discarded went to the same area for disposal irrespective of who had previously used them. One day Aboyo cut her foot on a piece of glass while collecting water bottles and was taken to the village clinic. Besides attending to Aboyo's cut, what should the nurse at the village clinic teach Aboyo? What else could the village nurse do besides working with Aboyo and getting her perspective? How could the Queen Mother (the most influential female in the village) and the village elders be involved to improve the health of the village children?

Economic Factors Affecting Health

Economic factors have a major impact on health and health promotion activities. For example, sometimes elderly patients on limited incomes have to decide which of their medications they will get refilled. Or, elderly clients only take half the medications prescribed by their physician or nurse practitioner because they can't afford to fill the entire prescription.

Think about Louise's situation. Her husband worked on and off as a carpenter in a state with 13% unemployment. For the last year he had been unable to find steady work due to a downturn in the construction industry. They did not have health insurance. Louise began having heavy menstrual periods at the age of 57, two years after she had gone through menopause. Her doctor determined that she had uterine cancer and performed a hysterectomy. The cost of the surgery, on top of the decrease in her husband's employment, resulted in the family losing their home to foreclosure. They had to move into a travel trailer on the property of one of their long-time friends. Two years after her surgery, Louise noticed a lump in her breast. Because she could not afford regular visits with her physician, and did not qualify for low-income medical care due to her husband's fluctuating income, she relied on the emergency room for her health care when absolutely necessary. After a needle biopsy determined the lump in her breast was not a cyst, Louise's doctor ordered a mammogram. The results came back indicating Louise now had breast cancer. If you were the emergency room nurse working with Louise, how would you approach her? What would you say to her? What economic factors influenced Louise's health and health promotion activities?

Consider how Thomas, a community health nurse, became involved in promoting the health of Oak Park, a low-income area where he worked. As Thomas made home visits, he was consistently frustrated by the lack of grocery stores that sold fresh fruits and vegetables in Oak Park. He attempted to do health education about nutrition with families on his caseload only to hear over and over that local convenience stores only stocked prepared foods, cigarettes, and alcohol. Most of his families did not own a car and had difficulty traveling the 5 miles to the nearest grocery store that stocked fruits and vegetables. Walking was out of the question as well, due to the active presence of gang violence in Oak Park. Finally, Thomas volunteered to participate in a community development task force that was being organized. The task force interviewed key community members and then presented their findings to the mayor. As a result of the key informant interviews, the Senior Gleaners (a community organization that harvests leftover vegetables from surrounding fields) partnered with a well-respected local church to use their parking lot to distribute free farm produce each Saturday. In addition, the task force successfully advocated for increased police presence in Oak Park. The task force also partnered with developers and submitted a grant to renovate a square block of buildings in a dilapidated Oak Park strip mall. Within two years the grant was funded and construction began for a library branch, a grocery store, and a healthcare complex surrounded by ample lighting within a park-like setting. Thomas concluded that the hours he had volunteered had a major impact on the daily life of the families that he worked with in the Oak Park community.

Sociocultural Factors Affecting Health

Sociocultural factors can have a major impact on health beliefs, health practices, health communication, and the trust that patients have in healthcare providers. Consider, for example, Oleg's perspective about taking medications. Oleg was a 45-year-old Russian male admitted to the hospital for a blood pressure of 215/110 mmHg. His nurse practitioner had prescribed a spectrum of blood pressure medications at increasing dosages over the last few months without seeing any change in his blood pressure. When Oleg was admitted to the cardiac floor, his inpatient nurse followed the written orders in his chart, which were based on the last dosage of blood pressure medication that his

NP had tried. Thirty minutes after the nurse gave him the medication, Oleg's blood pressure dropped so dramatically that he had to receive a bolus of fluid to bring it back within normal ranges. When a Russian-speaking nurse interviewed Oleg, he shared that he got the prescriptions his NP ordered filled because he worried that she would not continue to see him if he did not fill the prescriptions. However, Oleg did not take the medications because he shared a common view among Russian individuals that he was too young to have to take medication on a daily basis for the rest of his life. Which sociocultural factors should his NP and nurse have considered when working with Oleg? What else could the NP have done? What else should the staff nurse do in this situation?

Behavioral Factors Affecting Health

A variety of behavioral factors influence whether patients comply with their ordered treatments. Sometimes lack of compliance or adherence with ordered care is based on previous negative experiences with the healthcare system. Consider the example of Judy, a 350-pound, 84-year-old woman who had hip surgery the previous year. During that hospitalization, the lift team was delayed and the nurses who were moving her from the gurney to the bed dropped her. Her back was broken and required numerous painful injections to manage the fracture and the associated pain. When Judy left the hospital after that surgery she vowed to never return to any hospital. One year later her friend called on the phone and noticed Judy was confused. After arriving at her home, the friend called the paramedics because Judy was disoriented and had a fever of 103°F. When the paramedics arrived at her home Judy refused to go to the hospital. Finally, after almost 30 minutes, her friend persuaded Judy to go to the emergency room just long enough to get checked out and she consented. At the hospital it was determined Judy had a severe urinary tract infection. After one day in the hospital Judy insisted that she be discharged. Her temperature had gone down to 99°F and her mental status was back to normal. When Judy arrived home she got a call that her best friend had just passed away. In addition, the pharmacy employee who was supposed to deliver her antibiotics made a mistake and a day and a half went by before she was able to get her antibiotic prescription delivered. When Judy's friend called she said she felt too nauseated to eat or take her antibiotics. Judy said "when life isn't fun anymore there is no reason to be around." Which experiences, feelings, attitudes, behaviors, and medical conditions were influencing Judy at this moment? How might a visit by a home health nurse help Judy?

As the case studies here illustrate, health promotion requires empowerment, collaboration, and participation by the client. Sometimes health promotion requires community level intervention if effective health goals are to be accomplished. Health promotion can also require the nurse to take an active role in promoting environmental, organizational, or social change at the local, regional, or national level (Maben & Macleod-Clark, 1995).

THE RELATIONSHIP BETWEEN HEALTH, HEALTH PROMOTION, AND ILLNESS PREVENTION

Defining health as well-being laid the foundation for health promotion practice and expanded the role of nursing and medicine beyond just disease prevention and treatment (Saylor, 2004). Including a focus on well-being and wellness expanded health care from disease prevention and treatment to a consideration of the patient's capacity to cope with stress, choose healthy behaviors, recognize their health-related limitations, participate in lifestyle modifications, and manage changes in their health status (Manderscheid, Ryff, Freeman, McKnight-Eily, Dhingra, & Strine, 2010).

Wellness

Dunn (1959), the father of the wellness movement, advocated for maximizing human potential by simultaneously focusing on the mind, body, and spirit. He stressed the importance of personality, motivation, environment, and capacity for change. Dunn advocated for improving quality of life and active engagement of individuals and communities in health promotion, health maintenance, and disease prevention.

Primary, Secondary, and Tertiary Prevention

The terms primary, secondary, and tertiary prevention came from an epidemiological understanding of risks experienced by particular groups. Primary prevention has averting the occurrence of disease as its goal. Interventions occur before the disease process starts. Primary prevention includes health promotion and protecting at-risk individuals from threats to their health. Harris and Guten (1979) describe five dimensions of health protective behavior, including personal health practices, safety practices, preventive health care, environmental hazard avoidance, and harmful substance avoidance. Primary prevention and health promotion both focus on protecting individuals and communities from disease and increasing health and well-being. Disease prevention typically targets specific disease processes while health promotion is focused on general health and well-being, not necessarily one specific disease (King, 1994).

Secondary prevention aims to halt disease progression before it becomes more acute and is designed to lessen complications and disability (Breslow, 1999). Early diagnosis and prompt treatment are the priority. Tertiary prevention is often called rehabilitation. It begins once a disease has been stabilized and aims to restore the individual to their highest level of functioning (King, 1994).

Health promotion includes health education, health maintenance and protection, community and environmental development, and health policy advocacy (King, 1994). Given the provided definitions of health, health promotion, wellness, and primary prevention, which healthcare professionals are well prepared to implement these health promotion activities both at the individual and community level?

THE IMPORTANCE OF A TRAINED HEALTH PROMOTION WORKFORCE

Authors have argued for making health promotion a specialized practice and profession. Those who support this view argue that professions other than nursing, medicine, and health education should be trained in health promotion practices. They argue for a need for identifying health promotion competencies, accreditation standards for health promotion, and development of professional standards of practice.

Core competencies for such a role include the ability to: (1) catalyze change and empower individuals and communities to improve their health; (2) provide leadership in developing public health policy and building capacity in systems for supporting health promotion; (3) assess the needs and assets in communities to analyze the behavioral, cultural, social, environmental, and organizational determinants of health; (4) develop measurable goals after assessing needs and assets and identifying evidence-based interventions; (5) carry out efficient, culturally sensitive strategies to improve health; (6) evaluate the effectiveness of health promotion policies and disseminate results; (7) advocate on behalf of individuals and communities while building their capacity by incorporating an understanding of their assets; and (8) work collaboratively among varied disciplines to promote health (Barry, Allegrante, Lamarre, Auld, & Taub, 2009).

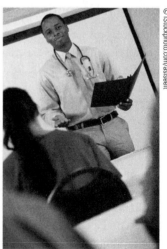

Given the scope and definitions of nursing practice, do you think health promotion competencies are part of the role of a nurse? The WHO in the Munich Declaration called for active involvement of nurses in health policy development. But as

Whitehead (2003c) stressed, nurses often struggle with finding the time and having the skills needed to take an active role in shaping health policy. As Smith and colleagues (1999) commented, the immediacy of the situation in most inpatient settings diverts nurses from participating in community-level interventions, environmental assessments, and health policy development. Most health policy design occurs with little input from nurses even though health policy has a profound influence on nursing practice (Whitehead, 2003c).

A number of nurses who work in the community in public health settings, nurse researchers, and some advanced practice nurses are engaged in health policy development and evaluation. However, many acute care nurses who work in busy inpatient settings do not see health promotion as part of their role. Activities such as political involvement, health policy development, and community advocacy are not typically easy to do in an inpatient setting (Casey, 2007a). In addition, within the literature too few examples are presented of how inpatient nurses might engage in these expanded activities that are part of health promotion.

A variety of authors have begun to describe how inpatient nurses might fulfill some of these broader health promotion–oriented roles. Wilson-Barnett (1993) suggested nurses need to view health promotion as a guiding philosophy about advocacy, participatory involvement, enhanced social support, and individualized care. By incorporating advocacy, considering social support, involving patients in care planning, and providing individualized care, nurses are promoting health. Casey (2007b) agreed that by engaging in active listening, checking with the patient and/or family, eliciting patient involvement in care planning and daily care, and individualizing care based on patient priorities, nurses are engaging in participatory care, an important component of health promotion. Since developing a therapeutic nurse–patient relationship requires patient participation, this too is part of health promotion. Nursing interventions that foster social support, decrease barriers to care, and improve self-efficacy are also health promoting. Determining the client's and family's perceived needs based on their societal position, along with developing realistic objectives and ways to monitor progress, is a vital part of health promotion (Whitehead, 2001). By mediating and advocating for a patient's rights or needs with other healthcare professionals or community organizations, especially during daily rounds or discharge planning activities, nurses are fulfilling these broader health promotion oriented roles (Casey, 2007a).

However, Whitehead (2001) has cautioned against busy inpatient nurses ignoring the complexity underlying health behavior by offering overly simplistic patient education without exploring barriers to behavior change or environmental/cultural influences. He argued that nurses must explore why patients adopt a particular lifestyle, what would work for them, and how to engage the patient in setting realistic goals.

DISCUSSION QUESTIONS

1. Do you think nurses should focus exclusively on health education for individual patients or should they also assess sociocultural, organizational, political, and environmental aspects of health promotion? Please explain your answer.
2. Do sociocultural factors like educational status, employment status, marital status, place/country of residence or birth, access to health care, and cultural beliefs/customs impact the health status of individuals? Please explain your answer.
3. Do you believe that individual health behaviors such as smoking, drinking, drug use, exercise/eating patterns, and access to preventative care primarily determine a person's health? Please explain your answer.
4. Should a separate health promotion practitioner role be created? Or should health promotion be retained as an integral part of nursing practice? Please explain your answer.
5. Do the definitions of health, health education, and health promotion have any influence on your nursing practice? Please explain your answer.
6. Imagine how health care will be provided 10 years from now. Describe how the different definitions included in this text could influence how you practice nursing 10 years into your professional career.

CHECK YOUR UNDERSTANDING

How many of these health promotion competencies do you see as being part of nursing practice? Complete the following chart by writing "yes" or "no" in the grid next to each competency. Provide in the middle column an example of a time you observed a nurse demonstrate the given competency at the local, national, or international level.

Is this competency an aspect of nursing practice? Write "yes" or "no" in this column next to the given competency.	Describe a scenario you have observed where a nurse demonstrated the given competency.	Health Promotion Competency
		1. Catalyze change and empower individuals and communities to improve their health.
		2. Provide leadership in developing public health policy and building capacity in systems for supporting health promotion.
		3. Assess the needs and assets in communities to analyze behavioral, cultural, social, environmental, and organizational determinants of health.
		4. Develop measurable goals after assessing needs and assets and identifying evidence-based interventions.
		5. Carry out efficient, culturally sensitive strategies to improve health.
		6. Evaluate the effectiveness of health promotion policies and practices and disseminate results.
		7. Advocate on behalf of individuals and communities by building their capacity and incorporating an understanding of their assets.
		8. Work collaboratively among varied disciplines to promote patient health.

In your list of scenarios where nurses performed these nursing competencies, did you include the following examples?

- For Competency 1, have you ever seen a nurse catalyze change in a community and empower individuals by offering a health screening fair in a local church to motivate individuals with high blood pressure to seek out a primary care physician or nurse practitioner to manage their blood pressure?
- For Competency 2, did you include a description of how nurses in California lobbied the governor to support the nurse–patient ratio law to increase the capacity of hospitals to provide quality health care?
- In terms of Competency 3, did you include an example of a nurse researcher who interviewed community members to determine the behavioral, cultural, social, environmental, and organizational determinants of childhood obesity and how to best prevent it?
- Did you include a description of your own clinical write-ups or concept mapping when listing examples of Competency 4? Have you developed measurable goals after assessing patient needs and assets by using evidence-based nursing interventions that you learned about in lecture?
- As an example of Competency 5, did you describe patient care that you have provided in an efficient and culturally sensitive manner? Have you ever allowed a Spanish-speaking or Hmong-speaking patient to have family visits beyond the scheduled visiting hours because it was more convenient for the families' schedule or needs? Have you ever altered your teaching method based on the patient's culture?
- In terms of Competency 6, did you describe a poster or a podium presentation from a professional nursing conference where the researcher was discussing the effectiveness of health promotion practices and disseminating the results?
- Did you describe a public or community health nurse who you observed demonstrating Competency 7 when advocating for a mother by building on one of her existing parenting strengths?
- In terms of health promotion Competency 8, did you mention that nurses work collaboratively with social workers, psychologists, occupational therapists, speech pathologists, physical therapists, physicians, and pharmacists when promoting patient health?

WHAT DO YOU THINK?

Think about what health means to you. Rank-order the concepts that others have identified as being central to definitions of health by placing a 1 next to the best definition of health from your point of view, placing an 11 next to the definition of health that is least meaningful for you, and numbering the remaining definitions accordingly. Look over the list and enter a "yes" or a "no" next to the aspects of health you would include in a definition. Describe your rationale for including or excluding the given aspect of health from a definition.

Rank Order	I would include this aspect in my definition of health— yes or no	Rationale	Defining Aspect of Health
			1. The absence of physical and mental disease.
			2. Living well despite illness or disability.
			3. A complete state of physical, mental, social, and emotional well-being, not merely the absence of disease.
			4. The capacity for living.
			5. Individualized fitness that allows one to live a full and creative life.
			6. Good quality of life.
			7. Actualization of inherent and acquired human potential through goal-directed behavior.
			8. Competent self-care and satisfying relationships with others while maintaining harmony with relevant environments.
			9. The state of optimum capacity to perform the roles and tasks one has been socialized into.
			10. A joyful attitude toward life and a cheerful acceptance of one's responsibilities.
			11. The capacity to maintain balance and be free from undue pain, discomfort, disability, or limitation of action including social capacity.

Review the common aspects of health in the grid presented. Are any of them unique to a given society and not a definition that would be acceptable in any society? Which aspect would not apply to all cultures and societies? For example, do all cultures value individualized fitness, self-care, and maintaining balance? Of individualized fitness, self-care, and maintaining balance, which aspect of health is typically least valued within the United States? In your view, which aspect of health is least valued in Asian countries?

Health is a phenomenon that most of us understand, yet it remains difficult to define. Imagine your health as a large soap bubble surrounding your body that goes everywhere you go. Also, think back to a time when your health was suffering for a short period. Now, write the title "Health," followed by seven sentences that describe your health on different days when you felt the healthiest during your life. Select specific phrases that capture what it means and what it is like to be healthy. Just write without censoring your thoughts and feelings. You can go back afterward to edit your responses.

REFERENCES

American Nurses Association. (1995). *Nursing: A social policy statement*. Kansas City, MO: Author.

American Nurses Association (2010). What is nursing? Retrieved from http://www.nursingworld.org/EspeciallyForYou/StudentNurses/WhatisNursing.aspx

Barry, M. M., Allegrante, J. P., Lamarre, M., Auld, E., & Taub, A. (2009). The Galway consensus conference: International collaboration on the development of core competencies for health promotion and education? *Global Health Promotion, 16*(2), 5–11.

Breslow, W. (1999). From disease prevention to health promotion. *JAMA, 281*(11), 1030–1033.

Brown, J., Kazi, L., Spitz, P., Gertman, P., Fires, J., & Meehan, R. (1984). The dimensions of health outcomes: A cross-validated examination of health status measurement. *American Journal of Public Health, 74*, 159–161.

Carlson, J. (2003). Basic concepts. In *Complementary therapies and wellness* (pp. 1–8). Upper Saddle River, NJ: Prentice Hall.

Casey, D. (2007a). Health promotion: Findings from non-participant observational data concerning health promotion nursing practice in the acute hospital setting focusing on generalist nurses. *Journal of Clinical Nursing, 16*, 580-592.

Casey, D. (2007b). Nurses' perceptions, understanding, and experiences of health promotion. *Journal of Clinical Nursing, 16*, 1039–1049.

Cribb, A., & Dunes, A. (1993). What is health promotion? In A. Dines & A. Cribb (Eds.), *Health Promotion Concepts and Practice* (pp. 20–33). Oxford, UK: Blackwell Scientific.

Diemert-Moch, S. (1998). Health-within-illness: Concept development through research and practice. *Journal of Advanced Nursing, 28*(2), 305–310.

Dunn, H. L. (1959). High-level wellness in man and society. *American Journal of Public Health, 49*, 786.

Eldh, A. C., Ekman, I., & Ehnfors, M. (2010). A comparison of the concept of patient participation and patients' descriptions as related to healthcare definitions. *International Journal of Nursing Terminologies and Classifications, 21*(1), 21–32.

Goldsmith, S. (1972). The status of health indicators. *Health Service Reports, 87*, 212–220.

Harm, T. (2001). Patient education in Estonia. *Patient Education and Counseling, 4,* 75–78.

Harris, D. M., & Guten, S. (1979). Health protective behavior: an exploratory study. *Journal of Health and Social Behavior, 20,* 17–29.

International Council of Nurses (2010) The ICN definition of nursing. Retrieved from http://www.icn.ch /definition.htm

King, P. M. (1994). Health promotion: the emerging frontier in nursing. *Journal of Advanced Nursing, 20,* 209–218.

Larson, J. S. (1999). The conceptualization of health. *Medical Care Research and Review, 56,* 123–136.

Larsson, G., Starrin, B., & Wilde, B. (1991). Contributions of stress theory to the understanding of helping. *Scandinavian Journal of Caring Sciences, 5,* 79–85.

Maben, J. & Macleod-Clark, J. (1995). Health promotion: A concept analysis. *Journal of Advanced Nursing, 22,* 1158–1165.

Mackintosh, N. (1996). *Promoting health: An issue for nursing.* Dinton, Nr. Salisbury, Wilts, Quay Books.

Manderscheid, R. W., Ryff, C. D., Freeman, E. J., McKnight-Eily, L. R., Dhingra, S., & Strine, T. W. (2010). Evolving definitions of mental illness and wellness. Preventing Chronic Disease. *Public Health Research, Practice and Policy, 7*(1), 1–6.

Morgan, I. S., & Marsh, G. W. (1998). Historic and future health promotion contexts for nursing. *Image: The Journal of Nursing Scholarship, 30,* 379–383.

Nightingale, F. (1859). *Notes on Nursing: What it is, and what it is not.* London, UK: Harrison and Sons.

Pender, N., Murdaugh, C., & Parsons, M. (2002). *Health promotion in nursing practice* (4th ed.). Upper Saddle River, NJ: Prentice Hall.

Robertson, A. (2001). Biotechnology, political rationality, and discourses on health risk. *Health, 5,* 293–309.

Saylor, C. (2004). The circle of health: A health definition model. *Journal of Holistic Nursing, 22,* 97–115.

Sullivan, M. (2003). The new subjective medicine: Talking the patient's point of view on health care and health. *Social Science and Medicine, 56*(7), 1595–1604.

Smith, P., Masterson, A., & Smith, S. L. (1999). Health promotion versus disease and care: Failure to establish blissful clarity in British nurse education and practice. *Social Science and Medicine, 48,* 227–239.

Tones, K. (1985). Health promotion a new panacea? *Journal of the Institute of Health Education, 23*(1), 16–21.

Tones, K. (2000). Evaluating health promotion: A tale of three errors. *Patient Education and Counseling, 39,* 227–236.

Tones, K., Tilford, S., & Robinson, Y. (1990). *Health education effectiveness and efficiency.* London, UK: Chapman & Hall.

Ware, J., Brook, R., Davies, A. & Lohr, K. (1981). Choosing measures of health status for individuals in general populations. *American Journal of Public Health, 71,* 620–625.

Whitehead, D. (2001). Health education, behavioral change, and social psychology: Nursing's contribution to health promotion? *Journal of Advanced Nursing, 34*(6), 822–832.

Whitehead, D. (2003a). Health promotion and health education viewed as symbiotic paradigms: Bridging the theory and practice gap between them. *Journal of Clinical Nursing, 12,* 796–805.

Whitehead, D. (2003b). Incorporating sociopolitical health promotion activities in clinical practice. *Journal of Clinical Nursing, 12,* 668–677.

Whitehead, D (2003c). The health-promoting nurse as a health policy career expert and entrepreneur. *Nurse Education Today, 23,* 585–592.

Whitehead, D. (2004). Health promotion and health education: Advancing the concepts. *Journal of Advanced Nursing, 47,* 311–320.

Whitehead, D. (2006). Health promotion in the practice setting: Findings from a review of clinical issues. *Worldviews on Evidence-Based Nursing, 3*(4), 165–184.

Whitehead, D. (2008). Health promotion: An international Delphi study examining health promotion and health education in nursing practice, education and policy. *Journal of Clinical Nursing, 17*, 891–900.

Williamson, D. L. & Carr, J. (2009). Health as a resource for everyday life: Advancing the conceptualization. *Critical Public Health, 19*(1), 107–122.

Wilson-Barnett, J. (1993). Health promotion and nursing practice. In A. Dines and A. Cribb (Eds.), *Health promotion: Concepts and practice* (pp. 195–204). Oxford, UK: Blackwell Scientific Publications.

World Health Organization [WHO]. (1948). *Preamble to the constitution of the WHO.* Official records of the WHO (No 2, p. 100). Entered into force April 7, 1948.

World Health Organization [WHO]. (1986). *The Ottawa charter for health promotion.* Ontario, Canada: Canadian Public Health Association, Health and Welfare Canada, and the World Health Organization.

For a full suite of assignments and additional learning activities, see the access code at the front of your book.

CHAPTER 2

The History of Health Promotion

Bonnie Raingruber

OBJECTIVES

At the conclusion of this chapter, the student will be able to:

- Describe the ancient Greek approach to health promotion.
- Discuss how the health promotion movement was influenced by historical developments, critical documents, and international conferences.
- Identify which perspectives about health promotion correspond to a given historical era, document, or organization.
- Analyze how historical developments in health promotion have influenced nursing practice.

INTRODUCTION

Numerous historical practices, key documents, important task forces, and international conferences have shaped the nature of health promotion practice as it exists today. Each period and accomplishment has helped delineate the breadth of health promotion practice. A number of key time periods, documents, and conferences are described in the next section. Although the latter part of the 20th century is typically viewed as being most critical in shaping the nature of health promotion practice (Tountas, 2009), we will first begin with an overview of older influences.

ANCIENT HEALTH PROMOTION PRACTICES: INDIAN, CHINESE, EGYPTIAN, AND HEBREW

Indian systems of medicine trace back to 5000 BC, where ayurvedic practices focused on personal hygiene, sanitation, water supply, and engineering practices that supported health. Chinese medicine dates back to 2700 BC and included attention to hygiene, diet, hydrotherapy, massage, and immunization. From 200 BC, the Egyptians developed community systems for collecting rainwater, disposing of waste, inoculating people against small pox, and methods of avoiding the plague by controlling the rat population. They also used mosquito nets, encouraged frequent bathing, and advocated against excess use of alcohol (Kushwah, 2007).

Early references to health promotion are found in the Code of Hammurabi and Mosaic Law. These references address disease prevention, disposal of waste, and segregation of infectious persons, including those suffering from leprosy. Mosaic Law encouraged a weekly day of rest for health as well as for religious reasons, and recognized that eating pork could result in illness (Moore & Williamson, 1984).

GREEK ANTIQUITY

The ancient Greeks (460 to 136 BC) were the first civilization to emphasize that health is a function of physical and social environments as well as human behavior. They empowered individuals and communities to establish conditions and practices that supported health since being strong and beautiful was highly valued in Greek society (Tountas, 2009).

The Pythagoreans suggested that harmony, equilibrium, and balance were key factors in maintaining health. They felt that living life in a way that minimized disturbance would promote health. The Pythagoreans also placed a great deal of emphasis on hygiene. They ate little meat, practiced moderation, and worked on maintaining self-control and calmness at all times. Plato suggested that health is a state of being in harmony with the universe and experiencing a sense of completeness and contentment. Hippocrates defined health as equilibrium between environmental forces (such as temperature, water, and food) and individual habits (diet, alcohol, sexual behaviors, work, and leisure). Health was seen as a matter of balancing the perpetual flux of the body. Hippocrates suggested that a person's most valuable asset was health, so knowing how to modulate one's thoughts to maintain health was a critical skill. An epidemiologist, Hippocrates coined the term "endemic" to describe diseases that were consistently present in a population and the word "epidemic" to describe diseases that occurred at select times.

A Greek physician was tasked with evaluating the season and climate; the location of a person's home; the wind; water sources; geography; and whether people ate well, drank to excess, got adequate rest, and exercised on a regular basis. The trainer, the physician, and the educator were closely linked roles in Greek society.

Social, political, and economic influences were seen as critical in Greek society in terms of achieving empowerment, autonomy, self-sufficiency, and health. Donations from the rich were used to subsidize health care for the poor. Physicians had an obligation to treat the rich and poor alike (Tountas, 2009).

Asklepieions, temples to the god of Medicine, were found throughout the country where Hippocratic medicine was practiced and were situated in beautiful areas next to rectangular pools of water, auditoriums where entertainment and oratory was available, and close to gymnasiums and stadiums. This proximity allowed for simultaneous attention to physical, psychological, social, and spiritual well-being (Tountas, 2009).

THE ROMAN EMPIRE

The Romans focused on community health measures including transportation of clean water, paved streets, street cleaning, and sanitary waste disposal. According to Roman philosophy, the state—not the individual—had the greatest influence on health. Public baths were provided to support community health. A census of both citizens and slaves was used to plan community health programs and structures. Ventilation and central heating were required by building codes of the day. A Roman physician, Galen, described health as "a condition in which we neither suffer pain nor are hindered in the functions of daily life such a taking part in government, bathing, drinking, eating, and doing other things we want" (Moore & Williamson, 1984, p. 196). He suggested that disease was caused by predisposing, exciting, and environmental factors (Kushwah, 2007).

THE MEDIEVAL PANDEMICS

Between 1000 and 1453 AD, bubonic plague (Black Death) and pulmonary anthrax moved from Asia to Africa, the Crimea, Turkey, Greece, and then Europe. Quarantine was used, in which travelers from plague-infested areas had to stop at designated spots and remain there for 2 months, without demonstrating any symptoms, before being allowed to continue their journey (Kushwah, 2007).

KEY ORGANIZATIONS, CONFERENCES, TASK FORCES, AND DOCUMENTS THAT HAVE INFLUENCED THE NATURE OF HEALTH PROMOTION IN MODERN TIMES

Next we will review a number of modern day organizations, movements, conferences, task forces, and documents that have helped shape the nature of health promotion. Many have argued that social and political developments such as civil rights, women's movements, self-care, and the human potential movement during 1960s influenced the onset of the health promotion era by advocating for increased knowledge, participatory control over one's life, and equal access for all (Morgan & Marsh, 1998). It is also likely that the greater than 50% increase in life expectancy that occurred during the 20th century helped fuel the health promotion movement: People were now living longer and a need existed to focus on improving quality of life (Breslow, 1999).

Many of the key organizations, conferences, and documents we will review have had global impact, influencing not only health promotion within one country but also around the world. Timeframes associated with each organization are provided in the headings so that you can gain a sense of the chronology of historical influences that have shaped health promotion practice.

The World Health Organization (1948–Present)

Since the United Nations created the World Health Organization (WHO) in 1948, it has been focused on global health promotion. The WHO advocates for legislation, fiscal change, and organizational and community efforts to promote health. In 1984, the WHO defined health promotion as the process of enabling people to take control over maintaining and improving their health. With the issuance of this definition, a decade of focus on the impact of lifestyle on health shifted to attention on the structural factors in society that support health. These societal factors included things such as income, housing, food security, employment, and working conditions.

In 2001, the WHO published an International Classification of Functioning, Disability, and Health (ICF) to encourage the attainment, monitoring, and enhancement of health and functioning. This document focuses on functional abilities, activities, participation levels, and environmental factors that contribute to health promotion. Self-determination and autonomy, as well as 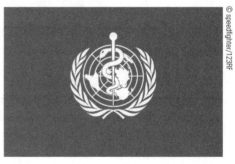 personal and environmental factors, are seen as key in shaping health, according to the ICF (Howard, Nieuwenhuijsen, & Saleeby, 2008).

The International Union for Health Promotion and Education (1951–present)

The International Union for Health Promotion and Education (IUHPE) is a global, professional, nongovernmental organization dedicated to advancing health promotion (Mittelmark, Perry, Wise, Lamarre, & Jones, 2007). Its mission is to promote global health and equity between and within countries around the world. Globalization, transboundary influences on health, urbanization, consumerism, chemical/radiological/biological threats to health, and population growth are issues of key interest to the IUHPE (Mittelmark, 2007). By partnering with Oxford University Press, the IUHPE currently publishes *Health Education Research* and *Health Promotion International* to support health promotion research and dissemination. In addition, the IUHPE publishes *Promotion and Education* along with sponsoring regional and global conferences dedicated to health promotion. They also maintain a health promotion website and sponsor health promotion research. Since 1998 IUHPE has been involved in lobbying for social clauses to be added to trade agreements in an effort to protect poor countries from exploitation.

A specific focus of the IUHPE is health impact assessment and evaluating the effectiveness of health promotion programs (Mittelmark et al., 2007). The IUHPE believes health promotion programs are best evaluated when linked to the daily life of communities, when the research is in sync with local traditions, and when it is led by community members (Mittelmark, 2007).

The IUHPE and the WHO coordinate the Global Programme for Health Promotion Effectiveness (GPHPE). The goals of the GPHPE are to: (1) improve standards of health-promoting policymaking; (2) review evidence of program effectiveness in terms of political, economic, social, and health impact; and (3) disseminate evidence to policymakers, teachers, healthcare practitioners, and researchers (Corbin & Mittelmark, 2008).

The Lalonde Report (1974)

The first authoritative policy statement to suggest that health promotion was determined by issues other than those associated with the healthcare system or medical care came from the Lalonde Report (Lalonde, 1974). As a result, Canada became recognized as a leader in the conceptual development of health promotion policy. This report is credited with bringing the term *health promotion* into prominence (Morgan & Marsh, 1998).

The Lalonde Report introduced the health field model, which emphasized that lifestyle/behavior, biology, environment, and healthcare organizations all impacted health. It advocated for viewing preventative care as important as treatment and cure. Mortality statistics were used to summarize the number of unnecessary diseases and illustrate that chronic disease, rather than infectious disease, accounts for the preponderance of disability and death.

Within Canada, the Lalonde Report influenced the government to shift public policy from a focus on disease treatment to health promotion. The Lalonde Report had the goal of prompting individuals and organizations to accept more responsibility for their health, and it resulted in interventions to decrease automobile accidents, eliminate drunken driving, increase seat belt use, and minimize alcoholism (MacDougall, 2007).

The Lalonde Report was used by the World Health Organization and numerous governments as the rationale for expanding the definition and understanding of health promotion to include both environmental and lifestyle factors. This report was the source of the best known definition of health promotion, which is that it is the art and science of helping people change their lifestyle and move toward an optimal state of health. Influential as the Lalonde Report was, it was criticized for emphasizing lifestyle issues more than environmental, economic, social, and health system–related influences. For example, it stressed the importance of self-imposed risks and individual blame associated with poor lifestyle choices (Raphael, 2008).

WHO: Declaration of Alma-Ata on Primary Health Care (1978)

In 1978, the WHO issued the Alma-Ata declaration in support of the idea that health promotion was not entirely in the purview of the healthcare sector. The Alma-Ata declaration also emphasized that (1) global cooperation and peace were vital, (2) local and community needs must drive health promotion activities, (3) economic and social needs shape health, (4) prevention must be an integral part of health care, (5) equity in terms of health status is needed, and (6) multiple sectors and players must be involved to improve health (Awofeso, 2004). It emphasized the need for health promotion as well as curative and rehabilitative services. The Alma-Ata declaration suggested that evidence indicates that healthcare resources are too concentrated in centralized, professionally-dominated, highly technological institutions, which limits care available at local and community levels (King, 1994). The Alma-Ata declaration put forth many ideas that later appeared in the Ottawa Charter.

The Alma-Ata declaration emphasized issues of particular importance to developing countries to a greater extent than other documents had done. For example, issues of food security, affordable health care, global peace, safe water, proper nutrition, and family planning were highlighted (Awofeso, 2004).

Healthy People (1979–2020)

Motivated by the Canadian Lalonde Report, the United States' Surgeon General developed a comprehensive public health policy with associated 10-year prevention strategies and outcome targets designed to decrease mortality and morbidity. Health promotion was separated from disease prevention and both targets were given priority

(Morgan & Marsh, 1998). This policy was called Healthy People 1979. Healthy People consists of national objectives for promoting health and preventing disease designed to encourage collaborations across sectors, to guide people in making healthy choices, and to measure the impact of U.S. policy. A unique aspect of Healthy People 1979 was establishing measurable target goals for improvements in population health, which resulted in improvements in seat belt use, decreased alcohol consumption, and lower rates of smoking (MacDougall, 2007).

"Healthy People 1979 argued that 50% of mortality in 1976 was due to unhealthy behavior or lifestyle, 20% to environmental factors, 20% to human biology, and 10% to inadequacies in health care" (MacDougall, 2007, p. 958). Healthy People 1979 became a roadmap for public health activities and prevention strategies across the United States. Prior to its issuance, no national guide for primary prevention had existed (Brown, 2009). Healthy People 1979 called for a reexamination of U.S. priorities for national health spending, since only 4% of funding was previously allocated to prevention. The report argued for the development of community-based and individual interventions to help develop healthy lifestyles and enhance a state of well-being.

The Healthy People 1979 Report was followed by the development of Healthy People 1990, 2000, 2010, and 2020, with each report building on the previous agenda. Healthy People 1990 focused on reducing mortality across the lifespan with priority being assigned to accident/injury prevention, control of stress/violent behavior, family planning, fluoridation of drinking water, high blood pressure, immunization, alcohol and drug abuse, physical fitness, pregnancy, sexually transmitted diseases, smoking, and toxic agents. In addition, in Healthy People 1990, it became clear that there were subpopulations within the United States who experienced greater health disparities and need for care. Equal access became a priority (Brown, 2009).

Can you think of a type of cancer that is related to a health disparity? If you mentioned (1) African American women are more likely to die from breast cancer and be diagnosed with cervical cancer, (2) African American men have the highest incidence of prostate cancer, (3) African Americans have the highest incidence and death rate for both colorectal and lung cancer, (4) Hispanic women have the highest incidence of cervical cancer, (5) Asian Americans and Pacific Islanders have the highest incidence of liver and stomach cancer, (6) American Indians have the highest incidence of kidney cancer, or (7) White women living in Appalachia have a higher risk of cervical cancer than other White women, then you would have correctly identified a cancer-related health disparity (National Cancer Institute, 2010).

Healthy People 2000 focused on increasing years of healthy life, reducing health disparities, and increasing access to preventative services. Priority areas were cancer, diabetes, community-based programs, environmental health, food and drug safety, heart disease and stroke, HIV infection, maternal and infant health, mental health, surveillance and data systems, and violent/abusive behavior, in addition to previously unmet target goals from 1990 (Brown, 2009).

During the period between 2000 and 2010, the Behavioral Risk Factor Surveillance System and the National Health Interview Survey were implemented so that quantitative data could be used to evaluate progress and shape future priorities of the Healthy People agenda (Brown, 2009).

Healthy People 2010 was based on the same goals as Healthy People 2000, with priority being given to access to health services, arthritis, osteoporosis, kidney disease, health communication, medical product safety, public health infrastructure, and respiratory diseases, in addition to all previously unmet target priorities (Brown, 2009). Another goal was increasing quality and years of healthy life by assisting people to gain knowledge, motivation, and opportunity to make informed decisions about their health. Eliminating health disparities or gaps between two or more groups in term of health outcomes continued to be a priority of Healthy People 2010. Healthy People 2010 includes a number of indicators, such as physical activity, obesity, tobacco use, and mental health, so that health promotion successes can be tracked (Howard, Nieuwenhuijsen, & Saleeby, 2008).

In order to provide a structure for integrating Healthy People 2010 objectives, the U.S. Department of Health and Human Services, the Centers for Disease Control and Prevention, the Office of National Drug Control Policy, and the Fordham Institute created a roadmap called Mobilizing, Assessing, Planning, Implementing and Tracking, or MAP-IT. The MAP-IT structure is available for use by anyone, including government officials, community leaders, and healthcare professionals, who want to create positive change in a community. There is a MAP-IT website, which includes action plans and successful models of using MAP-IT techniques. MAP-IT is designed to help groups map out, implement, and evaluate a community-level change. These techniques were created to help bring individuals and organizations into a coalition to improve health; to assess community needs, resources, and strengths; to plan interventions that are congruent with community needs and wants; to implement the plan using measurable goals; and to track process and report outcome measures (Jesse & Blue, 2004).

One example of a MAP-IT strategy described on the website involves a community task force organized in Lafayette, Louisiana after the Columbine school shootings. The task force consisted of school officials, psychologists, and community members. They proposed closer monitoring of indications of adolescent anger and provision of early professional intervention to defuse potentially dangerous situations (Healthy People, 2010).

An external advisory committee of 13 public health and healthcare delivery experts has provided input regarding the Healthy People 2020 goals. In addition, a public comment website (http://www.healthypeople.gov) was established for input from the public, although this phase of development has been completed and the comment period has ended. Determinants of health that will be addressed in Healthy People 2020 include: (1) social, economic, cultural, and environmental conditions and policies of global, national, state, and local levels; (2) living and working conditions; (3) social, family, and community networks; and (4) individual behaviors and traits, such as age, gender, race, and biological heritage, that shape health.

The priorities of Healthy People 2020 are to: (1) eliminate preventable disease, disability, injury, and premature death; (2) achieve health equity by eliminating health disparities; (3) create social and physical environments that promote health; and (4) support healthy development and behavior across the lifespan (MacDougall, 2007). Many of the objectives of previous years are retained along with a focus on disability and secondary conditions, community-based programs, genomics, and health care–associated infections.

The Healthy People initiative has been criticized for focusing excessively on individual responsibility for lifestyle choices while giving less credence to the ethnic, gender, environmental, and socioeconomic factors that influence health (MacDougall, 2007). Morgan and Marsh (1998) suggested this perspective, in which health promotion is seen as being based in personal behavior, and is a reflection of the strong current of responsibility and rugged individualism that is part of U.S. culture and history. There have also been concerns about the measurability of target indicators, the quality of data being collected, the lag time associated with data analysis, the reality that too many

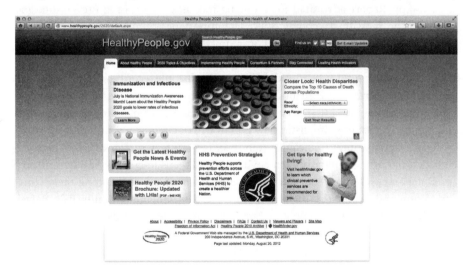

Image: U.S. Department of Health and Human Services. Office of Disease Prevention and Health Promotion. Healthy People 2020. Washington, DC. Available at http://www.healthypeople.gov /2020/default.aspx. Accessed 8-22-2012

objectives dilute the impact of the policy, and the fact that each priority is assigned an equal weighting.

Nonetheless, Healthy People was the first document to include outcomes that were designed to be measurable. Healthy People has played a major role in public health in the United States, and it has a major impact on federal and private funding for health promotion programs (Brown, 2009). Healthy People has helped increase public awareness and understanding of determinants of health, engaged multiple sectors to take action to promote health, and identified continuing research and data collection needs (Fielding & Kumanyika, 2009).

Achieving Health for All: The Epp Report (1986)

In 1986, the Canadian Minister of National Health and Welfare created a report titled "Achieving Health for All: A Framework for Health Promotion," which has come to be known as the Epp Report. This report documented that disadvantaged groups have lower life expectancies and poorer health than those with more resources. The Epp Report posited that self-care, mutual aid from others, and healthy environments were major influences on health promotion. Mutual aid included emotional support and the sharing of ideas, information, and experience in the context of a family, a neighborhood, a community organization, or a self-help group (Epp, 1986).

The Epp Report advocated for reducing inequities, increasing prevention, and enhancing an individual's coping skills. The importance of fostering public involvement in policymaking, strengthening community-based health services, and coordinating public policy were also stressed (McIntyre, 1992). Epp (1986) stated that all policies that impact health need to be considered, including income security, employment, education, housing, business, agriculture, transportation, criminal justice, and technology.

Epp (1986) asserted that "people often associate health promotion with posters and pamphlets but this simplistic view is akin to associating medical care with white coats and stethoscopes . . . health promotion is a strategy that synthesizes personal choice, social responsibility, and an environmental focus to create a healthier future" (p. 27). The Epp Report ended with an admonition to avoid "blaming the victim" and to stop underestimating social and economic determinants of health (Falk-Rafael, 1999; McIntyre, 1992). Although the Epp Report was released at the same time as the Ottawa Charter, it was never fully realized due to budget cuts in the 1980s and the new Canadian government that came to power in 1993.

WHO: Ottawa Charter for Health Promotion (1986)

The first international health promotion conference sponsored by the WHO was held in Ottawa, Canada in 1986. It resulted in the Ottawa Charter for Health Promotion, which is a quintessential document in the international health promotion arena. The Ottawa Charter emphasized that individuals need to have supportive environments and economic resources to lead healthy lives and experience well-being. It addressed the role of health inequalities and the importance of political, economic, and social influences on health (Scriven & Speller, 2007). This perspective expanded attention from individual lifestyles alone to the influence of groups.

The Ottawa Charter put forth the ideas that health promotion: (1) includes the concept of well-being; (2) rests on political, economic, social, cultural, environmental, behavioral, and biological advocacy; (3) necessitates attention be given to equity; (4) requires action by governments, voluntary organizations, local authorities, industry, health care, and the media; and (5) should be adapted to local needs and cultural/economic norms (Irvine, Elliott, Wallace, & Crombie, 2006). The Ottawa Charter asserted that to reach a state of complete physical, mental, and social well-being, "an individual or group must be able to identify and realize aspiration, to satisfy needs, and to change or cope with the environment . . . . Health is a positive concept emphasizing social and personal resources as well as physical capabilities" (WHO, 1987, p. iii).

This report was instrumental in stressing that health includes a state of physical, mental, and social well-being. It focused on caring, holism, advocacy, and mediation of differing social priorities as the cornerstones of health promotion (Falk-Rafael, 1999).

The Ottawa Charter stressed that health promotion is not the sole responsibility of the healthcare sector but rather requires political, economic, and social interventions as well as the involvement of voluntary organizations, local authorities, industry, and the media. The Ottawa Charter encouraged the use of community-based participatory research and the empowering of communities to take control of their own health (Scriven & Speller, 2007). An example of community involvement is including parents, youth, and community leaders in identifying health promotion strategies for youth at high risk of obesity, then involving those stakeholders in providing and evaluating the selected interventions.

It has been argued that involving diverse groups such as government, volunteer organizations, industry, community groups, and the media yields more creative, holistic, realistic, and relevant health promotion programs. Shared resources, relationships, and ideas result in outcomes that could not be achieved by any one group working alone. It is also true that maintaining effective multifaceted partnerships requires substantial communication, commitment, and time. Research has indicated that close to 50% of community-based partnerships dissolve within the first year. Issues of loss of focus, loss of control, consensus-building, and accountability are constant challenges that must be overcome (Corbin & Mittelmark, 2008).

Health promotion was defined by the Ottawa Charter as the "process of enabling individuals and communities to increase control over the determinants of health, thereby improving health to live an active and productive life" (Eriksson & Lindstrom, 2008, p. 194). The Ottawa Charter moved health promotion away from a focus on health education alone to increased attention to public policy, supportive environments, community action, personal skills, and the re-orientation of health-care services. The health promotion fulcrum shifted from an individual to a social, cultural, political, economic, and environmental perspective with this document (McQueen, 2008).

WHO: Adelaide Recommendations on Healthy Public Policy (1988)

The Second International Conference on Health Promotion was held in April 1988 in Adelaide, South Australia. It emphasized the necessity of supportive environments in promoting health. In addition, a call was issued for collaborations among governmental and private sector interests associated with agriculture, trade, education, industry, and communications to the extent that health was given priority over economic considerations. Conference presenters stressed that concern for equity in all areas of policy development results in substantial health benefits. They argued for equal healthcare access for indigenous peoples, ethnic minorities, and immigrants. They also stressed that education levels and literacy be taken into account when health policy is being designed. The importance of creating health information systems capable of evaluating the impact of policy change was highlighted. An argument was made for developing nationally-based women's health policies that supported women's choice in terms of birthing practices. They also advocated for parental/dependent healthcare leaves, and they created a larger role for women in the development of health policy. Issues such as the ecological impact of raising tobacco as a cash crop and how such practices limit food production were discussed (Kickbusch, McCann, & Sherbon, 2008).

The New Public Health Movement (1980s)

The New Public Health Movement (NPHM) was inspired by the Ottawa Charter on health promotion and by the growth of the field of population health. The NPHM embodies a number of the concepts just discussed, emphasizing that a socioecological rather than a biomedical approach is the most effective way to promote health. This socioecological view focuses on preventing rather than curing disease by examining root causes of disease such as economic inequalities, social problems, and environmental issues. The priority is on establishing health policy, services, and educational programs to prevent disease before it occurs.

The NPHM represents a shift from the "lifestyle" era in health promotion policy, where the focus was on individual behaviors, to a "public health" era where the primary focus is on population-level issues such as social, cultural, and environmental factors that affect health. Falk-Rafael (1999) suggested the new public health movement signals a return to the values and philosophy regarding health and health promotion that are consistent with a nursing paradigm.

WHO: Sundsvall Statement on Supportive Environments for Health (1991)

The Third International conference on health promotion was held in June 1991 in Sundsvall, Sweden. The conclusion of the conference was that a supportive environment is of paramount importance to health. Supportive environments meant both the physical and social aspects of where one lives, works, socializes, is educated, and seeks care. Four main aspects of supportive environments were emphasized: (1) the social dimension, including norms, customs, purpose, and heritage; (2) the political dimension, including participation in decision making and a commitment to human rights and peace; (3) the economic dimension, including sustainable development; and (4) the need to recognize and use women's skills and knowledge.

The conference highlighted growing inequities between rich and poor countries as well as the relationship between social justice and health. Creating equity was identified as a priority for creating supportive environments. There was also a focus on sustainable development and a call for the involvement of indigenous peoples in developing health promotion policies. The wisdom and spiritual relationship that indigenous peoples maintain with their environment was presented as a model for the rest of the world.

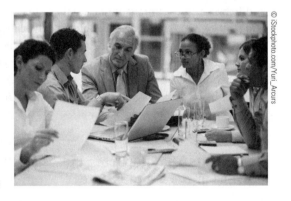

The conference also called for four key public health action strategies: (1) strengthening advocacy through community action, (2) empowering and educating communities to take control of their own health, (3) building alliances between environmental and health oriented groups, and (4) mediating conflict to ensure equitable access to healthy environments (WHO, 2010a).

WHO: Jakarta Declaration on Leading Health Promotion into the 21st Century (1997)

The Fourth International conference on health promotion was held in July 1997 in Jakarta, Indonesia. It was the first WHO conference to be held in a developing country and the first to involve the private sector. The Jakarta Declaration, which derived from that conference, emphasized that poverty is the greatest threat to health, while summarizing that peace, shelter, education, social relations, food, income, the empowerment of women, a stable ecosystem, sustainable resources, social justice, respect for human rights, and equity are requirements for health (WHO, 2010b).

The conference presenters highlighted the fact that transnational factors such as the global economy, financial markets, ease of access to communication technology, environmental degradation, and irresponsible use of resources also have a significant impact on health. A call for action to establish a global health promotion alliance was issued. Goals for that alliance were to: (1) raise awareness of changing determinants of health, (2) support collaborations dedicated to health promotion, (3) mobilize resources for health promotion, (4) accumulate best practice knowledge, (5) enable shared learning, (6) promote solidarity in action, and (7) foster transparency and public accountability in health promotion (WHO, 2010b).

WHO: Bangkok Charter for Health Promotion (2005)

In 2005, the WHO issued the Bangkok Charter, which built on the Ottawa Charter by adding a focus on coherence of health policy and a commitment to partnership within and between governments, international organizations, and the private sector. The Bangkok Charter encouraged people to "advocate for health based on human rights, invest in sustainable policies, actions, and infrastructure to address the determinants of health, target knowledge transfer and research, and address health literacy" (Howard, Nieuwenhuijsen, & Saleeby, 2008, p. 943). It advocated for equal opportunity for health and well-being for all people. Health was now seen as a critical part of foreign policy, national security, trade, and geopolitics.

Documents That Impacted Public Health and Health Promotion Practice in the United States

The majority of the documents we have discussed so far were global in their reach, but it is equally important to become familiar with historical documents within the United States that have shaped public health and health promotion practice. In 1850, Lemuel

Shattuck, the first president of the American Statistical Society and a member of the Massachusetts legislature, published "Report of a General Plan for the Promotion of Public and Person Health," which later became known as the Shattuck Report. The report reviewed mortality data and documented survival rates based on age and social class in Massachusetts. Dramatic differences by social class were used to support the conclusion that health status could be modified. The Shattuck Report included 50 recommendations addressing, among others, the organization of local health boards, town planning, and the need for national health education. Nineteen years after release of this report the Massachusetts legislature enacted a law based on the recommendations of the Shattuck Report that became a pattern for public health legislation across the United States (Winkelstein, 2009).

By 1932, the Committee on the Costs of Medical Care had been created. This committee commissioned a survey of health status and medical care utilization of 8,000 families nationwide who were followed for 12 months. The report of that study was titled "Medical Care for the American People" This report recommended that: (1) both preventive and medical care be provided for all citizens, (2) public health services be available to everyone based on need, (3) taxation and insurance should be used to ensure that medical care was based on group rates for all, (4) each state and local community health agency would evaluate their services, and (5) professional education of healthcare workers should include content on prevention and the social factors that influence health. The report was considered radical at the time: *The New York Times* claimed that it called for socialized medicine and the American Medical Association referred to it as incitement to revolution. This report served as the basis for President Franklin Roosevelt's failed attempt at passage of national health insurance (Winkelstein, 2009). Are any of these issues still being debated today in the United States?

In 1959, the U.S. Surgeon General wrote in the *Journal of the American Medical Association* that the weight of evidence implicated smoking as being the principal factor influencing the incidence of lung cancer. Following that commentary, presidents of the American Cancer Society, the American Public Health Association, the American Heart Association, and the National Tuberculosis Association contacted then-President Kennedy asking that a presidential commission be established to study smoking and health. A blue ribbon advisory committee was appointed. They issued a report that addressed biological effects of tobacco, epidemiological patterns, dose/response mortality ratios, and psychosocial implications associated with smoking. These documents had a major impact on tobacco-related advertising and taxation legislation while also serving as a model for future development of evidence-based health policy (Winkelstein, 2009).

SUMMARY OF HISTORICAL CHRONOLOGY

In the 1970s, the focus was on preventing disease and reducing risk behaviors through health education. Motivated by the Ottawa Charter, the 1980s saw increasing attention being given to the role of supportive environments, social influences, economic resources, health inequalities, and political action in creating health. During the 1990s, attention focused on the importance of setting and environment. Interventions within schools, workplaces, and community centers made it possible to reach large numbers of people and provide sustained interventions in a convenient location. Core values of the health promotion movement were identified as equity, participation, and empowerment (Eriksson & Lindstrom, 2008).

Specific capacity-building interventions focused on health promoting hospitals, health promoting universities, and health promoting prisons (WHO, 1986). Health promoting hospitals improve health by organizing rehabilitation efforts; empowering clients; encouraging links between community agencies, home health agencies, and hospital staff; and creating a healthy environment that supports a return to the highest level of functioning. An example of the latter is found in the adoption of smoke-free zones and healthy menus that support the health of both patients and staff.

Over the course of several decades, health promotion has shifted from the perspective that healthcare professionals need to educate individuals to a stance where involving people in decision making, program design, intervention, and evaluation is the priority. A 2007 synthesis of eight research reviews presented at the Bangkok WHO conference summarized that: (1) investing in public policy is key, (2) supportive environments are critical, (3) community-based action needs additional research, (4) personal skills development should be paired with other interventions, (5) multi-level interventions are most effective, and (6) collaborations and partnerships supported by political commitments, nongovernmental organizations, and local stakeholders are vital to the success of health promotion programs (Jackson, Perkins, Khandor, Cordwell, Hamann, & Buasi, 2007).

A 2008 summary of the literature (Howard, Nieuwenhuijsen & Saleeby, 2008) suggested that three themes are found in published studies on health promotion. Those themes are: (1) that health promotion is a broad and complex concept, (2) that health promotion requires addressing environmental factors with particular attention being given to barriers that interfere with health promotion, and (3) that focusing on the concepts of social capital, social support, and networking improves health. Barriers are a major predictor of involvement in health promotion activities. Barriers can include concerns over transportation, family responsibilities, language and cultural differences, and scheduling (Howard, Nieuwenhuijsen & Saleeby, 2008).

Social capital has been defined as "the features of social organization such as networks, norms, and trust that facilitate coordination and co-operation for mutual benefit" (Howard, Nieuwenhuijsen, & Saleeby, 2008, p. 944). Social capital includes peer support and professional support, as well as the input of family and friends.

SIX PHASES IN THE EVOLUTION OF PRIMARY CARE/PREVENTION

Awofeso (2004) suggested there have been six major historical approaches to providing primary health care. These approaches included attention to health protection, sanitary control, contagion control, prevention, primary health care, and health promotion. The health protection era, which continued until the 1830s, relied on religious and cultural rules, spiritual practices, community taboos, and quarantine of contagious individuals, including those with leprosy and Black Death.

The sanitary control era between 1840 and 1870 was ushered in following the Industrial Revolution, when filthy working conditions, unsafe water supplies, poor drainage systems, and inadequate sewage disposal resulted in deaths. During this period modern epidemiological methods were used to track disease outbreaks.

The contagion control era between the 1880s and 1930s followed on Robert Koch's publication on germ theory. Attention was on infectious diseases like cholera, and vaccination and improved water filtration processes were used to improve health.

The preventative medicine era between 1940 and 1960 brought awareness of disease vectors, an understanding that some microbes are necessary for healthy bodily function, and knowledge that nutritional deficiencies, such as inadequate intake of iodine, influenced health. High-risk groups such as pregnant women, the elderly, and factory workers were often target groups during this period. Disease vectors such as mosquitoes were researched. Advances in clinical pathology were used to design interventions.

The primary healthcare era of 1970–1980 saw a focus on preventive health care; an emphasis on equity, community participation, and access to services; and an understanding of the social determinants of health. Links were forged between health care and socioeconomic development. Multicultural and participatory, community-based interventions were priorities.

The health promotion era that began in the 1990s brought attention to advocacy efforts with individuals and communities. Economic and political interventions were used to create supportive environments, strengthen community action, and develop personal skills (Awofeso, 2004).

THE ROLE OF NURSING LEADERS IN HEALTH PROMOTION

In addition to examining historical documents, conferences, and organizations, it is also important to focus specifically on the role of nursing in shaping health promotion practice. In 1862, when Florence Nightingale established a school to educate district nurses, a full year was devoted to promoting the health of communities. Self-care and an emphasis on active involvement in social and health reforms were included in the curriculum. Training addressed how to "depauperize" individuals in poverty by addressing their self-image and by becoming involved in social reform designed to minimize economic disparities. Nightingale argued that health dollars would be better spent maintaining health during infancy and childhood than by building hospitals. She was active in health promotion activities and policy development related to air pollution reduction in factories (Falk-Rafael, 1999).

In the early 20th century Lillian Wald established the Henry Street Settlement. Nurses in the Henry Street Settlement were active in political lobbying to obtain health care for individuals living in poverty, establishing school nursing and rural nursing, and influencing the development of child labor laws. Wald supported the development of community coalitions to influence social and health policy. She felt nurses were in a pivotal position to link agencies and communities in an effort to support social betterment. Wald viewed nurses as the trusted partner of those in need and she saw nurses as being able to link community needs with resources in support of health (Falk-Rafael, 1999).

The Flexner report, distributed in 1910, promoted the adoption of a reductionist, biomedical, cause-oriented, disease-focused explanation of illness that moved away from a focus on the broad determinants of health. As a result public health nursing came to be viewed as outdated and out of step with scientific advances. Public health nurses found themselves operating under new philosophies and policies controlled by bureaucracies that were themselves under medical control. A reduction in public health nursing services followed, and a narrow, medicalized definition of health promotion as being exclusively focused on primary prevention was adopted (Falk-Rafael, 1999). Public health nurses who had previously treated individuals recovering from heart disease, stroke, and other chronic conditions were no longer allocated time on their caseloads to work with these clients.

Mary Breckinridge created the Frontier Nursing service to provide health care and health promotion in rural Kentucky. As a child she traveled to Russia when her father was appointed minister there. During those years she developed a sense of the challenges that come with poverty. As a young mother, she lost a daughter and son to illness, which motivated her lifelong interest in the health of mothers and children. Toward the end of World War I she worked as a volunteer in France. Between nursing school and midwifery school she spent a summer exploring the Appalachian

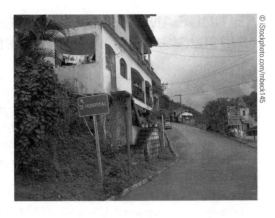

Mountains on horseback to learn about rural Kentucky health needs. In 1925 she created a nurse-managed midwifery service in Kentucky that provided prenatal care, attendance at births, vaccines, and health promotion. She involved the community in designing the model of care, based her midwifery service on community needs, and kept detailed statistical records. Her program exemplified a community-based participatory intervention and became a model for health professionals around the world.

In 1994 in Canada, a nursing union facing layoffs brought a lawsuit claiming that health promotion was exclusively nurses' work. The arbiter cited federal health policy documents to conclude that although nurses have always been involved in health promotion, current nursing practice did not support their claim that lesser skilled workers should not be assigned health promotion duties. Falk-Rafael (1999) emphasized that this decision, political pressures, global influences, and history itself provide evidence that it is critical for nurses to reclaim their health promotion legacy, become knowledgeable about all the factors that influence the field of health promotion, and educate the public about ways that nurses are involved in health promotion. Falk-Rafael argued that nurses must be attentive to whose voice is silent and whose voice is heard when health policy decisions are being made and restrictions are created about which clients can be served and by whom. Nurses must understand external influences that are shaping the way that health promotion is being practiced within and beyond the nursing profession if they are going retain health promotion as a dominant aspect of nursing practice. Otherwise, Falk-Rafael claims nurses who do not educate themselves and voice their opinions when political decisions are being made run the risk of seeing their practice confined by prevailing ideologies, administrative directions, economic cutbacks, and political pressures.

CRITIQUE AND PROMISE ASSOCIATED WITH NURSING'S ROLE IN HEALTH PROMOTION

Whitehead (2008), who has been active in the health promotion literature within nursing for over a decade, commented that nursing has continued to primarily rely on the traditional health education paradigm rather than the health promotion paradigm in guiding practice, research, and education. He cited the main reason for this being a lack of theoretical, educational, and conceptual clarity in the literature and within educational institutions. He also claimed that nurses continue to view health promotion as a single-discipline endeavor rather than view it as a multiagency intervention, a perspective consistent with current agendas (Whitehead, 2009).

Citing nursing's potential, Whitehead (2001) also argued that nursing is a sleeping giant, large enough to have a substantial impact on the health of people throughout the world if the profession adopts an active role in advocating for social change, returning to their humanistic roots, and promoting well-being. Nurses, because of their knowledge base, access to the community, sustained interaction with patients, experience working with underserved and vulnerable groups, and public trust/credibility, are well suited to become leaders in the new health promotion movement (Whitehead, 2009).

Morgan and Marsh (1998) emphasize that the nursing process is based on a medical model that supports providing generic health education rather than offering individualized care that builds on patient perspectives and goals. They argue for expanding the scope of nursing practice, incorporating an appreciation of sociopolitical and cultural environments that impact health, focusing on building social capital, providing individualized care, and increasing health equity. Doucette (1989) declared that nurses must shift from their traditional roles and adopt a greater responsibility in a wider arena of action that supports healthy people and healthy environments. She commented that nursing needs to focus on community equity, participatory involvement, and empowerment.

Butterfield (1990) stated that nursing has to adopt an upstream view in which a nurse works to understand and modify contextual factors that lead to poor health if nurses are to become leaders in health promotion. Maglacas (1986) highlighted how important it is that nurses understand the agendas and priorities of key decision makers and become involved in public policy as it relates to health.

Northrup and Purkis (2001) suggested that if nurses are to sustain their claim to having a unique role in promoting health, the discipline must clearly articulate the philosophical and theoretical underpinnings of their health promotion practice. Berg and Sarvimaki (2003) agreed that there "is a need to clarify, refine and redefine health promotion in nursing because the concept is partly non-specific and has not been used to identify a specific nursing focus" (p. 384).

WHAT ARE THE NEXT STEPS FOR NURSING?

Falk-Rafael (1999) argued that nursing voices should not be invisible, absent, or silent within public and academic discourse about health promotion. She stressed that nurses should maintain strong community ties, challenge administrative constraints, reclaim their legacy in terms of health promotion, remain current regarding forces that are shaping health promotion, and educate the public and other disciplines about the contribution of nurses.

At present, the American Association of Colleges of Nursing and the National Organization of Nurse Practitioner faculty are part of the Healthy People Curriculum Task Force. The aim of this task force is to increase the proportion of schools of nursing, medicine, and health professional training that are teaching health promotion based on Healthy People goals (Jesse & Blue, 2004). There are many other examples of the active presence of nurses in shaping health policy and advocating for the needs of individuals with fewer economic and educational resources.

WHAT WILL YOU DO?

The majority of this chapter has been devoted to describing documents and task forces that have had a major impact on health promotion practice. Consider how influential volunteering to belong to a committee, joining a task force, or authoring a report can be in shaping the nature of practice. Think about what it must have been like to attend and actively participate in one of the pivotal conferences that shaped the future of health promotion.

DISCUSSION QUESTIONS

1. When you graduate, what do you hope to accomplish in your career that could help shape the nature of health promotion practice? List both a short-term goal and a long-term goal related to health promotion that you have for yourself and your career.
2. Think of a statement or perspective you have heard expressed in the media during a commercial or a news program. Did any of the documents discussed in this chapter (Healthy People, U.S. Surgeon General's Report on Tobacco, The Lalonde Report, The Ottawa Charter, etc.) strongly influence that statement or perspective you noticed in the media?

3. As you look to the future, what constraints do you see limiting health promotion practice? What resources will those engaged in health promotion be able to use to support their work?

4. What group or sector has the greatest responsibility for health promotion? Talk about the role of the healthcare sector, the legislature, local governments, the federal government, the police, the military, local communities, school personnel, volunteer organizations, the media, industry, and other influential groups.

5. Identify one intervention that has been implemented to improve the health of U.S. citizens within the last decade. At the time that intervention was implemented, which of the following groups had the most influence on its adoption: (A) an international body, (B) the U.S. government, (C) a professional organization, (D) a politician or political party, (E) a healthcare profession or group of healthcare professionals, (F) a community-based organization, (G) experts in public health, (H) the media, (I) non-profit organizations, (J) private foundations that support health promotion, (K) citizen groups, (L) one committed citizen, or (M) industry/the business sector? If a coalition of interested partners helped implement your identified health promotion intervention, describe why a coalition was needed. Talk about what the vision was that motivated the individual or group, how need for the project was assessed, and how progress was measured.

CHECK YOUR UNDERSTANDING: EXERCISE 1

A list of activities designed to promote health follows. Please match the numbered items with the most appropriate entry on the alphabetized list of health promotion paradigms and documents. Select the health promotion document that first and most uniquely gave support to the given activity. For example, the Adelaide Recommendations (J) first introduced the concept of health literacy into the definition of health promotion, so the provision of language-specific educational handouts targeted to a person's reading level (4) would most appropriately be matched with this document, although the Bangkok Charter also later supported health literacy.

Activities designed to promote health

1. Billboards about the risks of drunk driving
2. Taking a yoga class to increase one's level of wellness
3. Lettuce recalls associated with *E. coli* infection reported on the nightly news
4. Providing educational handouts in a person's primary language targeted to a person's reading level

5. Taxation on cigarettes, creation of smoke-free areas, and bans on tobacco advertising
6. Having 98% of at-risk individuals obtain H1N1 vaccines in the upcoming year
7. Attending a diabetic self-help group and learning about how to count "carbs"
8. Posting calorie counts and fat/salt/carbohydrate contents in restaurants
9. Limiting high sugar beverages in school vending machines
10. Scheduling regular mammograms
11. Fluoridation of municipal drinking water
12. Conflict resolution in Nigeria to promote peace
13. Having the wealthy contribute to the healthcare of the poor
14. Tailoring health information to cultural norms
15. Making food stamps available to low income individuals
16. Using immunizations to protect against disease
17. Conducting a regular census to plan for health infrastructure needs
18. Supporting solar power and other interventions related to sustainable growth

Health promotion paradigms and documents

A. Greek philosophy
B. Healthy People
C. Ottawa Charter
D. The Lalonde Report
E. The Bangkok Charter
F. The Alma-Ata Declaration
G. Chinese medicine
H. The Roman Empire
I. The Epp Report
J. The Adelaide Recommendations
K. The Sundsvall Statement
L. The Jakarta Declaration
M. The U.S. Surgeon General's Report on Tobacco

CHECK YOUR UNDERSTANDING: EXERCISE 2

Review the following quotations from healthcare professionals and match them with the document that comes from the historical period in which the comment would have been likely to have been accepted/expected.

Quotes about Health Promotion and Health

1. "Providing health care for everyone from taxpayer dollars is the first step toward socialism."
2. "If health promotion is supposed to be focused on disease prevention and you serve people who have already had a stroke, that doesn't make sense."
3. "We need to decrease HIV exposure by 20% in the next year."
4. "Childhood obesity is caused by lack of access to healthy foods, safe places to exercise, and constant promotional exposure to television ads about high calorie food."
5. "We should focus on the causes of disease rather than a spectrum of health determinants if we are to be successful in increasing years of productive life."
6. "Young women must be able to walk to the market without being shot or blown up if we are going to achieve progress."
7. "Business leaders, governmental agencies, and communities must all work together to develop a coherent health policy and well-being for all."
8. "Women are the primary people who promote health. We need ensure that women are equal partners who participate in developing health promotion policy."
9. "Poverty is the most immediate and critical threat to health."
10. "Indigenous people have a unique wisdom and spiritual understanding that must be accessed if we are to create environments that support health and sustainable development."
11. "Maintaining balance and harmony is essential for health."
12. "Not wearing seat belts accounts for the majority of highway deaths."

Historical Period Dominated by the Following Documents

A. Greek philosophy
B. Healthy People
C. Ottawa Charter
D. The Lalonde Report
E. The Bangkok Charter
F. The Alma-Ata Declaration
G. The Adelaide Recommendations
H. The Jakarta Declaration
I. The Sundsvall Statement
J. Medical Care for the American People
K. The Flexner Report
L. The Greeks

WHAT DO YOU THINK?

Review the priorities of each of the Healthy People initiatives (1979, 2000, 2010, and 2020). Which priority do you see as being most critical to health promotion in the United States within the next decade? Jot down your reasons and how you would make progress toward that goal using a health promotion perspective.

Review the priorities of the WHO conferences on health promotion. Which priority do you believe is the most relevant to U.S. health promotion policy? Which priority do you believe is most relevant to global health promotion? Provide a rationale for each of your answers..

What do you think the differences would have been in your role had you been working as a health promotion practitioner in ancient Greece as compared to that same role in 2010–2020 in the United States?

Do you think health promotion is best accomplished by a single discipline or multiple agencies and groups working together? Explain your answer.

What do you think would need to happen to shift the focus more toward prevention within the U.S. healthcare system?

REFERENCES

Awofeso, N. (2004). What's new about the new public health? *American Journal of Public Health, 94*(5), 705–709.

Berg, G. V., & Sarvimaki, A. (2003). A holistic-existential approach to health promotion. *Scandinavian Journal of Caring Sciences, 17*, 384–391.

Breslow, L. (1999). From disease prevention to health promotion. *JAMA, 281*(11), 1030–1033.

Brown, D. W. (2009). The dawn of Healthy People 2020: A brief look back at its beginnings. *Preventive Medicine, 48*, 94–95.

Butterfield, P. (1990). Thinking upstream: Nurturing a conceptual understanding of the societal context of health behavior. *Advances in Nursing Science, 12*(2), 1–8.

Corbin, J. H., & Mittelmark, M. B. (2008). Partnership lessons from the Global Programme for Health Promotion Effectiveness: A case study. *Health Promotion International, 23*(4), 365–371.

Doucette, S. (1989). The changing role of nurses and the perspective of the medical services branch. *Canadian Journal of Public Health, 80*(2), 92–94.

Epp, J. (1986) Achieving health for all: A framework for health promotion. *Health Canada*, 23–33.

Eriksson, M. & Lindstrom, B. (2008). A salutogenic interpretation of the Ottawa Charter. *Health Promotion International, 23*(2), 190–199.

Falk-Rafael, A. (1999). The politics of health promotion: Influences on public health promoting nursing practice in Ontario, Canada from Nightingale to the nineties. *Advances in Nursing Science, 22*(1), 23–39.

Fielding, J., & Kumanyika, S. (2009). Recommendations for the concepts and form of Healthy People 2020. *American Journal of Preventive Medicine, 37*(3), 255–257.

Healthy People (2010). MAP-IT: A strategy for creating a healthy community. Chapter 2. Retrieved from http://www.healthypeople.gov/publications/HealthyCommunities2001/Chapter_2.htm

Howard, D., Nieuwenhuijsen, E. R., & Saleeby, P. (2008). Health promotion and education: Application of the ICF in the US and Canada using an ecological perspective. *Disability and Rehabilitation, 30*(12–13), 942–954.

Irvine, L., Elliott, L., Wallace, H., & Crombie, I. K. (2006). A review of major influences on current public health policy in developed countries in the second half of the 20th century. *The Journal of the Royal Society for the Promotion of Health, 126*(2), 73–78.

Jackson, S. F., Perkins, F., Khandor, E., Cordwell, L., Hamann, S., & Buasai, S. (2007). Integrated health promotion strategies: A contribution to tackling current and future health challenges. *Health Promotion International, 21*(S1), 75–83.

Jesse, E. & Blue, C. (2004). Mary Breckinridge meets Healthy People 2010: A teaching strategy for visioning and building healthy communities. *Journal of Midwifery and Women's Health, 49*(2), 126–131.

Kickbusch, I., McCann, W., & Sherbon, T. (2008). Adelaide revisited: From healthy public policy to health in all policies. *Health Promotion International, 23*(1), 1–4.

King, P. M. (194). Health promotion: The emerging frontier in nursing, *Journal of Advanced Nursing, 20,* 209–218.

Kushwah, S. S. (2007). Public health learning and practice from hygiene to community medicine, health management and beyond issues: Challenges and options. *Indian Journal of Community Medicine, 32*(2), 103–107.

Lalonde, M. (1974). *A new perspective on the health of Canadians.* Ottawa, Canada: Government of Canada.

MacDougall, H. (2007). Reinventing public health: A new perspective on the health of Canadians and its international impact. *Journal Epidemiology and Community Health, 61,* 955–959.

Maglacas, A. M. (1986). Health for all: Nursing's role. *Nursing Outlook 36*(2), 66–71.

McIntyre, L. (1992). The evolution of health promotion. *Probe, 26*(1), 15–22.

McQueen, D. V. (2008). Self-reflections on health promotion in the UK and the USA. *Public Health, 122,* 1035–1037.

Mittelmark, M. B. (2007). Shaping the future of health promotion: Priorities for action. *Health Promotion International, 23*(1), 98–102.

Mittelmark, M. B., Perry, M. W., Wise, M., Lamarre, M., & Jones, C. M. (2007). Enhancing the effectiveness of the International Union for Health Promotion and Education to move health promotion forward. *IUHPE Promotion and Education Supplement 2, 14*(33), 33–35.

Moore, P. V., & Williamson, G. C. (1984). Health promotion: Evolution of a concept. *Nursing Clinics of North America, 19*(2), 194–207.

Morgan, I. S., & Marsh, G. W. (1998). Historic and future health promotion contexts for nursing. *Image: Journal of Nursing Scholarship, 30*(4), 379–383.

National Cancer Institute (2010). *Cancer Health Disparities: How do incidence and death rates affect different racial or ethnic groups?* Pages 2–5. Retrieved from http://www.cancer.gov/cancertopics/factsheet/cancer-health-disparities

Northrup, D. T., & Purkis, M. E. (2001). Building the science of health promotion practice from a human science perspective. *Nursing Philosophy, 2,* 62–71.

Raphael, D. (2008). Grasping at straws: A recent history of health promotion in Canada. *Critical Public Health, 18*(4), 483–495.

Scriven, A. & Speller, V. (2007). Global issues and challenges beyond Ottawa: The way forward. *Promotion and Education, 14,* 194–198.

Tountas, Y. (2009). The historical origins of the basic concepts of health promotion and education: The role of ancient Greek philosophy and medicine. *Health Promotion International, 24*(2), 185–192.

Whitehead, D. (2001). Health education, behavioural change and social psychology: Nursing's contribution to health promotion? *Journal of Advanced Nursing, 34*(6), 822–832.

Whitehead, D. (2008). Health promotion: An international Delphi study examining health promotion and health education in nursing practice, education, and policy. *Journal of Clinical Nursing, 17,* 891–900.

Whitehead, D. (2009). Reconciling the differences between health promotion in nursing and general health promotion. *International Journal of Nursing Studies, 46,* 865–874.

Winkelstein, W. (2009). The development of American public health, a commentary: Three documents that made an impact. *Journal of Public Health Policy. 30*(1), 40–48.

World Health Organization [WHO]. (1986). *The Ottawa Charter for Health Promotion.* Copenhagen, Denmark: Author.

World Health Organization [WHO]. (1987). Ottawa Charter for Health Promotion. *Health Promotion, 1*(4), iii–v.

World Health Organization [WHO]. (2010a). *Sundsvall statement on supportive environments for health.* Retrieved from http://www.who.int/healthpromotion/conferences/prevous/sundsvall/en/index.html

World Health Organization [WHO]. (2010b). *Jakarta declaration on leading health promotion into the 21st century.* Retrieved from http://www.who.int/healthpromotion/conferences/prefious/jakarta/declaration /en/

For a full suite of assignments and additional learning activities, see the access code at the front of your book.

CHAPTER 3

Health Promotion Theories

Bonnie Raingruber

OBJECTIVES

At the conclusion of this chapter, the student will be able to:

- Compare and contrast nursing and non-nursing health promotion theories.
- Examine health promotion theories for consistency with accepted health promotion priorities and values.
- Articulate how health promotion theories move the profession forward.
- Discuss strengths and limitations associated with each health promotion theory or model.
- Describe the difference between a model and a theory.
- Identify theoretical assumptions and concepts within nursing and non-nursing theories.
- Develop his or her own health promotion model.

WHY SHOULD HEALTH PROMOTION BE THEORY-BASED?

A variety of authors have commented that health promotion programs typically lack a theoretical foundation or are based on a conceptual model that does not conform to the current values and norms of health promotion practice (Bauer et al., 2003; King, 1994; Stokols, 1996; Whitehead, 2004). Commonly, environmental, social, cultural, economic, and political influences are given scant or no attention within health promotion theories. These factors may well be some of the main reasons a health promotion program that has its design based on a particular theory is not as effective as the author hoped it would be.

Whitehead (2001a) commented that the reliance on health education theories and frameworks may actually pose a barrier to progress in the arena of health promotion.

He emphasized that if the confusion persists between health education and health promotion theories and models, it will be increasingly difficult for nurses to identify when they are implementing health promotion activities and programs. Whitehead (2006) suggested that without a clear theoretical basis, it would not be possible to move forward or ensure that the health promotion components of nursing practice are recognizable.

As we have seen, there has been a shift from individually focused health education to community and environmentally-based health promotion. There has also been a shift from illness-focused priorities, such as disease prevention and health protection, to a focus on complete physical, emotional, and social well-being. We will see if these new priorities show up in the theories and models that are currently providing guidance to practice, research, and education in the health promotion field.

Given the complexity of health promotion practice, multilevel, comprehensive interventions are needed to develop effective programs. It is vital to consider psychological, organizational, cultural, community-level, political, and policy-driven factors that influence health. Targeting one single pattern of unhealthy behavior such as smoking will not be effective if the person also drinks to excess, consumes large amounts of saturated fat, has an irregular sleep pattern, performs a stressful job, and works in an area that has poor air quality. Interventions that target unhealthy lifestyles by simultaneously focusing on multiple factors are more likely to be effective. Theories are needed to provide support for multilevel interventions that produce reliable outcomes. As we will see, not all existing health promotion theories support multilevel interventions.

Theories provide a roadmap and a step-by-step summary of what factors to consider when designing, implementing, and evaluating a health promotion program. It is vital to have a theoretical understanding of why people behave the way they do if nurses are to help a person, a family, a group, or a community improve their health status. Theories provide relevant clues as to why people and communities make health-related choices and offer a systematic way of understanding situations, examining relationships, and predicting outcomes. Theories help explain why an intervention is necessary, how to intervene, and how to evaluate success (Glanz & Rimer, 2005). Glanz and Rimer (2005) suggested that theory "helps practitioners to interpret the findings of their research and make the leap from facts on a page to understanding the dynamic interactions between behavior and environmental context" (p. 43).

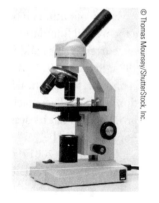

The succinct summary or graphic presentation provided by a theory makes complex interrelationships among multiple variables easier to understand (Healey & Zimmerman, 2010). As Green and colleagues (2010) commented, "the role of theory is to untangle and simplify for human comprehension the complexities of nature. Once the critical components of a complex problem are illuminated by theory, practical applications become possible" (p. 398). The job of a good theory is to present content in enough detail so that it describes the behavior of a large (generalizable) group of people, but also to be simple to understand, implement, and evaluate (Green et al., 2010). Theory provides a broad road-map that helps explain the dynamics of health behavior, identify effective interventions, select suitable target audiences, and evaluate outcomes (Glanz & Rimer, 2005).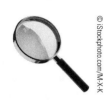

Cole (1995) stressed that all healthcare practitioners need to be introduced to theoretical concepts in their formal education because whether they are aware of it or not, they use theories and models to guide their practice and research efforts. Antonovsky (1996) suggested that without adequate theoretical guidance from a theory or model that is consistent with principles of health promotion, the field is at risk of stagnation. He emphasized that theory is needed to guide the field, provide direction to practice, and structure program evaluation, believing that good theories give birth to good ideas capable of being incorporated into practice.

As Best and colleagues (2003) commented, the field of health promotion has become too complex for any one theory to provide adequate guidance to education, practice, and research. Green et al. (2010) stressed that "there are different ways of knowing, different lenses for viewing reality, and different realities to be known" (p. 401). Different perspectives are needed for different health promotion issues and settings. Glanz and Rimer (2005) agreed that multiple theories are needed to address the varied challenges that arise in health promotion. They emphasized that "effective practice depends on using theories and strategies that are most appropriate to a given situation" (Glanz & Rimer, 2005, p. 6). The key is being able to analyze how well a theory or model fits the given situation, because different theories are needed for individual-level intervention, organizational-level intervention, and community-level intervention. In order to select the most relevant theory for a given situation, it is necessary to become familiar with the numerous multidisciplinary theories that have been used in health promotion practice.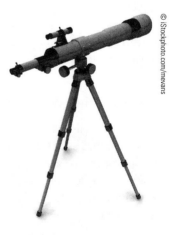

As we explore theories of health promotion, we will look at models that contain abstract, general concepts and do not yet have extensive research-based support as well as theories that have more clearly defined concepts and have been tested in a substantial number of studies. We will explore the assumptions or beliefs that were taken for granted by the theorist in creating the theory. We will pay attention to the concepts (set of elements or categories) that comprise and distinguish the theory. It may be helpful at times to examine the relationships (called propositions) between concepts within the theory.

In this chapter, we will examine behavioral theories, an intervention-based model, environmental theories, communication theories, and evaluation theories that come from a spectrum of disciplines. We will also review select nursing theories that have relevance to health promotion. It is important to examine the breadth of theoretical health promotion knowledge in order to identify the most practical theories that are able to provide guidance to practice, education, and research.

BEHAVIORAL CHANGE THEORIES

A number of behavioral change theories exist to explain why people do and do not adopt certain health behaviors. Often, these theories examine the predictors and precursors of health behavior. Many of these theories have common elements such as self-efficacy and motivation. Self-efficacy is one's belief in their ability to do something, such as change a health related behavior, and it is grounded in one's past success or failure in the given activity. One's self-efficacy is seen as predicting the amount of effort one will expend in trying to change (Bandura, 1977).

Criticism of many of the behavioral change theories focuses on their emphasis on individual behavior while excluding the influence of environment, sociocultural factors, economic issues, and policy level mandates. Constraints such as chronic exposure to violence, political upheaval, and poor sanitation are ignored in favor of paying greater attention to individual cognitive processes (Stokols, 1996).

Health Belief Model (1966)

The Health Belief Model (HBM) was developed by Irwin Rosenstock in 1966 and has been identified as one of the earliest and most influential models in health promotion. It was inspired by a study of reasons people expressed for seeking or declining X-ray examinations for tuberculosis. Initially the model included four constructs: (1) perceived susceptibility (a person's subjective assessment of their risk of getting the condition, as contrasted with the statistical risk), (2) perceived severity (the seriousness of the condition and its consequences), (3) perceived barriers (both those that interfere with and facilitate adoption of a behavior such as side effects, time, and inconvenience), and (4) perceived costs of adhering to the proposed intervention. Factors related to motivation were subsumed under susceptibility and fear of the disease (Rosenstock, 1966).

In the 1970s and 1980s, Becker and colleagues modified the HBM to include people's responses to symptoms and illness, and compliance with medical directives. The model was extended to include illness behaviors, preventative health, and health screening. Demographic variables (age, gender, ethnicity, occupation), sociophysiological variables (socioeconomic status, personality, coping strategies), perceived self-efficacy (ability to adopt the desired behavior), cues to action (factors that instigate preventive health such as information sought/provided, persuasive communication, and personal experience), health motivation, perceived control, and perceived threat were added to the model (Becker & Maiman, 1975). In recent years the model has been used to predict general health behaviors and positive health behaviors, although when it was originally proposed it was designed to predict actions by acutely or chronically ill clients. In the HBM a health-related action is seen as more likely when the action is viewed as being both cost effective and effective in terms of outcomes (Roden, 2004; Rosenstock, 1966).

Critique of the HBM has been based on the fact that not all health behavior is based on rational or conscious choice. It has also been critiqued for focusing on negative factors and ignoring positive motivations that prompt healthy behaviors (Roden, 2004; Rosenstock, 1974). The HBM also lacks concepts associated with strategies for change. The major complaint has been that the model focuses on individual factors rather that socioeconomic and environmental factors and, therefore, encourages victim-blaming (Roden, 2004).

Theory of Reasoned Action (1975)

The Theory of Reasoned Action (TRA) was developed by Martin Fishbein and Icek Ajzen in 1975. An assumption underlying the TRA is that people routinely consider the consequences of their behaviors before engaging in these behaviors. There are three constructs: behavioral intention, attitude, and subjective norms. In this model, a behavioral intention is a function of the person's attitude about the behavior and subjective norms. Subjective norms are the perceived expectations of key individuals such as significant others, family members, experts, and co-workers. Voluntary behavior is predicted by one's attitude toward the behavior and what important people would think if the behavior was not performed (Fishbein & Ajzen, 1975).

A critique of the TRA is that not all behaviors are under an individual's control, including spontaneous actions, habitual behaviors, and cravings. A second critique is that environmental, economic, and political factors are not part of the theory; like the HRA, it focuses on individual health behavior. The TRA has been tested in a large number of areas including dieting, condom use, and limiting sun exposure, and it has been found to have strong predictive utility.

Theory of Planned Behavior (1985)

Ajzen (1985) extended the Theory of Reasoned Action and developed the Theory of Planned Behavior (TPB) by adding a perceived behavioral control predictor. The concept of perceived behavioral control came from Bandura's work with self-efficacy, and it is used to account for times when people do not have conscious control over their actions as well as when they intend to carry out a behavior but they do not because they lack confidence or control. Ajzen's work emphasized the role of intention and suggested that the likelihood of behavior change is dependent on the amount of control a person has over a given behavior and the strength of their intent to change.

According to TPB, three factors influence intent: (1) the person's attitude toward the behavior, (2) the person's evaluation of how important significant others such as a partner or co-worker consider the behavior to be (subjective norms), and (3) the degree of perceived behavioral control or the perceived ease/difficulty associated with the behavioral change. Ajzen suggested that self-efficacy was a major factor in determining how successful a person will be in changing their behavior, as people who don't believe they have the assets, resources, or ability to change are not likely to do so (Ajzen, 1985). The TPB has been critiqued for focusing on cognitive elements and ignoring the role of emotion in behavioral change. However, it has proven to be an effective model for predicting health-related behavior.

Social Cognitive Theory (1989)

Social Cognitive Theory (SCT) is also known as Social Learning Theory (SLT). Developed by Bandura in 1989, this theory is based on vicarious learning. According to the theory, behavior is learned by observation, imitation, and positive reinforcement. Role models facilitate learning, in that individuals reenact behaviors they have observed directly or seen in the media. The theory also suggests people learn by noticing the benefits of actions that they observe other people performing (Bandura, 1989).

According to SCT, behavioral change is determined by environmental, social, personal, and behavioral elements. Each of these factors influences the other. Behavior is guided by expected consequences. There are six main concepts in Social Cognitive Theory:

1. Reciprocal determinism: the person, behavior, and environment influence one another
2. Behavioral capability: the knowledge and skill needed to perform a behavior
3. Expectations: anticipated outcomes
4. Self-efficacy: confidence in one's ability to take action
5. Observational learning: learning by observing others
6. Reinforcements: responses to a behavior that increase or decrease the likelihood of reoccurrence (Glanz & Rimer, 2005)

According to Bandura (1989), motivation and feelings of frustration associated with repeated failures influence behavior. Bandura discussed two types of expectations: self-efficacy and outcome expectancy. Because self-efficacy is needed to initiate change, it is the most crucial factor, while outcome expectancy is the person's evaluation that the behavior will lead to a positive outcome (Bandura, 1989). According to Macdonald (2000), the most widely recognized feeder theory for health education and health promotion programs is social cognitive theory.

Self-Determination Theory (1991)

Self-determination theory (SDT) is a personality theory that includes behavioral factors. It focuses on the motivation behind choices that individuals make. Self-determination theory was inspired by research into intrinsic motivation, which is the idea of engaging in an activity because it is interesting and satisfying rather than being motivated to achieve a goal or receive an external reward such as money. With intrinsic motivation, a person seeks out challenges that allow for growth. Intrinsic motivation flourishes if linked with a sense of security and relatedness (Deci & Ryan, 1991).

The need for competence, autonomy, and relatedness motivate self-initiated behavior and allow for optimal function and growth. These needs are not learned, but instead are innate and transcend gender and culture. Competence has to do with being effective in dealing with the environment and producing behavioral outcomes. Negative feedback decreases intrinsic motivation, while positive feedback increases intrinsic motivation. Relatedness involves the desire to interact with, be connected to, and care for others. It involves establishing satisfying relationships with others and society at large. Autonomy is the urge to have agency, initiate action, and regulate one's behaviors. It is undermined by offering external/extrinsic rewards and establishing deadlines, but increasing choices increases autonomy (Deci, 1971). Perspective taking, in which those in authority consider the perspective of the client on health-related matters, satisfies the client's need for relatedness and increases a sense of belonging. When healthcare providers offer meaningful and germane rationale for behavioral change, the client's sense of competence increases. Use of neutral language such as 'may' and 'could' instead of 'should' and 'must' increase client autonomy. People who operate autonomously freely choose to adopt a suggested behavior because they see that behavior as important and meaningful (Chatzisarantis & Hagger, 2009).

According to SDT, there are three ways people orient themselves to the environment and regulate their behavior; the orientations are autonomous, controlled, and impersonal. Autonomous orientations result from satisfaction of basic needs. Controlled orientations result from satisfaction of competence and relatedness needs, but not of autonomy needs; rigid functioning and diminished well-being result. Impersonal orientations result from a lack of fulfilling all three needs. Poor functioning and ill health result when a person has or experiences an impersonal orientation (Deci, 1971).

Life goals, according to SDT, include intrinsic aspirations and goals like affiliation, generativity, and personal development. Extrinsic aspirations include goals such as wealth, fame, and attractiveness. Research has shown intrinsic goals are associated with enhanced health and well-being (Deci, 1971).

Three important elements of SDT are that (1) humans desire to master their drives and emotions; (2) humans have an inherent tendency toward growth, development, and integrated functioning; and (3) optimal development actions are inherent but do not happen automatically. People need nurturing from their social environment (including healthcare professionals) to actualize their potential (Deci & Vansteenkiste, 2003).

Elsewhere in the text we will discuss motivational interviewing, a health promotion intervention that is derived from SDT. In motivational interviewing, the nurse explores ambivalent feelings clients have about a topic, such as stopping drinking, going on a diet, or exercising. The supportive atmosphere enhances autonomy and allows people to find their own source of motivation (Markland et al., 2005).

Self-determination theory has been confirmed in a number of correlational studies; however, few experimental studies have examined SDT in relation to promoting health behaviors (Chatzisarantis & Hagger, 2009). Additional experimental research on SDT is needed.

A study based on SDT was conducted with 215 pupils as part of a randomized school-based intervention to change physical activity intentions and self-reported leisure time physical activity behavior. Teachers in the intervention group provided positive feedback, gave rationale for becoming active, and acknowledged how hard it is to exercise. The pupils' sense of choice was enhanced by using neutral language such as "Physical education may be fun" (Chatzisarantis & Hagger, 2009, p. 34). The authors found that pupils who were taught by autonomy-supportive teachers reported stronger intentions to exercise and thus participated more often in leisure time physical activities than did those in the control group (Chatzisarantis & Hagger, 2009). Can you think of a time when someone gave you positive feedback that helped you change a specific behavior? Why does "neutral" language like "may" work better than more authoritarian language?

Transtheoretical Model or Stages of Change Model (1997)

James Prochaska and Carlo DiClemente (1992) posited that willingness or intention to change behavior varies among individuals and within individuals over time. Their Stages of Change Model (SCM) described a person's motivation and readiness to change a health-related behavior. Their initial work was based on experiences of smokers who quit without assistance and those who sought professional help. Prochaska and DiClemente described behavioral change as a five-step process: the stages of precontemplation, contemplation, preparation, action, and maintenance. In the precontemplation stage, the person may not even be aware of needing or wanting to change or they may be unwilling or uninterested in changing. It is in the contemplation stage that a person develops a desire to change. During the preparation stage, the person plans ways to change. When the new behavior appears on a regular basis, the person has moved to the action stage. After a person has consistently manifested the new behavior for 6 months, they are in the maintenance stage. It is possible for a person to relapse; this is not seen as a separate stage, but a return to a previous stage. In this model a person may cycle through the stages repeatedly before behavioral change finally occurs (Prochaska, DiClemente, Velicer & Rossi, 1992).

The Transtheoretical Model (TTM) evaluates a person's readiness to change their health-related behavior. Concepts such as self-efficacy, change processes, and decision criteria are considered. Some have called the TTM the dominant health promotion model because of the amount of research that has been conducted on it and the attention it has received from the media. The model was developed by analyzing a number of psychotherapy models. Originally the model consisted of four concepts: preconditions for therapy, processes of change, content to be changed, and therapeutic relationship. By 1997, the TTM model had been refined to include five core constructs: stages of change, processes of change, decisional balance, self-efficacy, and temptation (Prochaska & Velicer, 1997).

The TTM focuses more on health-related interventions than on individuals. You may wish to compare TTM with the Tannahill model, discussed next. The TTM is both an intervention and a behavioral model.

As seen in **Table 3-1**, Prochaska and colleagues assert that interventions to change behavior (processes of change) must be matched to the stage of change the person is experiencing. However, systematic reviews have shown that staged interventions are no more effective than non-staged interventions (Reimsma et al., 2003). Other authors have suggested the dividing lines between the TTM stages are somewhat arbitrary (West, 2005) and that there is insufficient evidence of sequential movement through discrete stages (Little & Girvin, 2002). Additionally, critiques have focused on the lack of attention to the environmental, economic, and political influences that impact health behaviors. Finally, instruments used to measure the stages of change have been criticized as not being adequately standardized or validated (Adams & White, 2005). Prochaska addressed these concerns by suggesting that future studies tailor interventions to all the core constructs of the model not just one stage of change (Prochaska, 2006).

The Precaution Adoption Process Model

The Precaution Adoption Process Model (PAPM) is similar to the Stages of Change Model, except that the PAPM focuses on the importance of educating people about health hazards and engaging them in behavioral change. In stage 1 of the PAPM, a

TABLE 3-1 Stages of Change Model: Match Between the Stage of Change and Process of Change

Stages of Change	Processes of Change	Decisional Balance	Self-Efficacy	Temptation
Moving from precontemplation to contemplation	Consciousness raising, dramatic relief, and environmental reevaluation	A person weighs the pros and cons of changing	Situation-specific confidence that people have that they can cope with high-risk situations without relapsing	The intensity of urges to engage in a given habit
Moving from contemplation to preparation	Self-reevaluation			
Moving from preparation to action	Self-liberation			
Moving from action to maintenance	Contingency management, helping relationship, counter conditioning, and stimulus control			

person is unaware of a health hazard. In stage 2, the person becomes aware of the hazard but is not engaged by it. In stage 3, the person decides whether to take action or not; stage 4 is reserved for those who decide not to act, while stage 5 focuses on those who have chosen to act. Stage 6 is acting on the health hazard, and stage 7 is maintenance. Unlike the SCM, in the PAPM one does not cycle back to previous stages (Glanz & Rimer, 2005).

AN INTERVENTION-BASED MODEL: THE TANNAHILL MODEL (1980)

In the 1980s, Andrew Tannahill created a health promotion model consisting of three overlapping spheres of activity: health education, prevention, and health protection (see **Figure 3-1**). He did so in response to a shift in focus within the literature from

FIGURE 3-1   Venn Diagram

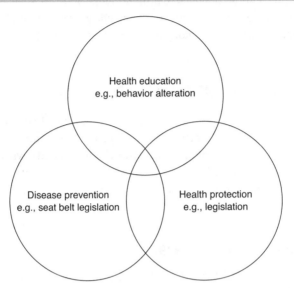

Source: Tannahill, A. (2009). Health promotion: The Tannahill model revisited. *Public Health, 123*(5), 397.

health education and prevention to health protection and health promotion. Health education is designed to change the knowledge, beliefs, attitudes, and behavior in a way that facilitates health. Disease prevention aims to decrease risk factors and minimize the consequences of disease; it includes primary, secondary, and tertiary prevention. Health protection focuses on fiscal or legal controls and policies and voluntary codes of practice aimed at preventing ill health and enhancing well-being. Tannahill (2009) asserts that health protection includes public policies that address fair access to housing, employment, education, and health care.

The Tannahill model has been criticized as being clearly within the reductionistic, medical model in that it pays insufficient attention to community-based factors. In response to these critiques, Tannahill (2009) proposed a new definition of health promotion as the "sustainable fostering of positive health and prevention of ill-health through policies, strategies, and activities in the overlapping action areas of: (1) social, economic, physical, environmental, and cultural factors; (2) equity and diversity; (3) education and learning; (4) services, amenities, and products; and (5) community-led and community-based activity" (p. 397). As we will see in the measurement/evaluation chapter, his new definition is consistent with evaluation methods described as action research and community-based participatory research. Education in his definition includes health education and interventions designed to promote empowerment, such as resilience, self-esteem, and life skills. Services and amenities include preventative care, while products include those that enhance health along with those that damage it.

ECOLOGICAL THEORIES AND MODELS

Ecological theories and models present health as an interaction between the person and their ecosystem or social web, which consists of their family, community, culture, and the physical environment. The interaction between behavior and environment contributes to both health and illness. There is a reciprocal influence in that people are affected by their ecosystem and environment and likewise people affect those systems (Glanz & Rimer, 2005).

Social Ecological Models (1979)

The Social Ecological Model (SEM) is derived from Systems Theory. It consists of person-focused and environment-focused interventions designed to promote health. The word *ecology* refers to interrelationships among intrapersonal factors, interpersonal connections, primary groups, institutional factors, community influences, and public policy. Social Ecological Models focus on how the environment and people influence one another. The SEM assumes that individual efforts at behavioral change will be more likely to succeed within supportive environments. The model targets social, institutional, and cultural environments in addition to biologic processes and geographic issues.

According to the SEM, human behavior is shaped by recurring patterns of activity that take place in structured environments; examples include residential, educational, occupational, recreational, religious, and healthcare environments. These environments have a cumulative and combined influence on well-being. Within these environmental contexts, social roles, personal behaviors, and situational conditions influence both personal and collective well-being. These social roles, personal behaviors, and situational conditions are leverage points that health promotion programs should target to accomplish the maximal amount of behavioral change possible (Stokols, 1996).

Several versions of the SEM have been developed. The initial and most commonly used model was authored by Urie Bronfenbrenner (1979) and is called Ecological Systems Theory. His work was influenced by Kurt Lewin's proposition that behavior is influenced by the person and the environment.

In Ecological Systems Theory, the primary influences are intercultural, community-level, organizational-level, and interpersonal/individual. In this theory the individual, the organization, the community, and culture are nested spheres like Russian dolls. Actions in one sphere can influence what happens in another sphere. There are micro and macro spheres of influence (Bronfenbrenner, 1979).

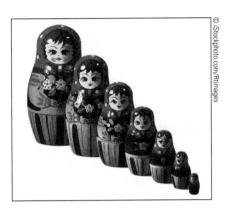

One interpersonal microsystem consists of the roles a person plays within his or her social context, such as mother, father, sister, brother, child, employee, friend, peer, or student. These microsystem influences can be learned but are also ingrained based on gender, ethnicity, generational influences, and culture. In this interpersonal sphere personality, knowledge, and beliefs are important in that they are continually shaped by the environment and other individuals with whom one comes into contact (Gregson, 2001).

Mesosystems are organizational or institutional factors that shape and structure one's environment. Policies, acceptable etiquette, and norms of behavior act at this level to shape individual behavior. Schools, companies, churches, sports teams, and community groups are examples of mesosystems (Bronfenbrenner, 1979).

Exosystems are community-level influences that include norms, standards, social networks, and the media. An individual does not have to be an active member in an exosystem for it to have an influence on him or her. For example, one can be influenced by Republican or Democratic initiatives without belonging to either political party, or one can be influenced by Southern culture even if a person recently moved to the South from, for example, California (Bronfenbrenner, 1979).

Macrosystems are cultural influences. Examples include Christianity, Islam, Western thought, the military, and communism, to name a few. Isomorphisms are impacts within one level that affect another level. The impact of an isomorphism is equal in effect in both magnitude and direction across spheres of influence. A discontinuity is an effect on one sphere that results in an unequal, opposite impact on another level. Top-down effects are how macrosystems and exosystems affect individual behavior (Oetzel, Ting-Toomey, & Rinderle, 2006). An example is the government requiring that restaurant menus post information on the fat, carbohydrate, and salt content of food. Bottom-up effects are how individuals or communities influence higher levels. An example of a bottom-up effect is when Mothers Against Drunk Driving helped shape health policy changes.

An advantage of environmental theories is that health promotion strategies that work at this level have the capacity to benefit a large number of people, not just one individual. Moreover, policy level interventions include passive interventions that do not require sustained effort on the part of an individual. An example of this would be use of child-resistant caps on medicine or the installation of air bags in automobiles; individuals are protected without having to take action themselves. Behavioral change models, on the other hand, target individual change and emphasize active interventions that require voluntary and sustained effort to accomplish behavioral goals (Stokols, 1996).

It is critical to examine barriers such as limited education, income, and geographic mobility when designing health promotion programs based on Ecological Systems Theory. It is also important to include multiple physical, social, and cultural factors that influence health outcomes, including such factors as developmental maturation, genetic heritage, psychological dispositions, behavioral patterns, emotional well-being, and social cohesion (Stokols, 1996). The focus in SEM is on the "congruence (or compatibility) between people and their surroundings as an important predictor of well-being" (Stokols, 1996, p. 286).

There are suggested guidelines for designing and evaluating health promotion programs that derive from the ecological principles within the SEM. Those guidelines suggest one should:

> examine the links between multiple facets of well-being and diverse conditions of the physical and social environment; examine the joint influence of behavioral, dispositional, developmental, demographic factors on people's exposure and responses to environmental hazards and demands; identify sources of person-environment and group-environment misfit and develop interventions that enhance the fit between people and their surroundings; identify behavioral and organizational leverage points for health promotion; consider both personal and other-directed health behavior as targets for change within community interventions; account for the moderating and mediating influences of physical and social conditions on health; design community interventions that span multiple settings and have enduring positive effects on well-being; integrate biomedical, behavioral, regulatory and environmental interventions for health promotion; and use multiple methods to evaluate the health and cost-effectiveness of community programs. (Stokols, 1966, p. 288)

The Salutogenic Theory (1996)

Antonovsky (1996) proposed the Salutogenic Theory (ST) as a conceptual basis for the health promotion movement while addressing concerns that previous models focused excessively on health education, rather than the broader perspective of health promotion. This theory was also designed to focus on health- enhancing (salutary) rather than risk factors for disease, to view the person in a holistic manner rather than as at risk for a particular disease, and to examine factors that bring a sense of meaning and coherence to life. The focus was on the health of the person (a salutogenic orientation), not the disease (a pathogenic orientation). Antonovsky (1996) emphasized that attention should be on the ease/dis-ease continuum and not the health/disease continuum.

Salutogenesis means the origins of health. Salutogenesis was described as "the process of enabling individuals, groups, organizations, and societies to emphasize abilities, resources, capacities, competences, strengths, and forces in order to create a sense of coherence and thus perceive life as comprehensible, manageable, and meaningful" (Lindstrom & Eriksson, 2009, p. 19).

Two central concepts in Antonovsky's (1996) theory are coherence and generalized resistance resources (GRRs) that help one avoid disease. Generalized resistance resources include external and internal resources that help one to cope with and manage life; they facilitate balance, shape health outcomes, create meaning, help one make sense of the world, and result in strong sense of coherence (SOC). This SOC results in seeing the world as comprehensible, manageable, and meaningful. Coherence is based on cognitive, behavioral, and motivational factors as well as by empowering relationships and meaningful pursuits. Antonovsky suggested that a strong SOC creates movement towards health. When confronted with stresses, people want to be motivated to cope (meaningfulness), to believe the present challenge can be understood (comprehensibility), and to recognize that resources exist that will help them cope with the challenge (manageability). The strength of a person's SOC is shaped by consistency of one's life experiences, underload–overload balance, participation in decision making, social standing, family structure, work type, gender, and genetics. A strong SOC allows one to reach out and use resources to minimize current stressors (Antonovsky, 1996).

The Salutogenic theory has been researched at the individual, group, and population levels (Lindstrom & Eriksson, 2009). A scale, the SOC Orientation to Life Scale, has been created in 29- and 13-item versions for both adults and adolescents. It has been translated into 15 languages and has proved to be a valid and reliable measure.

Antonovsky (1996) called for additional longitudinal research on the theory. He also suggested research attention be given to whether there is a stronger relationship between SOC and emotional, rather than physical, well-being. In addition, he emphasized the need for examining whether a SOC is mediated by emotions or by psychoneuroimmunology via the central nervous system.

The Salutogenic theory combines cognitive, behavioral, and motivational constructs. Antonovsky (1996) asserted that a SOC is not a culture-bound concept, although he acknowledged the research on the ST has primarily been conducted in Western countries.

The Life Course Health Development Model (2002)

The Life Course Health Development Model (LCHDM) aims to explain how health evolves over a lifetime. Halfon and Hochstein (2002), the authors of the LCHDM, suggest that knowing how health evolves as a person ages is crucial in developing health promotion policy and research. Similar to the Social Ecological Model, the LCHDM asserts that health is a result of multiple determinants operating in a nested genetic, biological, behavioral, social, and environmental context.

One way in which LCHDM differs from SEM is in suggesting these contexts change as a person grows and develops. Second, health development is seen as an adaptive process in which biological, genetic, behavioral, social, and economic contexts all have an influence. Third, critical developmental periods are seen as key to the health trajectory of individuals, as they can result in protective factors or health risks. Fourth, the timing and sequence of all of the factors that influence health shape both individual health and population-based health (Best et al., 2003; Halfon & Hochstein, 2002).

The main aspect of the SEM that was incorporated into the LCHDM was the idea that behavior is embedded within spheres of influence that are mutually reciprocal. However, the LCHDM adds a temporal dimension: Health is viewed as a lifelong adaptive process (Best et al., 2003; Halfon & Hochstein, 2002).

There are several key concepts in the LCHDM. Embedding is the process whereby experiences are programmed into the structure and functioning of the person. This concept has a number of policy implications in terms of critical periods for intervening in early childhood education, nutrition, and social skills training. It also has implications for policy-level intervention during key times for the elderly—who, for example, may become depressed or suicidal due to a decreasing social network, when this was not a problem earlier in life.

Another concept addresses risk and protective factors. An example of this is research on stress deregulation in adulthood, as stress has a demonstrated link to the development of cancer, hypertension, and cardiovascular disease. Another concept is that of extended timeframes.

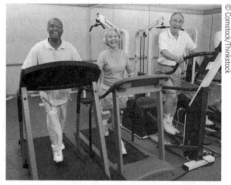

© Comstock/Thinkstock

Early experiences during childhood can influence outcomes in middle and later life. A final concept is that of functional trajectories. This concept highlights the importance of longitudinal research and examining changes in functional status over a lifetime. Policies that support early childhood growth and development are of critical importance within the LCHDM (Best et al., 2003; Halfon & Hochstein, 2002).

PLANNING MODELS

Planning models are designed for use in community-based settings, not for use with individual clients. They are useful in guiding community needs assessments, planning, implementation, and evaluation.

The Health-Promoting Self-Care System Model (1990)

Susan Simmons, a nurse, developed the Health-Promoting Self-Care System Model (HPSCSM) by drawing heavily on Orem's Self-Care Theory, Pender's Health Promotion Model, and Cox's Interaction Model of Client Health Behavior (which we will discuss later in the chapter). Assumptions of the theory are that "individuals are capable of developing the knowledge, attitudes, and skills necessary for deciding upon and performing health-promoting behaviors; and due to the value of self-care in health promotion, nursing practice is directed toward fostering self-responsibility in the acquisition and maintenance of health-promoting behaviors" (Simmons, 1990, p. 1164).

Basic conditioning factors (social, environmental, perceived health state, and healthcare experiences) and self-care requisites are described as influencing therapeutic self-care demand, exercise of self-care agency, health-promoting self-care, health outcomes, and nursing care. Nursing care also reciprocally influences each of the conditioning factors 1 through 4 (Simmons, 1990). The model includes both environmental and personal factors but it has been critiqued for the amount of emphasis it places on the need for clients to assume responsibility for their own self-care (Whitehead, 2001a).

A Stage Planning Program Model for Health Education/Health Promotion Activity (2001)

In 2001, Whitehead, a nurse, developed the Stage Planning Program Model for Health Education/Health Promotion Activity. It begins with identifying a target group or communities and then having the nurse reconcile their own health beliefs with those of the community they will be working with; identifying needs of the community with input from community members; collaborating with other disciplines to locate needed resources; empowering clients; and involving them in needed social, environmental, and political changes. The model concludes with participation of community members in evaluation activities (Whitehead, 2001a).

Another branch of the model, which is a variant of the just-described bottom-up approach, is the expert-driven approach. In this branch, community members are considered to be responsible for their own health and are expected to comply with treatment recommendations of the healthcare provider, while standard research approaches are used to evaluate results (Whitehead, 2001a).

The model, with its expert-driven and bottom-up branches, highlights the different planning approaches that are possible. One branch corresponds to the biomedical model while the other is consistent with values of the New Public Health Movement and community-based participatory research.

COMMUNICATION THEORIES

Communication theories are relevant when discussing health promotion because the Ottawa declaration (WHO, 1986) stressed the need for re-orientation of healthcare services. Theories that focus on provider–client communication, provider–provider communication, and the adoption of new technological advances contribute to the re-orientation of healthcare services.

Diffusion of Innovations Theory (1962)

Diffusion of Innovations (DOI) theory, although primarily a model describing the stages of change involved in adopting technological advances, is relevant to health promotion in two ways. First, as we will see in a later chapter, informatics and the use of electronic media has increasingly become a critical part of health promotion. Second, initial attempts at implementation do not always lead to sustained use of a health promotion program or behavior (Glanz, Rimer, & Lewis, 2002; Rogers, 1962). As you read the stages of change included in diffusion theory, ask yourself whether the concepts also describe how a behavioral change is adopted and sustained. Relevant stages of change according to the DOI theory include: knowledge (understanding), persuasion (developing a favorable attitude), decision (weighing benefits and barriers, then committing to adoption), implementation (action), and confirmation (reinforcement based on positive outcomes). Do you think these stages are relevant to behavioral as well as technological change?

To be adopted as an innovation or a planned health promotion, a program must have relative advantage (be better than other options), compatibility (be consistent with existing values, past experiences, and needs), trialability (the ability to be experimented with on a limited basis), and observability (be able to produce visible results). An innovation or health promotion program must also be easy to use, easily understood and communicated, able to be adopted with a minimal investment of time, able to be undertaken with minimal risk, and able to be used with only a moderate level of commitment (Glanz, Rimer, & Lewis, 2002; Rogers, 1962).

Important roles in the adoption of innovations and health promotion behavior include opinion leaders (those having informal influence over others), change agents (who mediate between the new change and relevant social systems), and change aides (trusted individuals who interact with clients) (Rogers, 1962). Diffusion theory has been used to study the dissemination of AIDS education curricula in schools; the use of new tests, technologies, and pharmaceutical agents as they are incorporated into practice by health professionals; workplace health promotion; and the adoption of safe sexual practices, among other topics (Glanz, Rimer, & Lewis, 2002).

Weick's Health Communication Theory (1969–1979)

Weick's theory (1979) emphasizes the central role of communication and information processing within social groups and institutions. The theory focuses on communication between healthcare providers within organizations as well as client–provider communication. Weick's work is important to consider as a health promotion theory based on the Ottawa declaration, which stated that there is a need for identifying group influences on health. Improving communication promotes the accuracy of information transfer and organizational adaptation (Kreps, 2009; Weick, 1979).

There are three phases in Weick's theory: enactment, selection, and retention. The enactment phase focuses on health-related challenges. In the enactment phase, consumers and healthcare providers must develop the best communication strategies and interventions for addressing the given health issue. In the selection phase, decisions are made about ways of increasing the understandability of communication. In the retention phase, processes are used to preserve what was learned by creating a repertoire of experience about what worked and what didn't. An example of the retention phase is a patient navigator program in which clients who have experienced a healthcare issue help other clients to navigate the healthcare system using their wisdom and past experience (Kreps, 2009, Weick, 1979).

Organizational rules and interaction patterns are used to increase equivocality (message understandability). Each level of organizational participant strives to transform equivocal messages into understandable and predictable messages. Because different individuals are able to manage different levels of equivocality, multiple communication strategies and cycles may be needed to make sense of the information being shared (Kreps, 2009; Weick, 1979). For example, a non-English speaking client who is presented with detailed information about a crucial diagnosis may feel confused. Rules and cycles are used to help individuals manage equivocal information. Health pamphlets and printed instructions are examples of rule-governed strategies, while examples of communication cycles include establishing a procedure for referring a client to a specialist, having a nurse explain information in the client's primary language, or referring a client to a support group that could help him or her gather needed information (Kreps, 2009, Weick, 1979).

EVALUATION MODELS

Both the RE-AIM framework and the PRECEDE-PROCEED model are useful in evaluating health promotion programs. These frameworks and models are helpful to researchers who are trying to measure the effectiveness of a health promotion program and also to practitioners who are designing interventions.

The PRECEDE-PROCEED Model (1992)

The PRECEDE-PROCEED Model (PPM) is a planning model that came from Johns Hopkins University and was designed as a way to teach students about health promotion. It was also created as a planning, intervention, and evaluation framework. The PPM is based on the assumption that interventions will be effective if they (1) come from the community, (2) are planned thoroughly, (3) are based on data, (4) include interventions the community sees as feasible, (5) include multiple strategies woven into a cohesive program, and (6) rely on feedback and progress evaluation. Green and Kreuter (1992), in developing the PPM, suggested that centrally packaged programs are difficult to adapt to unique settings. Each community must assess its own needs and priorities.

PRECEDE stands for Predisposing, Reinforcing, and Enabling Constructs in Educational/Environmental Diagnosis and Evaluation, while PROCEED stands for Policy, Regulatory, and Organizational Constructs in Educational and Environmental Development. Despite its long name the model is widely used in health promotion practice and community development activities. The PRECEDE portion of the model focuses on identifying educational factors that influence change. The PROCEED portion of the model was added in 1991 to acknowledge the importance that environmental, regulatory, policy, and organizational factors have in shaping health, and it focuses on identifying ecological factors that influence change. The goal of the PPM is to identify the most effective way to promote change by conducting local needs assessments and program evaluations. The model was based on epidemiology, social-cognitive psychology, education, and management principles (Green, Kreuter, Deeds, & Partridge, 1980).

The PRECEDE-PROCEED model is divided into phases and promotes identification of priorities for action (see **Figure 3-2**). The first step is to conduct a social assessment in which community members and involved participants identify their own health promotion needs. In step two, an epidemiological assessment is conducted using vital statistics and state or national surveys to identify the health problems that have the largest impact on the given community.

During step three, a behavioral and environment assessment is conducted to evaluate factors that contribute to the identified problem. These can be the lifestyles of individuals, environmental factors, or social influences. Each of the factors is ranked according to importance in terms of contributing to the selected health problem and is evaluated based on whether it can or cannot be changed. Those factors that are most important and most changeable are considered the priority targets.

FIGURE 3-2 The PRECEDE-PROCEED Planning Model

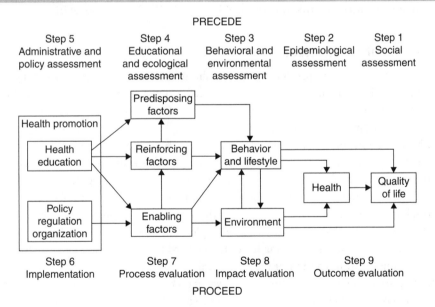

Source: Glanz, Rimer, & Lewis. (2002). *Health Behavior and Health Education: Theory, Research, and Practice, 3rd edition.* San Francisco, CA: Jossey-Bass. Reproduced with permission of John Wiley & Sons, Inc.

In step four, the antecedent, predisposing, reinforcing, and enabling factors are considered. Predisposing factors are antecedents that provide rationale or motivation for the health behavior. Reinforcing factors provide continuing reward and are things such as social support, peer influence, and vicarious reinforcement, while enabling factors include services and resources and policies necessary for health. Measurable objectives are also developed in step four.

In step five, intervention strategies are devised and policies, resources, and circumstances within the organizational contexts that influence the intervention are considered. Barriers at this level, such as staff commitment and lack of space, need to be considered. In steps six to nine, process impact evaluations are established to assess the changes in predisposing, reinforcing, enabling, behavioral, and environmental factors that determine the likelihood that change will happen. Outcome evaluations are also identified. Participatory approaches to planning that encourage individual and community-level involvement are key aspects of the model (Best et al., 2003; Glanz, Rimer & Lewis, 2002; Green & Kreuter, 1999).

The goal of the PRECEDE-PROCEED model is to describe proximal, intermediate, and distal outcomes associated with health promotion programs. It has been critiqued for being difficult to use; it is a highly structured, linear effect model, which at times has been implemented incorrectly because of its complexity (Whitehead, 2001a).

The RE-AIM Framework (1999)

The idea that a health promotion program should be efficacious (create a substantial amount of change) and reach a large number of people led to the development of the RE-AIM framework. RE-AIM stands for Reach, Efficacy or effectiveness, Adoption, Implementation, and Maintenance (Glasgow, Vogt, & Boles, 1999). Reach is a measure of how many people can be influenced by the health promotion program. Efficacious and effective programs produce positive outcomes along with few unintended consequences. Adoption focuses on the participation rate (number of people who engage in the health promotion behavior) and whether the setting is representative of a larger population. Implementation targets whether the health promotion program was employed as intended or whether, for example, multiple health educators presented content in different ways, making the outcome hard to evaluate. Maintenance focuses on the long-term utilization of the given health behavior. It also refers to whether a health promotion program is sustainable even if there is a change in available resources. The goal is not to have a health promotion program that is equally effective on all five dimensions; rather, these dimensions help to evaluate a program before it is adopted so that the characteristics that are most important in the given setting can be selected (Glanz, Rimer, & Lewis, 2002).

NURSING MODELS AND THEORIES

There are a vast number of nursing theories. While only those that are most relevant to health promotion are summarized next, it is likely that other nursing theories have some applicability to health promotion as well. Nursing models and theories that focus on health promotion have been critiqued for focusing on person-level issues rather than group or community level concerns (Whitehead, 2001a). However, a number of nursing theories, including Nightingale's, have included a community-oriented perspective. Two nursing models that included a focus on environment, authored by Simmons (1990) and Whitehead (2001a), were discussed earlier under the Planning Model section of this chapter and will not be summarized again in this section.

Nightingale's Environmental Theory (1859)

Florence Nightingale is credited with being the first nurse theorist. She proposed Environmental Theory, which aimed to restore the client to their optimal state of health. She asserted that the client's environment could be used to facilitate his or her recovery and that the nurse was responsible for helping configure the environment such that it supported recovery. Pure air, clean water, sufficient food, efficient drainage, cleanliness, and light were considered necessary for a healthy environment. A quiet, noise-free environment with adequate warmth during cold periods was also considered to be a priority (Nightingale, 1859). The practice of environmental configuration, based on client needs is still practiced today.

Leninger's Transcultural Care Theory (1968)

After completing a doctoral degree in anthropology, Madeleine Leninger spent more than a year with the Gadsup people of New Guinea, during which time she began to work on her theory of cultural care. Leninger's theory focuses on the ways in which cultures and subcultures differ in terms of caring behaviors, nursing care, health beliefs, and behavioral patterns and how caregiver and care recipient roles differ according to culture. Leninger emphasized that a nurse must discern the cultural values and beliefs of a client or family before intervening. She stated that social, religious, political, and economic factors influence how care should be provided (Alexander et al., 1986).

The major concepts of Leninger's theory are care, caring, culture, cultural values, cultural variations, and nursing. Assumptions include: 1) "care has biophysical, cultural, psychological, social, and environmental dimensions that must be explicated to provide holistic care" (Alexander, et al., 1986, p. 150), 2) care behaviors and goals vary with social structure, and 3) there is no curing without caring. Propositions include:

- "differences among caring values and behaviors between and among cultures leads to differences in the nursing care expectations of care-seekers" (Alexander et al., 1986, p. 150),
- the greater the reliance on technological caring approaches, the greater the interpersonal distance between nurse and client and the lower the satisfaction will be,
- "nursing care interventions that provide culture-specific caring practices result in greater satisfaction" (Alexander et al., 1986, p. 150), and
- the greater the gap between folk caring practices and nursing practice, the greater the level of stress that will be experienced by the client.

Leninger cautioned nurses to evaluate whether the client with whom they are working values self-care or not. The theory was developed specifically for use in cross-cultural contexts, so it does not attempt to be generalizable. It is relevant to this chapter in that cultural beliefs and practices are an integral part of health promotion practice. A criticism of the theory is that it relied heavily on anthropological research and theories (Alexander et al., 1986).

Goal Attainment Theory of Nursing (1981)

Imogene King (1981) created the Goal Attainment Theory of Nursing. Assumptions included the proposition that individuals are social beings, rational beings, reactive beings, perceiving beings, controlling beings, purposeful beings, action-oriented beings, and time-oriented beings. Other assumptions were that perceptions of the nurse and the client influence the nurse–client relationship and that clients have a right to information and should participate in decisions that influence their health (King, 1981).

King's theory is best described by defining the concepts which make up her theory. One concept, health, was defined as the life experiences and continuous adjustments to stressors in one's internal and external environment through optimal use of resources to achieve one's maximum potential. Another concept, environment, was defined as an open system with permeable boundaries permitting exchange of matter, energy, and information. Interaction was defined as "a process of perception and communication between a person and the environment and between person and person represented by verbal and nonverbal behaviors that are goal-directed" (King, 1981, p. 145).

The concept of transaction was defined as an interaction with the environment, while growth and development were defined as helping move from potential capacity for achievement to self-actualization. In King's theory, positive communication increases mutual goal setting between clients and nurses and leads to satisfaction. Goal attainment was seen as decreasing stress, increasing learning, and facilitating coping.

The theory has been critiqued for not defining terms such as controlling being. The theory places the nurse and client on the same level of responsibility for goal attainment and highlights the importance of participatory involvement in goal setting (King, 1981).

Pender's Health Promotion Model (1982)

Nola Pender, a nurse, developed this health promotion model in 1982 and revised it in 1987. This model, which had the aim of helping nurses educate clients with entrenched behaviors such as smoking and drug abuse, has been described as one of the predominant models of health promotion within nursing (King, 1994). Pender (1987) saw health promotion as comprised of activities designed to increase the level of well-being and self-actualization of individuals, families, communities, and society.

Pender's (1982) model consists of a decision-making phase and an action phase. Individual perceptions and modifying factors make up the decision-making phase. Individual perceptions include the importance of health to a person, perceived control, desire for competence, self-awareness, self-esteem, the person's definition of health, perceived health status, and perceived benefits of health-promoting behaviors.

When the desire for control is blocked, it can result in feelings of helplessness and frustration. The desire for competence can motivate a person to acquire knowledge about health. Self-awareness is a health-promoting factor seen in positive habits such as running and meditating. Self-esteem is important because it requires a feeling of self worth and a commitment to set aside time for health promotion (Pender, 1982).

Whether one defines health as an absence of illness or self-actualization influences whether one engages in health-protecting or health-promoting behaviors. Individuals with a poorer perceived health status are less likely to engage in health-promoting behaviors because they feel limited by their poor health; for example, symptoms of pain can interfere with an exercise program. The perceptions of long-term rather than short-term benefits from health-promoting behavior may influence the likelihood of continuing those behaviors. Each individual factor influences motivation and the readiness to engage in health-promoting behavior (Pender, 1982).

Modifying factors include demographic variables (age, ethnicity/race, education, income, gender), interpersonal variables (expectations of significant others, family patterns, interactions with health professionals) and situational variables (prior experience with health promotion and available options). The action phase consists of perceived barriers to action (unavailability, cost, inconvenience, extent of change needed), the likelihood of taking the health promotion action, and cues to action (feeling good as a result of the health promotion behavior, being aware of the potential for growth, advice from others, mass media advertising/campaigns) (Pender, 1982).

The constructs of perceived control of health and cues to action were removed from the revised model. In 1987, the client's history of prior health-related behavior was added to the model along with perceived self-efficacy and activity-related affect. These later concepts were included based on Bandura's theory (1986). Pender (1987) suggested that cognitive and perceptual factors provide motivation to engage in health-promoting behaviors.

One strength of the model is that a scale, the Health Promoting Lifestyle Profile, was developed to measure the dimensions of health-promoting behavior, including self-actualization, health responsibility, exercise, nutrition, interpersonal support, and stress management (Walker et al., 1987). Pender's model has been critiqued for focusing on cognitive and perceptual factors as influencing health while identifying environmental, situational, and interpersonal factors as only being important to the extent that they modify cognitive and perceptual influences. Pender emphasized the decision-making ability of individuals, their perception of control, and their definition of health as being critical factors. Scant attention was given in Pender's model to the importance of sociopolitical or economic context. In addition, whether perceptual factors precede behavioral change or result from change was not specified (King, 1994). The model has also been critiqued for being focused on preventative, disease-centered, behavioral, and lifestyle-oriented concepts of the health education paradigm rather than addressing broader concepts of the health promotion paradigm (Whitehead, 2009).

Theory of Humanistic Nursing Communication (1983)

Bonnie Duldt and colleagues (1983) developed a theory, called the Theory of Humanistic Nursing Communication (THNC) that focuses exclusively on interpersonal communication among the nurse, the client, peers, and colleagues. Although Duldt's theory is limited in that it focuses exclusively on interpersonal communication, the theory is being included in this chapter because it focuses to a great extent on the influence of bureaucratic and dehumanizing healthcare delivery systems. This is a unique aspect of the theory. As you will remember, a priority identified in the Ottawa Charter was on re-designing healthcare systems; examining factors that create the bureaucratic and dehumanizing aspects within those institutions may help in re-designing them.

One assumption in Duldt's theory that is not consistent with the Ottawa Charter is that growth and change arise from within an individual and are primarily dependent upon personal choice. Another assumption is that decision making is best achieved by communicating with other people. Duldt posits that communication can be either humanizing or dehumanizing. She assumes that the bureaucratic, complex nature of healthcare institutions can result in both clients and healthcare personnel being treated in a dehumanizing manner. Interpersonal communication is seen as the way a nurse becomes aware of and sensitive to the dynamic relationship among the client, the client's environment, and the client's potential. Health, in this theory, is assumed to be linked with feeling human and being treated in a humane way (Duldt et al., 1983).

The concept of nursing in the THNC is defined as an art and science of positive communication, caring, and coaching. Health as a concept is related to self-awareness, adaptation to one's environment, and one's state of being. The concept of a critical life situation is described as a situation in which a perceived threat to health and being occurs; examples include child birth, surgery, or the loss of a parent (Duldt et al., 1983).

The theory acknowledges that nurses have negative encounters with colleagues, administrators, and clients. It presents an approach based on dialogue, equity, and respect as a way to cope with and improve dehumanizing communications (Duldt et al., 1983).

Orem's Self-Care Theory (1985)

Orem's Self-Care Theory consists of three theoretical constructs, including self-care, self-care deficits, and nursing systems. The theory is based on the assumption that all clients wish to care for themselves and should be encouraged to engage in self-care to speed their rehabilitation. A person's self-care is seen as being influenced by developmental stages and life-stage-specific needs in addition to universal self-care needs that all people have (air, water, food, elimination, activity/rest, solitude/social interaction, hazard prevention, and promotion of normality).

Age, gender, living conditions, sociocultural orientation, and health state modify one's ability to perform self-care. Self-care agency, or one's belief that they can engage in self-care, influences those behaviors. Self-care agency is seen when a person seeks information about self-care and decides to undertake self-care behaviors. When clients are unable to care for themselves, they have a self-care deficit and the nurse needs to intervene to provide support until the clients can care for themselves (Orem, 1985).

Orem's theory has been widely researched and has resulted in the creation of three scales designed to measure self-care agency. Those scales include the Denyes self-care agency scale, the Kearney and Fleisher's exercise of self-care agency scale, and the Hanson and Bickel's perception of self-care agency scale (McBride, 1991). You may wish to research those scales in more detail elsewhere. A critique of Orem's theory is that not all cultures value self-care to the same degree.

The World Health Organization (WHO) (2009) conference, held in Bangkok, Thailand, suggested that self-care be incorporated into health promotion activities to a greater extent to revitalize primary care. The WHO encouraged member states to strengthen support structures, enact legislation, provide financing for self-care, and disseminate evidence-based self-care practices. They pointed out that in the information age in which we live, it is common for people to look online for health information, seek out their own resources to manage health-related problems, and to learn about health-promoting activities using technology.

A Social Cognitive Model for Health Promotion Practice in Nursing (2001)

Whitehead (2001b) proposed the Social Cognitive Model for Health Promotion Practice in Nursing (SCMHPPN). This was the second health promotion model created by Whitehead. Concepts in this model include cues to action, cues to non-action, the client's/nurse's reaction to the health threat, regulating factors, perceptions of the client/nurse, cost/reward calculations, and behavioral intent to change.

Cues to action include aspects such as motivation, pressure to succeed, influence of mass media, acceptance by significant others, and support systems, while clues to non-action are concepts such as anxiety, fear of failure, a non-conformist attitude, suspiciousness, and denial. Regulating factors include age, gender, personality, social status, health policies, economic factors, knowledge of the disease, and access to health care. Perceptions include self-efficacy, motivation, and locus of control. Costs of and rewards associated with changing are evaluated at four decision points in the model. Intention to change is not a firm indicator of "program success especially when strong external structural and socio-economic constraints are taken into consideration" (Whitehead, 2001b, p. 423).

The SCMHPPN is a cyclic model that considers the perspective of the nurse and the client. The model reinforces the idea that there may be rationale for a client deciding not to change. The model is unique in this aspect, in that it explicitly describes reasons for not pursuing health promotion activities. This addition could diminish the victim blaming that can occur in the health professions. Although it appears to have been designed for use with individual clients, the concepts presented are also relevant in working with families, groups, and communities.

Interaction Model of Client Health Behavior (2003)

The Interactional Model of Client Health Behavior (IMCHB) was developed by Cox (1982, 2003) because she felt other models did not address the dynamic nature of client–provider interactions and the effect of those relationships on health promotion. The theory is based on the assumptions that clients make competent health-related choices and that clients should be allowed as much control over their health decisions and actions as possible (Carter & Kulbok, 1995).

The first concept in the model, client singularity, focuses on the unique and holistic aspects of the client, including demographic variables, social influences, previous healthcare experience, and environmental resources. These demographic variables are considered to be antecedents to other concepts in the model, and therefore are pivotally important. Some authors have stressed that variables such as social influence, previous healthcare experience, and environmental resources need to be defined with greater specificity in the model (Carter & Kulbok, 1995).

Dynamic variables such as intrinsic motivation, cognitive appraisal, and affective response constitute the second concept within the model. Intrinsic motivation has been defined or operationalized as self-determination in health judgment and behavior, perceived competency in health matters, and internal/external cue responsiveness (Carter & Kulbok, 1995). The client's cognitive appraisal, not the healthcare professional's, is what is of interest in the model. Cognitive appraisal has been defined exclusively as perceived health status. Affective response includes emotions that promote or hinder behavioral change.

The third concept is client–professional interaction, which includes affective support, health information, decisional control, and professional competency. Client–professional interaction is seen as a reciprocal relationship within the model. The amount of health information that is provided must be consistent with the client's needs and must be understandable to the client.

The final concept, health outcome, includes topics such as utilization of healthcare services, clinical health status indicators, the severity of the healthcare problem, adherence to the prescribed regime of care, and satisfaction with care. Relationships between client–professional interaction, intrinsic motivation, cognitive appraisal, and affective response are reciprocal in that a change in one factor affects the others.

Although the IMCHB model has not been tested to the degree that it can be considered a theory, it has been studied in the elderly, women considering amniocentesis, school-aged children receiving diet and exercise interventions, and adolescent cancer survivors. Much of the research has focused on client singularity and health outcomes. Other concepts, including client–professional, interaction need additional study. Carter and Kulbok (1995) asserted that, after a decade of research, the IMCHB is ready for hypothesis testing, rigorous statistical analysis, and evaluation in additional populations. An advantage of the model is that it does focus on the domain concepts of nursing including client, nursing, health, and environment.

An instrument, the Health Self-Determination Index (HSDI) and a corresponding scale for children was developed from research on the IMCHB. This instrument is used to measure motivational components of health behavior. This instrument has been tested with a random sample from the general population, a community-based sample of the elderly, and mothers, and has been translated into Spanish, Chinese, Icelander, Kamir, Laotian, and Vietnamese (Carter & Kulbok, 1995).

An example of the application of the IMCHB model is described by Mathews and colleagues (2008). In this case, a single working mother comes to a dermatology clinic with a 5-month-old infant who has hives covering her face. The baby is in daycare but is cared for by the grandmother in the afternoons. The grandmother has tried various folk remedies including cream of tartar to treat the hives because of the limited financial resources within the family. The mother asks multiple questions about the cost of the office visit and prescriptions. She is concerned that the hives could spread to her other children. The nurse practitioner (NP) considers the economic situation of the single mother and provides her with free samples of the prescribed medication. A repeat visit to monitor the effectiveness of the medications is arranged, taking into consideration the mother's work schedule. The mother verbalizes understanding of the importance of taking the medication, maintaining proper hygiene, and avoiding allergens. The mother is satisfied with the care her baby received because she feels emotionally supported by the NP. This experience becomes part of her repertoire of healthcare experience, which in turn affects whether she will seek medical care in the future for her family.

Describe how future utilization of healthcare services, the severity of the health issue, adherence to the recommended regime of care, intrinsic motivation, and the mother's satisfaction with the care provided showed up in this case study.

The Self-Nurturance Model (2003)

Mary Ann Nemcek, a nurse, created the Self-Nurturance Model using aspects of the Health Belief Model and Pender's Health Promotion Model. She defined self-nurturance as the "feelings, attitudes, behaviors, and substances that stimulate, foster, and support life and growth of self" (Nemcek, 2003, p. 260). Dr. Nemcek suggested that self-nurturance includes nurturing physical, intellectual, social, emotional, and spiritual aspects of the self. Antecedents include knowledge, ability, and a sense of self. Contextual influences include culture, physiology, personality, demographics, social support, and illness. The model has been critiqued for adding little that is new, other than the concept of self-nurturance, and for needing additional research to support it.

HOW ARE THEORIES CONSTRUCTED?

The process of creating a theory begins with identifying concepts that influence health promotion by reviewing the literature or conducting research. The next step is to clus-ter related terms or concepts and eliminate any redundancy or overlap. Simultaneously, one considers whether there is any opposing or contradictory ideas within the concepts that have been identified, and it is best to eliminate contradictory ideas so the theory is internally consistent. Often sketching a picture, diagram, flowchart, or concept map helps to identify linkages between the concepts in the model. A list of assumptions that a person must believe to agree with the model are also provided. The final step needed to translate a model into a theory is to publish the model and design and conduct numerous research studies to test it.

Momentum Theory: An Example Of Theory Construction

I used the same approach just described to design my theory, which I have called Momentum Theory. Momentum Theory incorporates ideas from Newton's Second Law of Motion, the Health Belief Model, the Theory of Planned Behavior, the Transtheoretical Model, Ecological Systems Theory, Salutogenic Theory, the Life Course Development Model, Diffusion of Innovations Theory, and Pender's Health Promotion Model.

My theory is called Momentum Theory because most behavioral change (whether it is to modify an unhealthy behavior or to add a health-promoting behavior to one's life) requires substantial momentum and initial effort to get the ball rolling. When set in motion and rooted into daily life, habit patterns have their own sustaining force. Engrained habit patterns have a self-propelling nature, an ease of action associated with them. That momentum, once established, carries you along in a set direction or trajectory.

Assumptions of Momentum Theory include:

1. Health is a habit pattern that is shaped by one's daily activities, cultural background, family history, past experience, environment, economic situation, and future hopes.
2. A substantial amount of effort is required to adopt any new habit pattern.
3. Both external and internal forces motivate change.
4. Both pleasure and fear motivate behavioral change.
5. Habit patterns can be conscious or unconscious, health promoting or a detriment to health.
6. Sustained momentum requires balance between physical, mental, social, psychological, and spiritual factors.

Concepts within my theory include: (1) momentum, (2) roadblocks to change, (3) forces that get the ball rolling, (4) forces that provide ongoing impetus for change, (5) forces that help a person get past the plateaus where change seems to slow, and (6) habit patterns.

Momentum is defined as the amount, force, and duration of change required to sustain a new health habit. Engaging in healthy behavior on a regular basis has a self-sustaining aspect to it. It is also the case that, to initiate a behavior change, a substantial amount of effort is required to overcome past habit patterns.

Roadblocks to change are those things that interfere with, get in the way of, detour, or inhibit healthy habit patterns. Examples of roadblocks to change include; having to change rather than wanting to change; a lack of commitment to the planned change; time constraints; competing priorities; feeling overloaded or stressed; the amount of inconvenience associated with the change; a past history of not being successful with behavioral change; a staunch reliance on unhealthy comforting behaviors; policies, circumstances or laws that undermine health or interfere with change; environmental or psychological cues that tempt one to make unhealthy choices; and lack of money or resources.

A number of forces can either be a roadblock to or impetus to change depending on the person and their cultural, economic, environmental or family background. Therefore, change must begin with a through discussion of the person's or the community's history. Factors that can be either a roadblock or an incentive include: (1) engrained family patterns, cultural patterns, or learned behavioral patterns; (2) the perceived level of control over the given behavior; (3) the perceived threat (susceptibility and severity) associated with a particular health pattern that is being targeted; (4) the perceived health status of the person/community; (5) the person's or community's feeling of self-worth or lack thereof; (6) the degree to which the person/community intends to or wants to change; (7) past interactions with significant others, friends, co-workers, or healthcare providers related to the given behavior; (8) the person's/community's developmental stage of life; (9) the person's or community's narrative understanding (self image developed over time) and how that is shaped by the given health pattern; (10) unintended consequences of changing (side-effects); and (11) cultural, social, or gender-based norms and/or roles.

Forces that get the ball rolling are those factors that motivate one to initiate change. Examples include a perceived threat to one's health or daily routine associated with maintaining one's current habit pattern support, reinforcement, interest or coaching from significant others, healthcare providers or one's environment; clear benefits associated with the new habit pattern; or imaging positive future advantages associated with the change.

Forces that provide on-going impetus for change are those factors that help a person maintain behaviors that support their health-related goals. These forces include any of the listed forces that get the ball rolling or a sense of purpose, focus or meaning experienced during the process of changing.

Forces that help a person get past the plateaus where change seems to slow include the forces that provide impetus to stay the course and persist despite a lack of progress such as an ability to delay gratification; a strong investment in or commitment to the planned change; pleasure associated with the new habit pattern; skill in imaging future gratification that could result from the change; a strong investment in the new habit pattern; the ability to identify reasons for persisting with the new habit pattern; or the ability to identify small steps that indicate progress.

Habits patterns are attitudes or behaviors created from repetitive experiences or inherited from one's family or their social/cultural/environmental/economic background that affect your health. Habit patterns can be conscious or unconscious, health promoting or a detriment to health.

Several relational statements explain how these concepts are linked. Relational statements include:

1. larger habit pattern changes require greater effort
2. a substantial amount of effort over a short period, or a lesser amount of effort over an extended period, can both result in a new habit pattern (change can be radical or gradual)
3. the amount of pleasure one obtains from healthy habit patterns must exceed the amount of pleasure one obtains from unhealthy habit patterns,
4. the forces that provide impetus for change must be greater than the roadblocks that interfere with change if progress is to be made,
5. future anticipated gratification associated with maintaining one's health goals must exceed the gratification obtained from engaging in unhealthy habit patterns,
6. cultural, environmental, social, and economic factors can impede or support change,
7. balance (mental, physical, psychological, social, and spiritual) results in momentum,
8. imbalance (mental, physical, psychological, social, and spiritual) causes one to veer off center and detours health promoting action.

To understand Momentum Theory, imagine a car that has to accelerate over a small incline to begin its journey, and then gains speed as it travels down a long mountain road. Along the way, the car (representing the person experiencing change) can encounter unexpected roadblocks that derail its journey (such as a rock slide or detour). The car can also gain momentum from a strong tail wind or an open lane unblocked by other cars. The car can encounter a steep grade where little progress is being made (a plateau), and its speed drops unless extra gas is applied.

The main idea of Momentum Theory is that it requires effort to establish new habit patterns. Habit patterns have a driving force or thrust within them that structures life. Once a new habit has been established, the habit pattern itself has a momentum and an influence that is felt every day, whether one thinks about the habit pattern on a conscious level or not. Habit patterns actually define who we are in many ways. As Heidegger (1962) said one is what one does. Repetitive action has the power to shape a person's attitude, perception, hopes, and future action as well, unless a substantial amount of effort is devoted to changing one's habitual trajectory. One is pulled along by forces that facilitate change and pulled off track by roadblocks that impede changing. During plateau periods where little change seems to be accomplished, sustained motivation is needed before progress can be seen.

As you read through my theory, jot down a few notes about which parts of Momentum Theory derived from other theories that we discussed in this chapter. What is one unique aspect of Momentum Theory? Should Momentum Theory actually be called a theory or a model? Explain your answer.

Also, consider the following case about Vicki and how you would use Motivation Theory to help her. Vicki had lost 40 pounds on three different occasions in her life: once at the age of 25, again at 37, and finally at 45. Now, at the age of 58 she was having little success with her goal of losing 50 pounds. She mentioned that, in the past, "falling in love" always helped her lose weight but at this point in life she felt little motivation to discipline herself. She reminded herself that losing weight was an important goal since everyone in her family had been overweight and developed type 2 diabetes late in life. Vicki had a stressful job, a 3-hour commute per day, loved to cook, and expressed an avid disdain for exercise.

Which roadblocks interfering with Vicki's weight loss would you talk to her about first? What factors would you build on to help motivate Vicki to stick to her weight loss program? What else would you want to know about Vicki before you proceeded to coach her about weight loss?

CHAPTER EXERCISES

DISCUSSION QUESTION ONE

Which Theories Are the Best Fit for These Two Health Promotion Programs?

1. A nurse was working in an African American church helping to design a weight loss program for overweight female teens. She wanted to involve teens, parents, and church personnel in designing and implementing the program to ensure it would be supported by the community. The nurse believed that change is best designed by the community that will benefit from the health promotion program. She had a small grant to hire church members to help with data collection and dissemination of the study results. Which theories could she use in her grant and in the publications that are consistent with her assumptions and approach?

2. A nurse was working with a group of clients who had just received an organ transplant. The nurse wanted to encourage the clients to take their prescribed medications to ensure the transplant was a success. The nurse devised a program whereby in one group, medications were mailed to the client's home a week before their prescription ran out so that clients did not have to leave home to get their prescription refilled and risk exposure to a virus. In a comparison group, clients were given a wristband that beeped at preset intervals (corresponding to the client's medication schedule) to remind them when it was time to take their medications. The study also had a control group that received the

usual care without the medication mailing and wristband reminder. The nurse designed the study to evaluate the effectiveness of self-care interventions for transplant clients. Which theory or model should the nurse use in writing up the results of the study in a nursing journal?

DISCUSSION QUESTION TWO

Describe the similarities and differences between the two models that Whitehead developed namely: (1) The Social Cognitive Model for Health Promotion Practice and (2) The Stage Planning Program Model for Health Education / Health Promoting Activity. Why do you think Whitehead developed two health promotion models?

DISCUSSION QUESTION THREE

Think about the various health promotion values and consider whether the theories discussed in this chapter are consistent with these principles and values. List the names of the theories discussed in this chapter beside each value outlined below so you can track how many theories support each value or principle.

1. Views health as including well-being, not just the absence of disease

2. Considers social factors that influence health

3. Emphasizes cultural factors that influence health

4. Attends to economic factors that influence health

5. Considers environmental factors that influence health

6. Focuses on political or policy-level influences that shape health

7. Encourages a bottom-up or community-based participatory approach to promoting health

8. Includes interventions that are more broad ranging than just health education

9. Encourages multifactor and multidisciplinary research

10. Promotes client or community-level empowerment

11. Helps re-orient health systems

_____

12. Focuses on equity, health, disparities, and equal access

_____

13. Maintains consistency with the WHO settings–based focus on the workplace, hospital, university, school, prison, or church

_____

14. Testing of the theory has resulted in development of a standardized scale or method of evaluating health outcomes

_____

15. The theory is understandable, practical, and would be easy to use when designing a health promotion program

_____

DISCUSSION QUESTION FOUR

Compare and contrast nursing and non-nursing theories discussed within this chapter in terms of their strengths and limitations.

DISCUSSION QUESTION FIVE

Describe which theories summarized in this chapter would and would not provide a good framework for multilevel health promotion interventions.

DISCUSSION QUESTION SIX

Which theories described in this chapter target individual, group, and population level change?

CHECK YOUR UNDERSTANDING

Match the following statements with the theory that most accurately addresses the comment.

Quotes

1. "All my family smoke, so it seemed natural to start smoking."
2. "I trust my nurse practitioner because he understands how my knee pain affects my ability to exercise."

3. "I can't bring myself to start a diet because I always gain any weight that I lost back."
4. "Diabetes can cause you to lose your eyesight, so I need to keep my blood sugar under control."
5. "I worked around asbestos when I was in my 20s and I know that could lead to health problems down the road."
6. "I have appreciated the patient navigator program, it made dealing with my diagnosis of breast cancer much easier."
7. "I realize I need to start exercising if I want to have more energy."
8. "I am so tempted by Chardonnay, I can't avoid it."
9. "I can still sew, and that brings meaning to my life."
10. "You can't talk to me in that tone of voice just because you are a nurse and you think you know what is best for me!"
11. "I run because I enjoy running."
12. "Exercising to lose weight is a better way to go than dieting."
13. "You could think about ways to decrease your salt intake as one way to manage your blood pressure."
14. "I take calcium every morning to protect my bone density."
15. "Being a new mother at age 40, who was called to active duty military service in Iraq, hasn't been easy."
16. "It's important to begin with a needs assessment before planning or implementing a health promotion program."
17. "I have a goal now, I can begin my exercise program."
18. "I get depressed during the winter when I can't be out in the sun as much as my body seems to want."
19. "I saw gum advertised on TV that helps you quit smoking. I think that will work for me."

Theories

A. Theory of Reasoned Action (TRA)
B. Goal Attainment Theory of Nursing (GAT)
C. Theory of Planned Behavior (TPB)
D. Interaction Model of Client Health Behavior (IMCHB)
E. Social Learning Theory (SLT)
F. Transtheoretical Model or Stages of Change Model (TTM)
G. Self-Determination Theory (SDT)
H. Duldt's Theory of Humanistic Nursing Communication (THNC)
I. Health Belief Model (HBM)
J. Tannahill Model (TM)
K. A Social Cognitive Model for Health Promotion Practice in Nursing (SCMHPPN)

L. The Life Course Health Development Model (LCHDM)

M. Social Ecological Model (SEM)

N. Nightingale's Environmental Theory (NET)

O. PRECEDE-PROCEED MODEL (PPM)

P. Diffusion Theory (DOI)

Q. Weick's Health Communication Theory (WHC)

R. The Salutogenic Theory (ST)

Create Your Own Health Promotion Theory

Remind yourself of the definitions of health promotion, the principles of the new health promotion movement, and the concepts that were included in the health promotion theories. Also, think back to a time in your life when you made a major change that influenced your health. From these, create a list of the concepts that you believe contribute to health promotion. Cluster related terms (concepts) and eliminate redundancy. Next, sketch a picture, diagram, flowchart, or concept map that describes the linkages between the concepts in your model. Summarize the assumptions that one must believe to agree with your model. The final step needed to translate your model into a theory would be to conduct research studies and publish your results.

WHAT DO YOU THINK?

Provide Rationale for Your Answers.

1. Which theory do you see as most relevant to health promotion practice?
2. Which is your favorite theory? Why is it your favorite?
3. Which theory is the least likely to be of value in facilitating the promotion of health at the community level?
4. Which theory is most relevant for an acute care, inpatient setting such as a hospital?
5. Which theories are not well supported by research?
6. Which models are well-situated to become theories in the near future?
7. Which theory provides the best guidance in terms of creating measurable health outcomes that can be researched and evaluated?
8. Is there a need for additional health promotion theories? Why or why not?
9. Which theory contains concepts or language that is difficult to understand?
10. Which theory is the most pragmatic and would be easiest for clinicians and community members to use?
11. Which theory includes assumptions (taken for granted beliefs) that you disagree with?

12. Which theory would you use to guide your thesis work in the area of health promotion?
13. Describe which disciplines have contributed models or theories that are still being used in health promotion practice today.
14. Do you agree with Antonovsky (1996) that good theories give birth to good ideas that can be incorporated into health promotion programs? Please explain your answer.
15. Should health promotion theories and models be stage-based? Do you think health promotion occurs in stages? Explain your answer.
16. Discuss key similarities you have noticed among some of the theories in this chapter. Name the theories that are similar and describe any areas of commonality.
17. Which theories or models built on work that had been done by another theorist?
18. What is the difference between self-efficacy and self-determination in the theories described in this chapter?
19. Think of a health-related behavior you would like to change or have changed in the last year. Which of the models or theories would provide the best guidance to you in implementing that change?
20. What is an assumption? What is a concept? What is the difference between a model and a theory?
21. Do you agree or disagree with the statement that the field of health promotion has become too complex to be guided by any one theory? Explain your answer.

REFERENCES

Adams, J. & White, M. (2005). Why don't stage-based activity promotion interventions work? *Health Education Research*, *20*(2), 237–243.

Alexander, J., Beagle, C. J., Butler, P., Dougherty, D. A., & Andrews-Robards, K. D. (1986). Madeleine Leninger: Transcultural Care Theory. In Ann Marriner (Ed.). *Nursing theorists and their work* (pp. 144–160). St. Louis, MO: The C.V. Mosby Company.

Antonovsky. A. (1996). The salutogenic model as a theory to guide health promotion. *Health Promotion International*, *11*(1), 11–18.

Ajzen, I. (1985). From intention to actions: A theory of planned behavior. In J. Kuhl and J. Beckman (Eds.). *Action-control: From cognition to behavior* (pp. 11–39). Heidelberg, Germany: Springer.

Bandura, A. (1977). Self-efficacy: Toward a unifying theory of behavioral change. *Psychological Review, 84*, 191–215.

Bandura, A. (1989). Social cognitive theory. In R. Vasta (Ed.). *Annals of child development. Vol 6. Six theories of child development* (pp. 1–60). Greenwich, CT: JAI Press.

Bauer, G., Davies, J. K., Pelikan, J., Noack, H., Broesskamp, U., & Hill, C. (2003) Advancing a theoretical model for public health and health promotion indicator development. *European Journal of Public Health*, *12*(3), 107–113.

Becker, M. H., & Maiman, L.A. (1975). Socio-behavioral determinants of compliance with health and medical care recommendations. *Medical Care*, xiii, 10-24.

Best, A., Stokols, D., Green, L. W., Leischow, S., Holmes, B. & Buchholz, K. (2003). An integrative framework for community partnering to translate theory into effective health promotion strategy. *American Journal of Health Promotion, 18*(2), 168–176.

Bronfenbrenner, U. (1979). *The ecology of human development.* Cambridge, MA: Harvard University Press.

Carter, K. F. & Kulbok, P. A. (1995). Evaluation of the Interaction Model of Client Health Behavior through the first decade of research. *Advances in Nursing Science, 18*(1), 62–73.

Chatzisarantis, N. L. D., & Hagger, M. S. (2009). Effects of an intervention based on self-determination theory on self-reported leisure-time physical activity participation. *Psychology and Health, 24*(1), 29–48.

Cole, A. (1995). A model approach to health promotion. *Healthlines, 26,* 14–16.

Cox, C. L. (1982). An interaction model of client health behavior: Theoretical prescription for nursing. *Advances in Nursing Science, 5*(1), 41–56.

Cox, C. L. (2003). A model of health behavior to guide studies of childhood cancer survivors. *Oncology Nursing Forum, 30,* 92–99.

Deci, E. L. (1971). Effects of externally mediated rewards on intrinsic motivation. *Journal of Personality and Social Psychology, 18,* 105–111.

Deci, E. & Ryan, R. (1991). A motivational approach to self: Integration in personality. In R. Dienstbier (Ed.), Nebraska symposium on motivation, Vol 38. *Perspectives on motivation* (pp. 237–288). Lincoln, NE: University of Nebraska Press.

Deci, E. L. & Vansteenkiste, M. (2004). Self-determination theory and basic need satisfaction: Understanding human development in positive psychology. *Ricerche di Psicologia, 27,* 17–34.

Duldt, B. W., Giffin, K., & Patton, B. R. (1983). *Interpersonal communication in nursing: A humanistic approach.* Philadelphia, PA: F.A. Davis.

Fishbein, M. & Ajzen, I. (1975). *Belief, attitude, intention and behavior: An introduction to theory and research.* Menlo Park, CA: Addison-Wesley.

Glasgow, R. E., Vogt, T. M., & Boles, S. M. (1999). Evaluating the public health impact of health promotion interventions: The RE-AIM Framework. *American Journal of Public Health, 89,* 1322–1327.

Glanz, K., Rimer, B. K., & Lewis F. M. (2002). *Health behavior and health education: Theory, research and practice* (3rd ed.). San Francisco, CA: Jossey-Bass.

Glanz, K., & Rimer, B. (2005). *Theory at a glance: A guide for health promotion practice* (2nd ed.). Bethesda, MD: U.S. Department of Health and Human Services, National Institute of Health.

Green, L. W., Glanz, K., Hochbaum, G. M., Kok, G., Kreuter, M. W., Lewis, F. M., . . . Rosenstock, I. M. (2010). Can we build on, or must we replace, the theories and models in health education? *Health Education Research, 9*(3), 397–404.

Green, L. W. & Kreuter, M. W. (1992). CDC's planned approach to community health as an application of PRECEDE and an inspiration for PROCEED. *Journal of Health Education, 23*(3), 140–147.

Green. L. W. & Kreuter, M. W. (1999). *Health promotion planning: An educational and ecological approach.* Mountain View, CA: Mayfield.

Green, L. W., Kreuter, M. W., Deeds, S. G., & Partridge, K. B. (1980). *Health Education Planning: A Diagnostic Approach.* Mountain View, CA: Mayfield.

Gregson, J. (2001). System, environmental and policy changes: Using the social-ecological model as a framework for evaluating nutrition education and social marketing programs with low-income audiences. *Journal of Nutrition Education, 33*(1), 4–15.

Halfon, N. & Hochstein, M. (2002). Life course health development: An integrated framework for developing health, policy and research. *Milbank Quarterly, 80*(3), 433–479.

Healey, B. J. & Zimmerman, R. S. (2010). Program development. In *The new world of health promotion: New program development, implementation, and evaluation* (pp. 57–71). Sudbury, MA: Jones and Bartlett.

Heidegger, M. (1962). *Being and time.* New York, NY: Harper and Row.

King, I. (1981). *A theory for nursing: Systems, concepts, process.* New York, NY: John Wiley.

King, P. M. (1994). Health promotion: The emerging frontier in nursing. *Journal of Advanced Nursing, 20,* 209–218.

Kreps, G. L. (2009). Applying Weick's model of organizing to health care and health promotion: Highlighting the central role of health communication. *Patient Education and Counseling, 74*, 347–355.

Lindstrom, B. & Eriksson, M. (2009). The salutogenic approach to the making of HiAP/healthy public policy: Illustrated by a case study. *Global Health Promotion, 16*(1), 17–28.

Little, J. H. & Girvin, H. (2002). Stages of change. A critique. *Behavior Modification, 26*(2), 223–273.

Macdonald, G. (2000). A new evidence framework for health promotion practice. *Health Education Journal, 59*, 3–11.

Markland, D., Ryan, R. M., Tobin, B., & Rollnick, S. (2005). Motivational interviewing and self-determination theory. *Journal of Social and Clinical Psychology, 24*, 811–831.

Mathews, S. K., Secrest, J. & Muirhead, L. (2008). The interaction model of client health behavior: A model for advanced practice nurses. *Journal of the American Academy of Nurse Practitioners, 20*, 415–422.

McBride, S. H. (1991). Comparative analysis of three instruments designed to measure self-care agency. *Nursing Research, 40*(1), 12–16.

Nemcek, M. A. (2003). Self nurturance: Research trends and wellness model. *AAOHN Journal, 51*(6), 260–266.

Nightingale, F. (1859). *Notes on Nursing: What it is, and what it is not.* London, UK: Harrison and Sons.

Oetzel, J. G., Ting-Toomey, S., & Rinderle, S. (2006). Conflict communication in contexts: A social ecological perspective. In J. G. Oetzel & S. Ting-Toomey (Eds.). *The SAGE handbook of conflict communication* (pp. 727–739). Thousand Oaks, CA: Sage.

Orem, D. E. (1985). *Nursing concepts of practice* (3rd ed.). New York, NY: McGraw-Hill.

Pender, N. J. (1982). *Health promotion in nursing practice.* Norwalk, CT: Appleton-Century-Crofts.

Pender, N .J. (1987). *Health promotion in nursing practice* (2nd ed.). Norwalk, CT: Appleton-Century-Crofts.

Prochaska, J. O. (2006). Moving beyond the transtheoretical model. *Addiction, 101*(6), 768–774.

Prochaska, J. O, DiClemente, C. C. Velicer, W. R. & Rossi, J. S. (1992). Criticisms and concerns of the transtheoretical model in light of recent research. *British Journal of Addiction, 87*(6), 825–828.

Prochaska, J. O, & Velicer, W. F. (1997). The transtheoretical model of health behavior change. *American Journal of Health Promotion, 12*(1), 38–48.

Riemsma, R. P., Pattenden, J., Bridle, C. Sowden, A. J., Mather, L., Watt, I. S. & Walker, A. (2003). Systematic review of the effectiveness of stage based interventions to promote smoking cessation. *BMJ, 326*(7400), 1175–1177.

Roden, J. (2004). Revisiting the health belief model: Nurses applying it to young families and their health promotion needs. *Nursing and Health Sciences, 6*, 1–10.

Rogers, E. M. (1962/1983). *Diffusion of Innovations* (3rd ed.). New York, NY: The Free Press

Rosenstock, I. M. (1966). Why people use health services. *Milbank Memorial Fund Quarterly, 44*(3), 94–127.

Rosenstock, I.M. (1974). Historical origins of the Health Belief Model. In Becker, M. H. (ed.). *The Health Belief Model and Personal Behavior.* Thorofare, NJ: Charles B. Slack.

Simmons, S. J. (1990). The health promoting self care system model: Directions for nursing research and practice. *Journal of Advanced Nursing, 15*, 1162–1166.

Stokols, D. (1996). Translating social ecological theory into guidelines for community health promotion. *American Journal of Health Promotion. 10*(4), 282–298.

Tannahill, A. (2009). Health promotion: The Tannahill model revisited. *Public Health, 123*(5), 396–399.

Walker, S. N. Sechrist, K. R., & Pender, N. J. (1987). The health promoting lifestyle profile development and psychometric characteristics. *Nursing Research, 36*, 76–81.

Weick, K. E. (1979). *The social psychology of organizing* (2nd ed.). Reading, MA: Addison-Wesley.

West, R. (2005). Time for change: Putting the Transtheoretical (Stages of Change) Model to rest. *Addiction, 100*(8), 1036–1039.

Whitehead, D. (2001a). A stage planning programme model for health education/health promotion practice. *Journal of Advanced Nursing, 36*(2), 311–320.

Whitehead, D. (2001b). A social cognitive model for health education/health promotion practice. Journal of Advanced Nursing, 36(3), 417–425.

Whitehead, D. (2004). Nursing theory and concept development or analysis: Health promotion and health education: Advancing the concepts. *Journal of Advanced Nursing, 47*(3), 311–320.

Whitehead, D. (2006). Health promotion in the practice setting: Findings from a review of clinical issues. *Worldviews on Evidence-based Nursing, 3*(4), 165–184.

Whitehead, D. (2009). Reconciling the differences between health promotion in nursing and general health promotion. *International Journal of Nursing Studies, 46*, 865–874.

World Health Organization [WHO]. (1986). The Ottawa charter for health promotion. Ontario, Canada: Canadian Public Health Association, Health and Welfare Canada, and the World Health Organization.

World Health Organization [WHO]. (2009 January). *Regional consultation on self-care in the contest of primary health care* [Symposium], Bangkok, Thailand.

For a full suite of assignments and additional learning activities, see the access code at the front of your book.

CHAPTER 4

Genetic and Social Determinants of Health: An Ecological Perspective

Michelle T. Dang

OBJECTIVES

After reading this chapter and completing the case study, you should be able to:

- Identify the major determinants of health.
- Explain the ecological model and its application in health promotion.
- Apply the ecological model to a health promotion program.
- Explain the stress–diathesis model and how it affects health outcomes.
- Define epigenetics and its mechanisms.
- Explain the significance of both genetics and environmental factors on health.
- Develop health promotion strategies using the ecological framework.

Over the past 100 years, advances in public health in nutrition, vaccines, and sanitation have greatly improved quality of life and increased life spans. Deaths during infancy have also dramatically decreased. During the early 20th century, approximately 100 infants out of 1,000 live births died before the age of 1 year, and the average life span was only 47 years (Centers for Disease Control and Prevention [CDC], 1999; Turnock, 2004). Since then, the rate of infant mortality has declined by more than 90%, with an estimated rate of infant mortality in the United States of 6.8% (Mathews & MacDorman, 2007). Yet, not all individuals and populations benefitted equally from these advances (Marmot & Wilkinson, 2006). For example, African American infants are 2.4 times more likely to die before their first birthday than non-Hispanic white infants (The Office of Minority Health, 2010). The reason for this disparity is not completely clear, but it points to the importance of multiple biological and environmental factors that influence health.

As research in biomedicine and genetics proliferated in recent years, it became apparent that health is not as straightforward or as simple a concept as one may think.

There is no doubt that factors such as nutrition and vaccines are critical components to keeping individuals and populations healthy. However, a large body of evidence from various disciplines indicates that health and health behaviors are determined by multiple intertwining factors (Hernandez & Blazen, 2006). How healthy or susceptible people are to illness and disease depends on a combination of biological and social factors such as their genetics, social status, the extent and influence of their social networks, and the environment where they live and work. Together, the complex interactions between biological and social elements and their influence on health are termed the *determinants of health*.

The World Health Organization (WHO) (2010) has identified several important biological and social factors that can greatly affect people's health. **Table 4-1** lists some of the determinants of health as identified by WHO and how each factor influences health.

TABLE 4-1 Determinants of Health (World Health Organization, 2010)	
Factors That Influence Health	**Outcomes**
Socioeconomic status	Higher income is associated with better health.
Employment	Employed individuals and those who have more control over their working conditions are healthier.
Education	Lower educational attainment is associated with poorer health, higher stress, and lower self-confidence.
Physical environment	Safe homes and communities, clean air and water, and healthy workplaces contribute to good health.
Social networks	Greater support from friends, families, and communities is linked with better health.
Culture	Family and community customs, beliefs, and traditions all affect health.
Genetics	Inheritance plays a role in lifespan, health, and susceptibility to developing certain illness.
Gender	Men and women experience different types of diseases at different ages.
Health services	Access to services that prevent and treat diseases influences health.
Personal behavior and coping skills	What we ingest (eat, drink, smoke) influences our health. How we respond to stressful circumstances also affects our health.

THE ECOLOGICAL FRAMEWORK

This chapter uses the ecological model to discuss how nurses need to consider biological, social, cultural, and environmental determinants of health in understanding health behavior and health outcomes within and across populations (Sallis, Owen, & Fisher, 2008). It is critical that nurses examine the different determinants of health as part of health promotion planning and activities. The ecological model is an excellent framework for exploring the different determinants of health because the model posits that no one factor is responsible for one's health status. Our health is determined by multiple interacting factors at the individual, family, community, societal, and cultural levels. The model can be visualized as each system being nested within other systems, starting with the individual level in the center, followed by the policy level, interpersonal/social level, the institutional/environmental level, the community/cultural level, and finally the public policy level. These systems interact with and influence each other. No single factor, whether at the individual, policy or societal level, is considered more important than the other. It is the interaction of these multiple factors over time that affects our health and behaviors. The word *ecology* itself implies the interrelations between organisms and their environments (Sallis et al., 2008).

Sallis and colleagues (2008) reported four core principles of the ecological model in terms of health behaviors. These principles should be key components in any health promotion project that targets change at several levels of influence (p. 466):

1. Specific health behaviors are influenced by multiple factors at the intrapersonal, interpersonal, organization, community, and public policy levels.
2. Influences interact across different levels.
3. The most potent influence at each level and the specific behavior should be identified.
4. Multi-level interventions are most effective at changing behavior.

The ecological model reflects a departure from past dichotomies about whether nature or nurture determines our health and behavior. It also deflects the focus and blame on person-based variables such as individual behaviors, skills, and social influences in the immediate environment. The ecological model explicitly considers both proximal (i.e., individual, families) and distal (i.e., community, social policies) contexts and the bidirectional relationships from the different spheres of influence.

In the 21st century, we have witnessed amazing progress in the area of genetics as a result of the successful sequencing of the human genome (Lander et al., 2001). Advances in the field of genetics and genomics have further expanded our ability to hypothesize and seek connections among genes, behavior, and the social environment and explore how these factors influence health in ways that we have only imagined. For example, Caspi and colleagues (2003) discovered that a genetic variation of the serotonin transporter (5-HTT) gene can moderate or buffer against stressful life events and reduce one's risk of developing depression. Based on animal models that demonstrated the influence of the neurotransmitter serotonin on mood regulation, Caspi and colleagues conducted an investigation of gene by environment interaction. They looked at stressful life events and individuals with either short or long alleles (variants) of the 5-HTT gene; this gene has been implicated in the regulation and production of serotonin, which moderates the psychological reaction to stressful events. The results revealed that stressful life events predicted depression in individuals with the short alleles, not for individuals with the long alleles. Furthermore, subjects with the short alleles also had more suicidal ideation. Overall, individuals with the long version of the 5-HTT gene were less likely to develop depression from adverse life events, and individuals with the short version were more likely to develop depression *only* if they experienced adverse life circumstances. Before we can completely embrace the 5-HTT gene as being the target for causing depression in at-risk individuals, the authors cautioned that other genes may be involved where a gene by gene interaction could have occurred. Nevertheless, this study's findings provide remarkable evidence that genes and environment are intricately linked in influencing health and development.

Application of the Ecological Model

Consider this example: A nurse wants to promote a healthful diet for her client and the client's family. Using the ecological model, what factors should the nurse be considering and what information should she obtain before implementing her interventions? Some ecological factors that the nurse may consider, in addition to educating her client about healthy foods, are the availability of certain foods in the client's neighborhood, the cost or affordability of such foods, how foods are marketed and advertised, and the client's cultural and religious preferences and norms about food choices and preparation. The client's social network (e.g., family and friends) can also greatly influence her decision about what foods to buy and how to prepare them. It has been shown that people are more likely to change their behavior if the environment where they live supports the desired behavior. People are also more likely to change if they feel empowered to make their own decisions about their health (Minkler & Wallerstein, 2008). For example, clients who wish to increase the amount of fresh fruits and vegetables in their diet based on a nurse's recommendation will face difficulty achieving this goal if their neighborhoods lack venues where fresh fruits and vegetables are sold, but yet have an abundance of fast-food restaurants.

In summary, the ecological approach seeks a broader perspective to examining contributing factors that influence health. Substantial change in health behavior requires such an approach. The model's comprehensive approach to understanding health behavior has been used by the CDC, the Institute of Medicine (IOM), the U.S. Department of Health and Human Services (*Healthy People 2010*), and the World Health Organization (WHO). See **Box 4-1** for a successful application of the ecological model.

Box 4-1   Using the Ecological Model to Reduce the Rate of Smoking

In 1998, the California Department of Public Health established the California Tobacco Control Program (CTCP) with funding from the landmark Tobacco Tax and Health Protection Act (Proposition 99), which imposed a tax on sales of cigarettes (California Department of Public Health, 2009). Since its inception, the CTCP has successfully reduced per capita cigarette consumption by 69% and substantially decreased tobacco-related diseases and deaths. The CTCP's success derived from its comprehensive ecological approach to smoking and the use of tobacco products. The CTCP sought to change the social norms on smoking by "indirectly influencing current and potential future tobacco users by creating a social milieu and legal climate in which tobacco becomes less desirable, less acceptable, and less accessible." (California Department of Public Health, 2009, p. 3). In essence, they wanted to (and did) implement interventions at multiple levels of influence.

At the policy and community levels, the CTCP countered the tobacco industry's well-funded and aggressive marketing campaigns through their mobilization of communities to implement local policies that restricted tobacco sales and certain tobacco marketing practices; in addition, they implemented their own marketing campaign that increased public awareness about the tobacco industry's deceptive marketing tactics (e.g., that smoking is attractive) and created negative public attitudes about the tobacco industry. To further reduce acceptability and exposure to tobacco use, the CTCP promoted initiatives that banned indoor smoking. In 1995, California became the first state to pass a smoke-free indoor workplace law. The restriction has since been expanded to include certain public beaches and parks, entrances to public buildings, and vehicles with any youth under 18. Another tobacco restriction was the CTCP's efforts in the enforcement of existing laws that prohibited tobacco sales to minors, the elimination of sampling of free tobacco products, and the requirement that tobacco retailers be licensed.

The CTCP's attempt at changing social norms about tobacco use had an indirect effect at the individual level. Smokers who had a positive view of policies aimed at curbing secondhand smoke were much more likely to have made attempts to quit and their desire to quit smoking was more likely to be supported by their workplace and people in their social networks. The CTCP also collaborated with healthcare providers to spread the word about a free helpline to support people who wanted to quit smoking. The Helpline was culturally and linguistically appropriate and available in six different languages, including service for the hearing impaired. The CTCP became a model program for other public health programs.

The CTCP considered multiple levels of influence in health behaviors related to smoking and implemented interventions at these levels. In addition to the mentioned interventions, the CTCP established partnerships with numerous public health agencies, community coalitions, and the film industry. It is unlikely that the CTCP would have had the same level of success if they did not use an ecological approach to the complex issue of tobacco use.

THE STRESS–DIATHESIS MODEL

Within the ecological framework, the stress–diathesis model has been used to examine how social circumstances and individual responses to stressful events affect health (Repetti, Taylor, & Seeman, 2002). This model exemplifies how external environmental situations can influence health at the cellular and physiological level. Repetti and colleagues (2002) proposed that a stressful family environment creates a cascade of risk that "create[s] vulnerabilities and may exacerbate certain genetically based vulnerabilities, which not only put children at immediate risk for adverse outcomes, but lay the groundwork for long-term physical and mental health problems" (p. 330). The main mechanism in how the family environment predicts health and mental health outcomes involves the sympathetic-adrenomedullary (SAM) reactivity, hypothalamic-pituitary-adrenocortical (HPA) reactivity, and serotonergic functioning. Growing up in families that experience chronic psychosocial and environmental stress puts children at risk for experiencing major disruptions in their defensive systems and possibly impairing their normal response to stress. The nervous system and the endocrine system are two highly complex systems that are involved in response to stress, and both systems need to work synergistically in a delicate balance in order to maintain homeostasis in the organism while it interacts with the environment.

Research has also demonstrated that one's current health status is a reflection of physiological responses to past experiences (Sapolsky, 2004). It is now a well-known fact that the brain regulates hormonal production, and hormones in return influence the nervous system and cellular function; too much or too little hormones could prohibit optimal function of an organism. In fact, there is a dose–response relationship between the stress and the hormones being released. In addition, different stressors release different sets of hormones. Stress, whether real or anticipated, provokes a physiological response in the body through its release of specific hormones that target certain cells and tissues in the body. This influx of hormones creates behavioral and physical responses, such as increased energy, alertness, and vascular tone that allow the organism to respond to the stressor. When a stimulus is detected, the hypothalamus releases stimulatory hormones called corticotrophin releasing factor (CRF). Within 15 seconds of its release, CRF triggers the anterior pituitary gland to release adrenocorticotropic hormone (ACTH), which then triggers the adrenal glands to release the potent glucocorticoids, a class of steroid hormones, whose concentrations rise within minutes to exert its effects on the body. Because of its lipophilic characteristics, glucocorticoids can easily cross the cell membrane and continue its path directly to the cell's nucleus, where they can regulate genetic transcription. To prevent the hormones from creating an infinite stressed-out state, this hypothalamus-pituitary-adrenal pathway, more commonly referred to as the HPA axis, has a negative-feedback loop which turns on or off hormonal release depending on the circulating levels of the different hormones, similar to a thermostat that is set to maintain a certain temperature. Given the potency of these hormones, the stress–diathesis model speaks to this mechanism. Since these stress hormones are meant to temporarily heighten the body's defense system to stress, chronic production of these hormones, particularly glucocorticoids, can have deleterious effects on the body, eventually causing disease (McEwen, 2002). Chronic stress can result in stress-induced immunosuppression, a condition in which the body becomes more vulnerable to disease due to a disruption in immune functions. Diseases that have linked with stress include depression, ulcers, colitis, heart disease, and adult-onset diabetes (Sapolsky, 2004).

Application of the Stress–Diathesis Model

Access to health care is considered a vital commodity in preventing and treating illness, yet this is not always enough. Consider for a moment a client who has health insurance through his employment, but who feels that he has very limited or no control over his work condition. From an ecological perspective, what potential impact does employment have on this person at the individual, family, and community levels? Systematic reviews about the impact of work on health and well-being revealed that increased job control consistently had positive health benefits, whereas, low job control had negative health effects (Bambra et al., 2010).

GENETIC DETERMINANTS OF HEALTH AND GENE–ENVIRONMENT INTERACTIONS

In the post-genomic era, the search for genetic causes to health conditions has moved beyond the traditional model of Mendelian patterns of inheritance—the inheritance of genetic disorders from our parents (e.g., autosomal dominance, autosomal recessive, and X-linked). Even though it is recognized that Mendelian disorders such as cystic fibrosis and Tay-Sachs disease are serious health conditions, diseases with simple patterns of Mendelian inheritance are usually rare (see the *Online Mendelian Inheritance in Man*, http://www.ncbi.nlm.nih.gov/omim, for a comprehensive database about all known Mendelian disorders). Advances in molecular technology have permitted scientists to search for causative factors for more common diseases such as cancer, cardiovascular disease, diabetes, and Alzheimer's disease. This is significant as these diseases account for most of the morbidity and mortality in our society.

These diseases do not fit the Mendelian patterns of inheritance because they are caused by both hereditary and nonhereditary factors. Health conditions caused by a combination of both genetic and other factors such as aging, diet, lifestyle, and exposure to chemicals or toxins have what is known as multifactorial inheritance (Barlow-Stewart, 2007). Multifactorial inheritance also means that an individual who inherits the "faulty" gene will not necessarily develop disease unless other genetic and environmental conditions are in place. This approach to studying variations in genes among populations acknowledges the fact that development is a complex process where we not only inherit genetic materials from our parents but we also inherit their cultural and social experiences.

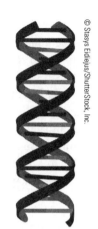

GENE REGULATION AND MUTATIONS

The human genome is estimated to have between 20,000 and 25,000 genes. Gene expression occurs through two critical cellular processes: transcription and translation, often referred to as the "central dogma" of molecular biology (Strachan & Read, 2004). In transcription, DNA serves as a template for the synthesis of RNA, including messenger RNA (mRNA). The mRNAs are subsequently "read" and "translated" into sequences of amino acids that make up proteins. The process of turning genes "on" or "off" is called gene regulation. Although not yet fully understood, gene regulation is critical to maintaining life. For example, liver cells function very differently than brain cells. To maintain this sense of order and balance, it is vital that our genes translate and transcribe appropriate proteins that serve specific functions. Gene regulation also permits our bodies to respond to sudden changes in the environment.

One of the mechanisms that can change gene regulation is mutation. A gene mutation causes a permanent change to a DNA sequence that makes up a particular gene. The rate of mutations in humans is considered low and can be a result of mistakes in the DNA upon replication. For example, new mutations can occur and cause significant changes to the phenotype as seen in Down syndrome, or mutations from excessive repeats of a certain DNA sequence that cause changes to the offspring. The same mutation but with less frequency does not cause phenotypic abnormality in the parent, as in the case of Fragile X. Mutations are not always harmful to an organism and are considered to be the driving force of evolution. However, some mutations can be quite pathogenic (Strachan & Read, 2004). For example, cystic fibrosis is caused by mutations in the cystic fibrosis transmembrane conductance regulator (CTFR) gene. Mutations can occur in a single DNA sequence, also known as a nucleotide, or a large segment of the chromosome. Mutations can be inherited from our parents (inherited mutations) or acquired during one's lifetime (somatic mutations). Acquired (somatic) mutations cannot be passed on to the next generation, and they can be caused by environmental factors such as exposure to ultraviolet rays and smoking (Strachan & Read, 2004). Many types of cancers, including certain types of neurofibromatosis, are caused by acquired mutations (National Institute of Health, 2010).

GENE–ENVIRONMENT INTERACTION

It is now accepted among the scientific community that development, including our health, is a co-action of genes and the environment. Gene–environment interaction can even be noted at the cellular level. The interactions of cells and how cells are differentiated during embryology depends heavily on their interactions with neighboring cells, as well as interactions within the cells themselves (Harper, 1995). The relationship between gene and environment in health outcomes can be compared to the relationship between the chromosome and cytoplasm. At the molecular level, this gene–environment interaction provides some flexibility to the developing organisms as cells differentiate before ending in their committed states as, for example, skin cells or liver cells. Genes themselves do not operate in isolation. Development is an interplay of genetic potentials and the environment. Even in prenatal development, the relationship of the fetus with its mother is bidirectional. It is well established that certain substances, such as alcohol, can have devastating effects on the fetus if ingested during pregnancy (Smotherman & Robinson, 1996). In this example, we can easily see how the genetic potential of the fetus whose mother regularly ingests alcohol can be altered due to this environmental effect. Another example of an environmental trigger that is preventable is the intake of folic acid during pregnancy. Lack of folate has been linked with neural tube defects during fetal development; as a result, women who supplement their diets with folic acid early in pregnancy can significantly reduce the incidence of neural tube defects.

Gene–environment interactions can also be illustrated through risk behaviors such as smoking, unhealthy diets, and physical inactivity. These environmental factors are the underlying forces behind the leading causes of death in the United States. Despite well-publicized facts about the positive health benefits of exercise and extensive public health efforts in increasing physical activity among the general public, only 49% of American adults meet the American College of Sports Medicine's recommendation for physical activity (cited in Haskell et al., 2007). It is clear that social determinants such as lifestyles and built environments (e.g., shopping malls) have a major influence on people's level of engagement in physical activities (Hernandez & Blazer, 2006). However, evidence suggests that physical activity may also be controlled by intrinsic biological processes. Studies have indicated that heritable factors account for the differences in people's levels of physical activity and sports participation. For example, in a study with 669 participants, Loos and colleagues (2005) found a significant association between individuals with a variant of the melanocortin-4 receptor (MC4R) gene and physical activity, suggesting a genetic underpinning to people's propensity for exercise. The MC4R gene plays a key role in regulating feeding behavior and energy homeostasis. Mutations in the human MC4R gene were first described in some patients with childhood obesity (Vaisse et al., 1998; Yeo et al., 1998). From a gene–environment perspective, genetic susceptibility related to low physical activity could be reinforced by a social environment that encourages sedentary activities such as television, computers, and video games. With the dramatic rise in the rate of obesity over the past 20 years, it is obvious that environmental factors contribute significantly to physical activity and dietary intake. Given the slow rate of mutations, genetic factors alone cannot account for the rapid increase in obesity.

EPIGENETIC MECHANISMS

An important mechanism where gene and environment interact to influence gene expression is epigenetics, which literally translates to mean "above the genes." Riggs and colleagues defined epigenetics as "the study of mitotically and/or meiotically heritable changes in gene function that cannot be explained by changes in DNA sequence" (cited by Bird, 2007, p. 396). Allis, Jenuwein, & Reinberg (2007) provided a more molecular perspective to the definition: They defined epigenetics as "the sum of the alterations to the chromatin template that collectively establish and propagate different patterns of gene expression (transcription) and silencing from the same genome" (p. 29). Others have provided a literal translation of epigenetics to mean "outside conventional genetics" (Jaenisch & Bird, 2003, p. 245). Moffitt, Caspi, & Rutter (2006) reported epigenetic programming along the line of the gene–environment interplay where "environmental effects on an outcome such as health or behavior are mediated through altered gene expression" (p. 5). Despite the differences in how epigenetics is defined, a clear common denominator to these definitions is that certain heritable changes are *not* explained by changes in the DNA. James Watson (cited by Allis et al., 2007), co-discoverer of the structure of DNA, alluded to epigenetics when he stated, "You can inherit something beyond DNA sequence. That's where the real excitement in genetics is now" (p. 25).

How epigenetics differs from genetics is that gene expression as a result of epigenetics is not due to any novel alterations to the DNA, the inheritance of ancestral DNA, or allelic differences caused by mutations that survived from selective pressure.

In epigenetics, gene expression is controlled by mechanisms that are interconnected to the complex process of gene translation but are separate from the actual genes themselves. These mechanisms are also highly influenced by the internal and external cellular environment. All cells carry the same DNA, but how genes express themselves in the form of mRNA has been attributed to mechanisms of epigenetics (Rutter et al., 2006). Researchers have known for many years that a pair of identical twins, who possess the exact same genes, can experience very different trajectories in the expression of disease (Fraga et al., 2005). Epigenetics phenotypes and nongenetic differences have been reported on a variety of organisms and cell types, which include human monozygotic twins, tumor tissues, mutant plants, and even cloned animals (Allis et al., 2007). The quest in finding specific genes that contribute to specific physical or psychological disorders is challenging due to the epigenetic effects that clearly have an influence in gene function but cause no visible changes to the genetic sequences themselves.

To have a clear understanding of how epigenetics influences gene expression, it is important to understand its mechanism. Research in this area is still emerging, but there is ample evidence to establish epigenetics as a specialty within the field of genetics. Epigenetic research revealed that DNA by itself is not solely responsible for gene expression, but has a very intimate relationship with specialized proteins and enzymes in the important work of coding for proteins. Two main mechanisms being credited for epigenetic regulation are DNA methylation and histone modification.

DNA Methylation

The oldest known mechanism of epigenetics is DNA methylation (Allis et al., 2007). The mechanism of DNA methylation occurs as a result of an extra methyl group on the DNA template where methylation is often found, at the cytosines of the dinucleotide sequence CpG. There is an inverse relationship between the level of DNA methylation and gene expression. To put it simply, methylation generally turns genes "off" and no methylation turns genes "on." Convincing evidence on the impact of methylation and gene expression can be found in a study on the modification of methylation in agouti mice (Jaenisch & Bird, 2003). This alteration in methylation induced by diet changed the phenotypes of the mice, which caused variations in coat color, cancer, and obesity. This remarkable discovery revealed that dietary intake can change gene expressions without any alteration to the actual DNA, as well as cause significant changes to the phenotype of the organism. A phenotype is an observable characteristic of an organism, such as hair color, and the not-so-observable traits such as temperament. Higher levels of DNA methylation are correlated with an increase in the noncoding regions of the genome. Only 4% of the DNA is coded for proteins. It is now recognized that the noncoding regions also play a significant role and may not be all that silent. Research in this area is starting to surface on the importance of the noncoding regions; it has been suggested that this correlation of DNA methylation with noncoding regions serves as a defense mechanism, where DNA methylation silences foreign genomes such as viral sequences. It has also been suggested that the integrity of the genome is highly dependent on DNA methylation, where deregulation of DNA methylation can cause instability in the genome that leads to chromosomal abnormalities and cancer progression (Chen et al., 1998). Hypermethylation has been found to inactivate tumor suppressor genes from being expressed and consequently cause cells to proliferate out of control. This proliferation is considered to be a major event in the cause of many cancers (Estellar, 2008).

Histone Modification

Human DNA is comprised of 23 chromosomes, which contain thousands of genes and 3 billion nucleotide bases. In order for the approximately 2-meter-long DNA to fit inside the very small nucleus, it is wrapped around "spools" of proteins called histone proteins. Histone proteins are amino acid sequences and, from yeast to humans, they remain fairly constant. This suggests that they have very important functions. The structure that organizes the histone proteins is called a nucleosome. Repeating units of nucleosomes make up the chromatin template. DNA does not vary in its structure, but chromatin varies from cell to cell, depending on the signal it receives from the intra- and extracellular environment. Because it responds to the environment, chromatin is highly dynamic and varies in its density in different areas of the chromosome. It can be silent indefinitely or expressed only during certain periods of development. Ultimately, it determines which genes get expressed and which genes should be silenced (Allis et al., 2007).

Numerous biochemical and genetic studies have revealed that histone modifications are achieved through chromatin-modifying enzymes. The enzymatic actions respond to external and intrinsic signals. The catalytic actions of the enzymes can also *reverse* modification, creating a steady-state balance. However, it is not completely clear how these enzymes are regulated or how sites are targeted. Histone modification has the ability to change the chromatin template and hence its influence on gene expression; for example, certain histone modifications permit transcription while others suppress transcriptional activities.

Epigenetics and the Stress Response

Given the intricate relationship between biological responses and environmental input, it is not surprising that response to stress is a highly focused area in the field of epigenetics (Anisman, Zaharia, Meaney, & Merali, 1998; Meaney, Aitken, Bhatnagar, & Sapolsky, 1991; Weaver, Meaney, & Szyf, 2006). Due to obvious ethical reasons, controlled experiments on stress responses are primarily based on animal models. Animal research by Meaney and colleagues (2001) has illuminated important clues about how the stress response system can be permanently altered as a result of variations in maternal care. The physiological and observable changes associated with the stress response can even be passed down to the next generation, without any mutations or changes to gene patterns. It was found that rats who exhibited high levels of attentive maternal behaviors of frequent licking and grooming (LG) of their pups and an arched back nursing (ABN) position (this position permits easier access to the breasts) had pups with reduced plasma levels of stress-related hormones, increased feedback of the HPA axis, and increased glucocorticoid receptor (GR) expression in the hippocampus compared with pups who were with mothers that demonstrated lower levels of such behaviors (licking/grooming and arched back nursing) (Liu et al., 1997). To control for possible genetic influences on parenting behavior, pups were cross-fostered with pups whose mothers had the opposite parenting style as their own biological mothers (Francis et al., 1999). Fostered pups, regardless of their biological mothers' parenting style, resembled their foster mothers. Again, pups with attentive mothers had lower levels of stress-related hormones and less reactivity to stress. The reverse was also true for the biological offspring of high LG-ABN pups who were raised by low LG-ABN mothers. Molecular examinations revealed that increased maternal LB-ABN caused modifications in DNA methylation and histone acetylation. These epigenetic modifications subsequently created marked changes in the expression of GRs (McCormick et al., 2000), and these changes remained stable even when the pups became adults. These important findings provide evidence for maternal "programming" of gene expression in their reared offspring, regardless of the biological connection between the mother and offspring—that is, maternal behavior modified gene expression without changes to the DNA, and these changes were heritable. Meaney (2001) suggested that the ability of organisms to alter their stress responses from early environmental effects provides a sort of plasticity for the animal to appropriately respond to threatening stimuli based on the biological programming from maternal behavior. In a sense, this kind of plasticity allows animals to be adaptive to the unique demands of their environment. This gene–environment interaction helps explain some of the differences in individual behaviors.

Summary

In summary, epigenetic changes allow the organism to change its gene expression in response to the environment, and they can even be inherited through mitosis. Since the alterations in gene expression do not require alterations in the DNA itself, it is likely that the modifications are short term and dependent on the environments of subsequent generations. Some of the current trends in epigenetics include searches for more mechanisms related to epigenetics (Martin & Zhang, 2007). Just as there are exceptions to Mendel's laws, it is highly possible that there are exceptions to current rules about epigenetics. On a broader perspective, scientists are actively searching for an "epigenetic code." Another active area of epigenetics research is in the area of human cancer and treatment. As noted, hypermethylation activity is associated with many cancers; therefore, knowing specific genetic regions for methylation could have great clinical significance in changing the methylation patterns and subsequently changing how proteins are created. It is now known that genes, even genes that cause cancer, can be turned on or off through epigenetic mechanisms (American Institute for Cancer Research [AICR], 2007; Robertson, 2005). This important discovery has led scientists to actively seek a cure for cancer in humans through an epigenetic lens. These exciting developments will make it easier for healthcare providers to tailor treatments to a person's epigenetic code. Several human epigenome projects with a focus on finding treatments for clinical disorders are already actively underway (Bradbury, 2003). An example is the Human Epigenome Project (HEP) (http://www.epigenome.org), which is a multinational study funded by both public and private organizations. Their primary focus is to map methyl groups in order to understand how they affect our DNA and the development of disease.

THE NURSE'S ROLE

Contemporary nursing practice demands that nurses are educated about genetics and possess an understanding of genetic influences on disease in order to convey genetic information and disease risks to patients and to effectively participate in disease management (Greco & Salveson, 2009). In 1997, the American Nurses Association established genetics nursing as an official nursing specialty with its own scope and standards of practice. This movement was a result of efforts begun by the International Society of Nurses in Genetics (ISONG) to increase genetics and genomics content in nursing curricula and nursing practice. Genetics is the study of single genes and their effects, whereas genomics is the study of all genes in the human genome and their interactions with the environment. Nurses who specialize in genetics are now able to obtain genetics nursing credentials through the Genetic Nursing Credentialing Commission (Greco & Salveson, 2009).

Nurses have an important role in assessing patients for familial patterns of disease that may have a genetic link. A complete history includes information from three generations of relatives, including children, brothers and sisters, parents, aunts and uncles, nieces and nephews, grandparents, and cousins. The National Coalition for Health Professional Education in Genetics recommends that health professionals create a pedigree, also referred to as a genogram, of the client's family using standard symbols and lines to demonstrate the relationships (Bennet et al., 1995). Conducting a family history can identify individuals who are at risk for rare diseases as well as those who are at risk for chronic diseases. Such individuals should be counseled about their risks and ways to reduce these risks, such as more frequent screenings or changing one's lifestyle, and possibly be referred for genetic counseling. Nurses should be alerted to genetic red flags such as family members with known or suspected genetic conditions, clusters of the same or related disorder (e.g., depression and alcoholism), earlier onset of disease than expected, and developmental delays or intellectual disabilities. It may be necessary for nurses to obtain additional information from medical records and having patients talk with their family members.

In addition to genes, families share many similar characteristics, such as lifestyle and environment. Therefore, nurses need to also consider the more distal factors within the ecological framework when conducting family histories. Nurses should also advise clients that just because they have family members with certain conditions, it does not mean that the clients are guaranteed to develop the same conditions, or that not having a family history of a condition precludes an individual from developing that condition. For example, it has been reported that the risk for Alzheimer's disease (AD) significantly increases with age. Scientists have also discovered that several genes, particularly the apoliprotein E (APOE) gene, are associated with AD. There appears to be a familial risk associated with AD as noted by a high concordance rate of AD among monozygotic twins; however, lower cholesterol and estrogen therapy have been associated with a lower risk of cognitive impairment, but *only* for those who do not carry the allele for the APOE gene (Gatz, 2007). This example demonstrates that we have come a long way in understanding the complex interactions of genes and environment, but we still have much more to learn about the specific mechanisms and how they are translated to disease management and clinical practice.

SOCIAL DETERMINANTS OF HEALTH

This section focuses on nongenetic, or social, conditions that are linked to health outcomes and their implications in health promotion. According to the WHO (2010), social determinants of health are defined as "the circumstances in which people are born, grow up, live, work, and age, as well as the systems put in place to deal with illness. These circumstances are in turn shaped by a wider set of forces: economics, social policies, and politics." (p. 1). We need very little explanation to understand why social conditions such as safe neighborhoods, quality education, equitable health care, and absence of personal harassment and violence would be more conducive to good health than the alternative. Unlike genetic determinants of health, social determinants of health are relatively more amenable to change if we have a solid understanding of the driving forces behind these factors and how they can be altered. This understanding will help identify specific health promotion strategies that will result in realistic and meaningful interventions for the targeted populations. Actions such as having equitable health systems, relieving poverty, improving circumstances in which people live and work, and addressing social issues such as violent deaths can significantly change social conditions for the promotion and maintenance of good health (Marmot, 2005). Such actions are also the foundation to eliminating health disparities.

The social determinants of health are considered such critical factors to overall health that the WHO created an independent Commission on Social Determinants of Health (CSDH) to address this issue at the global level (further information about the CSDH can be found at http://www.who.int/social_determinants/en/). The CSDH supports countries and health agencies in addressing the structural and daily life conditions that contribute to poor health and health inequities (Blas & Kurup, 2010). The social forces that contribute to differences in health outcomes do not just occur within countries; they also occur across boundaries. It has been reported that the life expectancy for men in Russia is about 20 years less than men in Sweden (WHO, 2005). In addition, there can be stark differences in the life expectancies between social groups within a country. For example, there could be as much as a 20-year difference in life expectancy between African American males who live in "unhealthy" counties of the United States and White males who live in the "healthiest" counties. The difference is even more alarming when considering that African American males in certain counties in the United States have life expectancies shorter than that of men in Bangladesh (Marmot, 2001).

The call for action by the WHO to address the social determinants of health is based on considerable evidence that the social forces around us, such as employment and social networks, can make substantial differences in our longevity and quality of life. More importantly, certain social conditions that place people at risk for poor health are often avoidable. For example, lead can cause significant neurodevelopmental harm in children and was a common ingredient in household paint. Children can have toxic blood levels of lead through ingestion of paint chips or exposure to household dust that contains remnants of lead-based paint. To minimize the risk of lead poisoning, the United States federal government banned lead-based paint in 1978. This preventive environmental action greatly reduced the risk of young children being exposed to lead-based paint. However, the risk for lead toxicity can still occur if children live in older homes where disclosures are not made about the presence of lead-based paint or where homes are not adequately updated to prevent lead exposure.

THE SOCIAL GRADIENT OF HEALTH

One of the suggested pathways to disparities in health outcomes and mortality is the powerful social phenomenon known as the social gradient of health (Blane, 2006). It has been confirmed for quite some time that there is a significant relationship between income/education and health (Marmot, 2006). On the surface, the link seems obvious, in that higher income is associated with better health, perhaps due to higher-income individuals having more resources and easier access to health care. However, the mechanism as to why people with higher incomes enjoy better health is more complex than just absolute wealth. Over the past several decades, evidence from large epidemiological studies (Marmot et al., 1978, 1991) has clearly indicated that the association between income and health is not just between low and high socioeconomic positions. There is actually an *incremental* increase in wealth and the rate of mortality—that is, mortality increases with decreasing socioeconomic position. People second from the top in terms of income fare worse than those at the very top of the social ladder, people third from the top fare worse that those at the second level, and so forth.

From their landmark study, the Whitehall study of British Civil Servants, Marmot and colleagues (1978) found an inverse relationship between people's grades of employment and their risk for coronary heart disease (CHD). People in the lowest grade positions (unskilled manual workers) had more than three times the risk of death from CHD than people in the highest grade positions (administrators). Furthermore, they found that there was a stepwise relationship in mortality from CHD; clerical workers had a higher risk than professionals and professionals had a higher risk than administrators. Therefore, manual labor alone did not explain the differences in mortality rate. Employment grades were also associated with health-related behaviors. People in the lowest employment grade reported smoking more and had less leisure time; both are possible contributing factors to CHD. However, when CHD risk factors (e.g., blood pressure, cholesterol, smoking) were controlled in the analysis, employment grade as a predictor for mortality remained strong, implicating a significant relationship between social circumstances such as employment and health. Marmot and colleagues (1991) conducted another study 20 years later and continued to find a steep inverse association between social status (as measured by employment) and health risks. Since then, the social gradient of health has been demonstrated worldwide and among diverse medical care systems (Mackenbach et al., 2003; McDonough, Duncan, Williams, & House, 1997). Moreover, the social gradient of health does not apply to just CHD, but also to all other major causes of death (Marmot, 2006).

How is it that people who are wealthy don't enjoy the same longevity and health as the "super" wealthy? Poverty is a well known contributor to poor health and shorter life spans, but the fact that people who live well above the poverty threshold still experience the social gradient of health suggests another mechanism besides income. This does not negate the fact that we should continue to pay attention to the people most deprived of basic needs as a result of poverty, but it illustrates for us that we are all part of this social gradient, regardless of whether or not we are poor (Marmot, 2007). From an ecological perspective, the relationship between employment/income and health is most likely not causative but reciprocal. Evidence suggests that social hierarchy is an important factor in the social gradient of health.

A suggested pathway for the interaction between social status and disease is the stress response that involves the neuroendocrine, endocrine, and immune systems (Brunner & Marmot, 2006) (see section on the stress–diathesis model of this chapter). It is hypothesized that the stress associated with work, the daily hassles of meeting life's demands, and the psychological perception of having low control can create a cascade of negative psychobiological responses that eventually lead to disease or exacerbate existing conditions. Therefore, it is suggested that those occupying the highest level of the social ladder experience the least hassles and enjoy the most autonomy and control. It is logical then to hypothesize that those societies with a more unequal distribution of power and prestige will more likely experience stark differences in health outcomes among its citizens; research has supported this hypothesis (Marmot, 2006). Marmot posits that the social gradient of health is not due to just differences in medical care or health behaviors related to one's socioeconomic position—it is also due to the fundamental human needs for autonomy and full social participation. He further emphasizes that it is not what people have that matters, it's what people are capable of doing with what they have that is key. For example, it would do little good for children to receive education about the importance of participating in physical activities if their neighborhoods lack safe sidewalks, parks, and community programs or their schools do not sponsor sports leagues. These barriers pose limitations on children in particular neighborhoods from fully participating in activities that are conducive to good health. Our standing in the social hierarchy may also impose psychosocial stressors such as a lack of control or outlets for frustration or perceived threat. These stressors are different than physical stressors, but they nevertheless activate endocrine and neural adaptations (Sapolsky, 2005). The stress response is vital for short-term survival but can be deleterious to health if it is chronically activated. Further support for the stress response as a contributing factor to the social gradient of health can be found in studies involving primates. Baboons of lower social rank (subordinate baboons) were found to have higher resting cortisol levels than the higher ranking baboons, suggesting a significant relationship between social status and stress (Sapolsky, 2005).

CULTURAL PERSPECTIVES

Understanding cultural diversity and the complex and multifaceted nature of culture is the cornerstone of health promotion. Culture influences how we perceive health and illness and our personal healthcare practices. The American Nurses Association (ANA) emphasizes the importance of cultural diversity by acknowledging that "knowledge about cultures and their impact on interactions with health care is essential for nurses, whether they are practicing in a clinical setting, education, research, or administration. Cultural diversity addresses racial and ethnic differences, however, these concepts or features of the human experience are not synonymous" (ANA, 1991).

Culture is inextricably linked to one's worldview and perception about health. As humans, we are cultural beings who require social interactions for growth and development and even to thrive (Rogoff, 2003). In short, we are very much a product of our culture. However, the analysis of how culture could interact with the individual to shape health outcomes is sometimes overlooked. Healthcare professionals may not consider different assumptions about health due to their own regularities and norms, their own cultural upbringing, and their healthcare practices. For example, the Hmong beliefs about illness and disease are tightly interwoven with their spiritual beliefs (Cha, 2003). As such, it would be ill advised to only use the biomedical framework and not acknowledge the spiritual aspect of health and illness in health promotion activities that involve the Hmong population. For example, a qualitative study revealed that Hmong parents who have children with developmental disabilities may not seek treatment or public assistance for their children's disabilities because of the cultural belief that their child's disability reflects a punishment or a "spiritual curse" from past mistakes by the family or their ancestors; therefore, it would be inappropriate for the family to seek outside assistance (Baker, Miller, Dang, & Hansen, 2010). As such, nurses who work with Hmong families need to recognize these cultural implications when advising Hmong families about obtaining health care and support for their children's disabilities. Families who do not follow through with recommendations about their children's disabilities may be wrongly perceived as noncompliant or apathetic. In certain cultures, it may be necessary to work with spiritual leaders to jointly develop strategies that will accommodate traditional cultural beliefs. Furthermore, it is important not to assume that certain cultural regularities apply to all individuals of the same ethnic background. For example, many cultures combine traditional healing practices, such as the use of shamans, with Western healthcare practices, and these patterns may reflect a combination of family care patterns, cultural values, and religious beliefs.

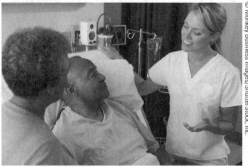

The first step in understanding how culture can influence is to take a step back and examine our own cultural assumptions and biases. It is also important to be cognizant of common stereotypes about certain cultures and how these perceptions may influence decisions about health promotion activities. To gain information about a family or a social group's perspective about an illness or disorder while minimizing cultural imposition (which is to impose our own beliefs, values, and patterns of behavior), Fadiman (2000) developed three questions that all health professionals should ask when seeking information: "What do you think caused this illness? What do you call it? What are you most afraid of?" (p. S7). These basic yet profound questions could give crucial information about the cultural perception and meaning of an illness, and can provide guidance for health promotion.

Leininger's theory of culture care diversity and universality is one framework for nurses to use in understanding how different cultural dimensions such as religious/philosophical factors, kinship factors, cultural values and lifeways, and social economic status (SES) factors can influence care expression, patterns, practices. and, ultimately, health outcomes (Leininger, 1995). Similar to the ecological model, these dimensions can be examined at the individual, family, community, and institutional levels. Leininger coined the term culturally congruent care to indicate that nurses need to practice in a manner that explicitly considers the client's cultural values, beliefs, and worldviews. Such practice not only respects each individual's unique history, but it also enables the nurse to bridge the mainstream healthcare system and the client's cultural practice of care. Professionals sometimes overlook the client or specific social groups as being experts about their own health and, therefore, may encounter resistance or negative attitudes toward certain health promotion activities because people's cultural norms are not recognized and acknowledged. The view of the client is so essential that it is considered a vital component of evidence-based practice. Sackett and colleagues (1996) argue that evidence should integrate "the best external evidence with individual clinical expertise and patient's choice" (p. 72).

CULTURE AND THE SOCIAL GRADIENT

In addition to cultural regularities, cultural determinants of health, particularly in the United States, are very diverse and often intertwined with the complex issues related to the social gradient of health. **Table 4-2** presents the latest figures of a few major indicators from the U.S. Census (2000). The data reflects demographic and socioeconomic diversity, but also illuminates the inequalities that may exist among major ethnic groups. These issues should be considered when planning health promotion activities, particularly if social equity is the ultimate goal. For instance, the data clearly show that African Americans have the highest rates of poverty and unemployment while

TABLE 4-2 Demographic and Socioeconomic Characteristics by Race/Ethnicity (U.S. Census, 2010).

	White	Black/African American	Asian/Pacific Islander	Hispanic/Latino
% high school graduate	87.6	84.2	88.9	62.9
% college graduate	30.3	19.8	52.4	13.9
% unemployed	7.5	13.4	6.8	10.8
% below poverty level	9.9	27.4	11.9	26.6
% management or professional occupations	40.9	31.5	48.6	20.4
% without insurance	14.5	19.1	17.6	30.7

Source: Census data can be found at http://www.census.gov/

Hispanics/Latinos have the second highest rate of poverty and the lowest rate of high school graduates. Whites and Asians have the highest rates of educational attainment and management or professional occupations, but Asians are more likely than Whites to live in poverty and not have health insurance. Hispanics and Latinos are the least likely to hold management or professional positions and most likely to not have health insurance. Based on what we know from the social gradient of health and the clear link between income and health, we can see how certain ethnic/racial groups are at a much higher risk for ill health and a poor quality of life. Therefore, it is vital that nurses not just consider the cultural values of particular individuals and social groups, but they also need to examine demographic factors such as income and education of certain populations and how these factors interact with other influences in the ecological environment to contribute to the determinants of health.

CONCLUSION

It is abundantly clear from current research that health is a multidimensional concept that cannot be attributed to any one factor. The ecological framework has practical application in health promotion activities because it requires careful examination of various contributors, such as genetic vulnerability, social support, socioeconomic position, distribution of health care, and policies, to health or illness. Research also reveals that genes and environment are intrinsically linked and that our genes are not necessarily our destiny. However, we also know that our environment can have a long-lasting impact on our health. Because of its comprehensive nature, the ecological approach can be challenging to implement, as it would most likely require extensive resources, time, and meaningful collaborations among different organizations. However, not factoring in these additional determinants of health will most likely result in only short-term outcomes or limited effectiveness on targeted behaviors.

Even though the ecological model requires a broad perspective to health behaviors, it is, nevertheless, critical that nurses first identify the *behavior* that influences a specific health outcome. For example, reducing sexually transmitted infections (STIs) among teens may be a goal for a health promotion activity, but it is important to first target the behavior that can lead to a reduced rate of STIs, such as the use of condoms or regular STI screenings. Once a behavior is determined, nurses can then map out individual and ecological factors that have significant influence on such behaviors. For example, what factors influence teen sexual behavior? The answers should encompass factors from the different levels of the ecological framework. These factors can be ascertained from the following sources: the scientific literature, professional experience, community assessment, focus groups, and epidemiological data. Having a specific behavior in mind will guide the health promotion process and help nurses stay focused on the outcome. Also, it is important that nurses consider the unique characteristics of the community when considering a specific health promotion activity. Not all communities have the same assets and barriers that influence health behaviors; just as individuals are unique in their attributes, so too are communities.

CASE STUDY

Lisa Lopez is a public health nurse who works in an ethnically diverse urban community of approximately 500,000 residents. She has worked in the community for 5 years and has developed a positive working relationship with several local community agencies and community leaders. She regularly attends community meetings and stays abreast of current events and health trends in the community. Recently, Lisa was asked by the public health agency to establish an adolescent health program at a drop-in community agency for homeless and marginalized youth. Many of these youth also came from the foster care system. As Lisa spent time at the agency and became familiar with the staff and youth at the center, she noticed that many female adolescents who came to the agency were either pregnant or parenting. She also noticed that many of these adolescents have unstable housing, limited or no income, inconsistent school attendance, and barriers to regular health care such as having neither insurance nor a primary care provider. Lisa recognized that these factors place the pregnant adolescents at high risk for poor pregnancy outcomes and put their children at risk for poor health and developmental outcomes.

Using the ecological model as a framework for health promotion, write a response to how Lisa should approach the issue of teen pregnancy in this community. Include the following components in the response.

1. What type(s) of data should Lisa gather?
2. Who should be key partners in this project and why?
3. Identify factors from the different levels in the ecological model that could influence the rate of teen pregnancy.
4. Develop health promotion strategies that encompass factors at the intrapersonal, interpersonal, organization, community, and public policy levels.

Note: The United States has one of the highest rates of teen pregnancy among any industrialized nation (CDC, 2009). Teen mothers are less likely to complete their high school education and more likely to live in poverty. Teen pregnancy is considered risky, as pregnant teens have higher rates for both preterm births and giving birth to low birthweight infants; both of these factors can lead to chronic health problems and developmental disabilities (CDC, 2009).

DISCUSSION QUESTIONS

1. Assess your own family background and the community where you live (and work if you are currently employed). What are some genetic, social, and cultural factors that have influenced your current health status and how may these factors influence your health in the future? What factors do you think are modifiable and why?
2. Interview a nurse who works in a hospital setting and a nurse who works in a community health setting, and ask each nurse what he or she thinks the determinants of health are. Do you suspect their responses to be similar or different and why?

CHECK YOUR UNDERSTANDING

1. _____ infants are more likely to die at _____ times the rate as that of White infants.
2. According to the WHO, which of the following are considered the determinants of health? Choose all that apply.
   a. Gender
   b. Education
   c. Employment
   d. Sexual orientation
   e. Health insurance
   f. Genetics
3. True or False: The ecological model of health posits that our health is determined by multiple factors, such as individual, family, community, and policy factors, and that each of these factors makes a unique contribution and does not overlap with over factors.
4. _____ stress can result in stress-induced immunosuppression, a condition in which the body becomes more vulnerable to disease due to a disruption in immune functions.
5. Two main mechanisms in epigenetics are _____ and _____.
6. True or False: In general, individuals with more wealth enjoy better health because they have easier access to healthcare services.

WHAT DO YOU THINK?

1. Should we screen individuals for certain genetic vulnerabilities (such as those with the short alleles of the 5-HTT gene) and provide early interventions in order to prevent ill health or psychopathology? Why or why not?
2. Do you think it is possible to have a more egalitarian society in the United States? Why or why not?
3. Do think health disparities in the United States (such as the higher infant mortality rate among African Americans) would be eliminated if we used more funding to target interventions for groups at high risk for poor health outcomes? Why or why not?

REFERENCES

Allis, C. D., Jenuwein, T., & Reinberg, D. (2007). Overview and concepts. In C. D. Allis, T. Jenuwein, & D. Reinberg (Eds.), *Epigenetics* (pp. 23–62). New York, NY: Cold Spring Harbor Laboratory Press.

American Institute of Cancer Research [AICR]. (2007, Spring). Epigenetics: A new frontier in cancer research. Retrieved from http://www.aicr.org/site/News2?abbr=res_&id=11800&page=NewsArticle

American Nurses Association (1991, October). Cultural diversity in nursing practice. American Nurses Association Position Statement. Retrieved from http://www.nursingworld.org/EthicsHumanRights

Anisman, H., Zaharia, M. D., Meaney, M. J., & Merali, Z. (1998). Do early-life events permanently alter behavioral and hormonal responses to stressors? *International Journal of Developmental Neuroscience, 16,* 149–164.

Baker, D. L, Miller, E., Dang, M. T., Yaangh, C-S, & Hansen, R. L. (2010). Developing culturally responsive approaches with Southeast Asian American families experiencing developmental disabilities. *Pediatrics, 126,* S146–150.

Bambra, C., Gibson, M., Sowden, A., Wright, K., Whitehead, M., & Petticrew, M. (2010). Tackling the wider social determinants of health and health in equalities: Evidence from systematic reviews. *Journal of Epidemiology and Community Health, 64,* 284–291.

Barlow-Stewart, K. (2007). Environmental and genetic interactions – complex patterns of inheritance. Centre for Genetics Education. Retrieved from http://www.genetics.edu.au

Bennett, R. L., Steinhaus, K. A., Ulrich, S. B., O'Sullivan, C. K., Resta, R. G., Lochner-Doyle, D., ... Hamanishi, J. (1995). Recommendations for standardized human pedigree nomenclature. Pedigree standardization task force of the National Society of Genetic Counselors. *American Journal of Human Genetics, 56*(3), 745–752.

Bird, A. (2007). Perceptions of epigenetics. *Nature, 447,* 396–398.

Blane, D. (2006). The life course, the social gradient, and health. In M. Marmot & R. G. Wilkinson (Eds.), *Social determinants of health* (2nd ed.) (pp. 54–77). New York, NY: Oxford University Press.

Blas, E., & Kurup, E. A. (Eds.) (2010). *Equity, social determinants, and public health programmes.* Geneva, Switzerland: World Health Organization.

Bradbury, J. (2003). Human epigenome project—up and running. *PLoS Biology, 1*(3), e82.

Brunner, E., & Marmot, M. (2006). Social organization, stress, and health. In M. Marmot & R. G. Wilkinson (Eds.), *Social determinants of health* (2nd ed.) (pp. 31–53). New York, NY: Oxford University Press.

California Department of Public Health (2009). *California tobacco control update 2009: 20 years of tobacco control in California.* California Department of Public Health, California Tobacco Control Program. Retrieved from http://www.cdph.ca.gov/programs/tobacco/Documents/CTCPUpdate2009.pdf

Caspi, A., Sugden, K., Moffitt, T. E., Taylor, A., Craig, I. W., Harrington, H., & Poulton, R. (2003). Influence of life stress on depression: Moderation by a polymorphism in the 5-HTT gene. *Science, 301,* 386–389.

Centers for Disease Control and Prevention [CDC]. (1999). Births, marriages, divorces and deaths: Provisional data for January-December 2000. DHHS PubNo (PHS) 2001-1120. National Vital Statistics Reports 49(6). National Center for Health Statistics, Department of Health and Human Services. Centers for Disease Control and Health Statistics. National Center for Health Statistics, Hyattsville, Maryland. Retrieved from http://www.cdc.gov/nchs/data/nvsr/nvsr49/nvsr49_06.pdf

Centers for Disease Control and Prevention [CDC] (2009). Preventing teen pregnancy: An update in 2009. Retrieved from http://www.cdc.gov/reproductivehealth/AdolescentReproHealth/AboutTP.htm

Cha D. (2003). *Hmong American concepts of health, healing, and conventional medicine.* New York, NY: Routledge.

Chen, R. Z., Pettersson, U., Beard, C., Jackson-Grusby, L., & Jaenisch, R. (1998). DNA hypomethylation leads to elevated mutation rates. *Nature, 395,* 89–93.

Estellar, M. (2008). Epigenetics in cancer. *New England Journal of Medicine, 358,* 1148–1159.

Fadiman, A. (2000). The spirit catches you and you fall down: Epilepsy and the Hmong. *Epilepsy & Behavior, 1*(1), S3–S8.

Fraga, M. F., Ballestar, B., Paz, M. F., Ropero, S., Setien, F., Ballestar, M. L., ... Esteller, M. (2005). Epigenetic differences arise during the lifetime of monozygotic twins. *Proceedings of the National Academy of the Sciences of the United States of America, 102*(30), 10604–10609.

Francis, D. D., Diorio, J., Liu, D., & Meaney, M. J. (1999). Nongenomic transmission across generations in maternal behavior and stress responses in the rat. *Science, 286,* 1155–1158.

Gatz, M. (2007). Genetics, dementia, and the elderly. *Current Directions in Psychological Science, 16*(3), 123–127.

Greco, K. E., & Salveson, C. (2009). Identifying genetics and genomics nursing competencies common among published recommendations. *Journal of Nursing Education, 48*(10), 557–565.

Harper, L. V. (2005). Epigenetic inheritance and the intergenerational transfer of experience. *Psychological Bulletin, 131*(3), 340–360.

Haskell, W. L., Lee, I.-M., Pate, R. R., Powell, K. E., Blair, S. N., Franklin, B. A., . . . Bauman, A. (2007). Physical activity and public health: Updated recommendation for adults from the American College of Sports Medicine and the American Heart Association. *Circulation, 116*(9), 1081–1093.

Hernandez, L. M., & Blazer, D. G. (Eds.) (2006). *Genes, behaviors, and the social environment: Moving beyond the nature/nurture debate.* Washington, DC: The National Academies Press.

Jaenisch, R., & Bird, A. (2003). Epigenetic regulation of gene expression: How the genome integrates intrinsic and environmental signals. *Nature Genetics, 33*, 245–254.

Lander, E. S., Linton, L. M., Birren, B., Nusbaum, C., Zody, M. C., Baldwin, J., & Chen, Y. J. (2001). Initial sequencing and analysis of the human genome. *Nature, 409*, 860–921. doi:10.1038/35057062

Leininger, M. (1995). *Transcultural nursing: Concepts, theories, research, and practice.* Columbus, OH: McGraw-Hill College Custom Series.

Liu, D., Diorio, J., Tannenbaum, B., Caldji, C., Francis, D., Freedman, A., . . . Meaney, M. J. (1997). Maternal care, hippocampal glucocorticoid receptors, and hypothalamic-pituitary-adrenal responses to stress. *Science, 277*, 1659–1662.

Loos, R. J. F., Rankinen, T., Tremblay, A., Perusse, L., Chagnon, Y., & Bouchard, C. (2005). Melanocortin-4 receptor gene and physical activity in the Quebec Family Study. *International Journal of Obesity, 29*, 420–428.

Mackenbach, J. P., Bos, V., Anderson, O., Cardano, M., Costa, G., Harding, S., & Kunst, A. E. (2003). Widening socioeconomic inequalities in mortality in six Western European countries. *International Journal of Epidemiology, 32*, 830–837.

Marmot, M. (2001). Inequalities in health. *New England Journal of Medicine, 345*(2), 134–136.

Marmot, M. (2005). Social determinants of health inequalities. *The Lancet, 365*(9464), 1099–1104.

Marmot, M. (2006). Introduction. In M. Marmot & R. G. Wilkinson (Eds.), *Social determinants of health* (2nd ed.) (pp. 1–5). New York, NY: Oxford University Press.

Marmot, M. (2007). Achieving health equity: From root causes to fair outcomes. *The Lancet, 370*(9593), 1153–1163.

Marmot, M., & Wilkinson, R. G. (2006). Social determinants of health (Eds.) (2nd ed.). New York, NY: Oxford University Press.

Marmot, M. G., Adelstein, A. M., Robinson, N., & Rose, G. (1978). The changing social class distribution of heart disease. *British Medical Journal, 2*, 1109–1112.

Marmot, M. G., Davey Smith, G., Stansfeld, S. A., Patel, C., North, F., Head, J., . . . Feeney, A. (1991). Health inequalities among British civil servants: The Whitehall II study. *Lancet, 337*, 1387–1393.

Martin, C., & Zhang, Y. (2007). Mechanisms of epigenetic inheritance. *Current Opinion in Cell Biology, 19*(3), 266–272.

Mathews, T. J., & MacDorman M. F. (2007). Infant mortality statistics from the 2004 period linked birth/infant death data set. *National Vital Statistics Reports, 55*(15). Hyattsville, MD: National Center for Health Statistics.

McCormick, J. A., Lyons, V., Jacobson, M. D., Noble, J, Diorio, J, Nyirenda, M., & Chapman, K. E. (2000). 5'-heterogeneity of glucocorticoid receptor messenger RNA is tissue specific: Differential regulation of variant transcript by early life events. *Molecular Endocrinology, 14*(4), 506–517.

McDonough, P., Duncan, G. J., Williams, D., & House, J. S. (1997). Income dynamics and adult mortality in the United States, 1972 through 1989. *American Journal of Public Health, 87*, 1476–1483.

McEwen, B. S. (2002). Sex, stress, and the hippocampus: Allostasis, allostatic load and the aging process. *Neurobiology of Aging, 23*, 921–939.

Meaney, M. J. (2001). Maternal care, gene expression, and the transmission of individual differences in stress reactivity across generations. *Annual Review of Neuroscience, 24*, 1161–1192.

Meaney, M., Aitken, D. H., Bhatnagar, S., & Sapolsky, R. M. (1991). Postnatal handling attenuates certain neuroendocrine, anatomical, and cognitive dysfunctions associated with aging in female rats. *Neurobiology of Aging, 12*, 31–38.

Minkler, M., & Wallerstein, N. (Eds.) (2008). *Community-based participatory research for health: From process to outcomes* (2nd ed.). San Francisco, CA: Wiley & Sons.

Moffit, T. E., Caspi, A., & Rutter, M. (2006). Measured gene-environment interactions in psychopathology: Concepts, research strategies, and implications for research, intervention, and public understanding of genetics. *Perspectives on Psychological Science, 1*(1), 5–27.

National Institute of Health [NIH]. (2010). What are genetic disorders? Retrieved from http://www.genome.gov/19016930

Repetti, R. L., Taylor, S. E., & Seeman, T. E. (2002). Risky families: Family social environments and the mental and physical health of offspring. *Psychological Bulletin, 128*(2), 330–366.

Robertson, K. D. (2005). DNA methylation and human disease. *Nature Reviews Genetics, 6*, 597–610.

Rutter, M., Moffitt, T. E., & Caspi, A. (2006). Gene–environment interplay and psychopathology: Multiple varieties but real effects. *Journal of Child Psychology and Psychiatry, 47*, 226–261.

Sallis, J. F., Owen, N., & Fisher, E. B. (2008). Ecological models of health behavior. In K. Glanz, B. K. Rimer, & K. Viswanath (Eds.), *Health behavior and health education: Theory, research, and practice* (4th ed.) (pp. 465–486). San Francisco, CA: Jossey-Bass.

Sapolsky, R. M. (2004). *Why zebras don't get ulcers: The acclaimed guide to stress, stress-related diseases, and coping* (3rd ed.). New York, NY: Henry Holt and Company.

Sapolsky, R. M. (2005). The influence of social hierarchy on primate health. *Science, 308*, 648–652.

Smotherman, W. P., & Robinson, S. R. (1996). The development of behavior before birth. *Developmental Psychology , 32*, 425–434.

Strachan, T., & Read, A. P. (2004). *Human molecular genetics 3*. New York, NY: Garland Science.

The Office of Minority Health (2010). Infant mortality and African Americans. Retrieved from http://minorityhealth.hhs.gov/templates/content.aspx?ID=3021

Turnock, B. J. (2004). *Public health: What it is and how it works* (3rd ed.). Sudbury, MA: Jones and Bartlett.

United States Census (2000). Retrieved from http://www.census.gov/

Vaisse, C., Clement, K., Guy-Grand, B., & Froguel, P. (1998). A frameshift mutation in human MC4R is associated with dominant form of obesity. *Nature Genetics, 20*, 113–114.

World Health Organization [WHO]. (2010). Social determinants of health. Retrieved from http://www.who.int/social_determinants/en/

Yeo, G. S. H., Farroqi, I. S., Aminian, S., Halsall, D., Stanhope, R. G., & O'Rahilly, S. (1998). A frameshift mutation in MC4R associated with dominantly inherited human obesity. *Nature Genetics, 20*, 111–112.

For a full suite of assignments and additional learning activities, see the access code at the front of your book.

CHAPTER 5

Health Disparities

Bonnie Raingruber

OBJECTIVES

At the conclusion of this chapter, students will be able to:

- Define a health disparity.
- Describe how quality of care and access to care affect health disparities.
- Discuss how health disparities are determined and monitored.
- Identify various health disparities that impact diverse populations.
- Articulate which factors and policies contribute to health disparities.
- Discuss effective ways to intervene to decrease health disparities.
- Discuss the role of governmental organizations in decreasing health disparities.
- Describe why it is crucial to increase the involvement of diverse populations in health promotion research.
- Evaluate policy recommendations for reducing health disparities and identify policies that are most likely to have substantial benefit.

INTRODUCTION

Overall, the health, average life span, and quality of life of Americans have improved since the beginning of the 19th century. However, not all individuals have enjoyed these improvements to the same degree. Select populations experience a disproportionate disease burden. Significant health disparities in health outcomes, healthcare access, and healthcare delivery have been documented (Chin, Walters, Cook, & Huang, 2007; Center to Reduce Cancer Health Disparities [CRCHD,] 2004).

As you begin this chapter, consider for a moment the health trajectories of four women, each of whom were 45 years old, lived within a block of one another, and jogged together three times a week. The four women included a Black woman with three children and an 11th grade education, a White woman with two children and a high school education, a Hispanic woman with four children and a community college degree, and a Filipino woman with one child and a bachelor's degree. All of the women had either publicly-funded or privately-funded health care. Which women would be most at risk of problems associated with diabetes, heart disease, cancer, and asthma? Which diseases are most affected by genetic rather than lifestyle factors? In terms of life expectancy and quality of life, which women could expect to be the healthiest 30 years from now? You can check your answers by reviewing content summarized in this chapter.

Health disparities often are reported based on racial and ethnic groups; for example, Blacks, Hispanics, Native Americans/Alaskans, and Asians/Pacific Islanders have higher incidences or mortality rates for given conditions than do Whites. However, health disparities can also be associated with a geographic area (such as a rural area or inner city), gender, age, income, education, disability, or cultural and/or linguistic barriers to care. Other priority populations who are at-risk include those who lack a medical home (one consistent healthcare provider), those in need of long-term care, and individuals whose chronic disease is not well managed (Agency for Healthcare Research and Quality [AHRQ], 2003).

Disparities exist across the continuum of care in terms of prevention, access to care, and treatment. Failure to screen for risk, lack of primary prevention, failure to detect a disease, lack of follow-up for abnormal test results, nonadherence to treatment plans, unequal access to effective treatments, and lack of adequate palliative care resources are all common disparities. These disparities lead to higher incidence rates for a spectrum of diseases, delayed diagnosis, poorer response to treatment, and disease re-occurrence. Treating disease later in its progression typically results in higher healthcare costs and always results in higher emotional and social costs (CRCHD, 2004). A report of the Joint Center for Political and Economic Studies estimated the combined costs of health inequities and premature death in the United States to be 1.24 trillion dollars in 2006; these estimates were based on lost productivity and increased healthcare costs associated with delayed treatment (La Veist, Gaskin & Richard, 2009).

"Race and ethnicity have been found to influence quality of care, service delivery, disposition after treatment, . . . and intensity of care provided to hospitalized patients" (Shavers & Brown, 2002, p. 335). Treatment location and insurance coverage are also major factors that influence health disparities. Physician recommendations also are important and are shaped by "stage of disease, prognostic indicators, perception of the patient's willingness to comply with treatment recommendations," and various other factors (Shavers & Brown, 2002, p. 335). Patient decision making also influences health disparities. Patient participation in care is impacted by factors such as family and provider beliefs about treatment approaches, the ability to navigate the medical system, language barriers, cultural differences, and lack of transportation (Shavers & Brown, 2002).

DEFINITIONS OF HEALTH DISPARITIES

In 1999, one of the first definitions of health disparity arose from a White House initiative. At the request of the White House, the National Institute of Health (NIH) convened a working group that included representatives from all of their institutes. The resulting working group definition stated that "health disparities are differences in the incidence, prevalence, mortality, and burden of diseases and other diverse health conditions that exist among specific population groups in the United States" (CRCHD, 2011a).

United States Public Law 106-525, the Minority Health and Disparities Research and Education Act, was enacted in 2000 and authorized the National Center for Minority Health and Disparities at NIH to provide a legal definition of a health disparity. This definition stated that:

> A population is a health disparity population if there is a significant disparity in the overall rate of disease incidence, prevalence, morbidity, mortality, or survival rates in the population as compared to the health status of the general population . . . Included are populations for which there is a considerable disparity in the quality, outcomes, cost, or use of healthcare services or access to, or satisfaction with such services as compared to the general population. (CRCHD, 2004, p. 13)

Health equity was emphasized in this definition, as was the right that everyone has to conditions, resources, and supports needed to ensure health.

HOW DISPARITIES ARE DETERMINED

To determine if a health disparity exists or whether improvement is being made in eliminating that disparity, it is common to look at three health statistics: incidence (the number of new cases), mortality (the number of deaths), and survival rates (length of survival following diagnosis). When any one group of people has a higher incidence of a given disease, a higher mortality rate, or a shorter survival time following diagnosis, that discrepancy constitutes a health disparity (CRCHD, 2004).

> Both prevalence and incidence rates are considered when evaluating health disparities. The *prevalence* method estimates the consequences and costs incurred during a year . . . . This approach tallies all healthcare costs in a year . . . . The *incidence* method sums the direct and indirect costs of disease from its onset in a base year and for every subsequent year over the natural course of the disease. The total cost of disease

equals the discounted sum of illness-related events over the lifetime of each individual with the disease. Incidence-based costing is based on life-cycle costs and therefore provides a more complete picture of the patient-level costs and baseline total costs against which new interventions can be assessed. But the incidence-based method requires a considerable amount of data, such as disease incidence, survival rates, long-term morbidity, and lifetime impact on employment. (CRCHD, 2004, p. 30)

Therefore, the *prevalence* method is the more commonly used approach because it requires less data.

TYPES OF HEALTH DISPARITIES

There are myriad health disparities, including those related to asthma, cancer, cardiovascular disease, diabetes, obesity, low birth weight, infant mortality, HIV/AIDS, mental health, and violence. Any listing of health disparities will inevitably be incomplete long before a book can be published; nevertheless, becoming familiar with common health disparities is a necessity. It is imperative that healthcare providers continually update their knowledge regarding which disparities affect which populations at any given point in time. A summary of several important health disparities are presented in **Table 5-1**, although the list is not meant to be all-inclusive. The data presented were extracted from profiles on the Office of Minority Health in the U.S. Department of Health and Human Services. All data are presented in comparison to non-Hispanic Whites and represent 2007–2008 figures.

After examining Table 5-1, imagine you are a legislator or on the board of a private health foundation that wants to allocate financial resources to decrease health disparities. Where would you allocate funds based on the highest health disparities? If you were considering the most costly health disparities in terms of lost productivity or overall healthcare costs, where would you focus the funding? In allocating funding, would you attempt to eliminate disparities for a particular disease or focus on improving education, income, or access to health care? Are there ethnic/racial groups who performed better on any of the given indicators than Whites or the U.S. population as a whole? What were those groups and indicators? Why are the disease incidence and mortality rates for White populations the norm against which other populations were compared? Is comparing incidence rates to White populations consistent with the NIH definition of health disparities? Why does Table 5-1 from the Office of Minority Health at the NIH include factors such as income, education, and insurance coverage? Provide a rationale for each of your answers.

TABLE 5-1 Health Disparities (2007–2008) Office of Minority Health, U.S. Department of Health and Human Services

Racial/ Ethnic Group	Income	Insurance Coverage	Education	% of Population	Cancer	Diabetes	Heart Disease	HIV/AIDS	Infant Mortality	Stroke
Black	Median income = $33,916. 24.5% living at the poverty level.	49% have employer sponsored insurance. 23.8% have public insurance. 19.5% were uninsured.	80% complete high school and 15% have a bachelor's degree.	13.5%	Males are 1.3 times as likely to have lung and prostate cancer and have lower survival rates; they are also twice as likely to have stomach cancer. Women are 34% more likely to die from breast cancer and twice as likely to have stomach cancer.	Adults are twice as likely to have diabetes and have 2.2 times as likely to die from it. Males are 2.1 times more likely to have end-stage renal disease.	Men are 30% more likely to die from heart disease. Adults are 1.5 times more likely to have high blood pressure.	Males have 7 times the rate of AIDS and are 9 times more likely to die, while females have 22 times the rate and are 20 times more likely to die.	The infant mortality rate is 2.3 times higher. SIDS deaths are 1.8 times higher and mothers are 2.5 times more likely to not have prenatal care or to not begin to receive it until the third trimester.	Adults are 1.7 times as likely to have a stroke and are 60% more likely to die from it. Survivors are more likely to be disabled from the stroke.

(continues)

TABLE 5-1 Health Disparities (2007–2008) Office of Minority Health, U.S. Department of Health and Human Services
(continued)

Racial/ Ethnic Group	Income	Insurance Coverage	Education	% of Popu-lation	Cancer	Diabetes	Heart Disease	HIV/AIDS	Infant Mortality	Stroke
American Indian/ Alaska Native	Median income is $33,627. 25% live at the poverty level.	36% have private insurance, 24% have public insurance, and 33% are without insurance.	76% have a high school education, 14% have a bachelors degree.	1.6%	Men are twice as likely to have liver or Intrahepatic Bile Duct (IBD) cancer. They are 1.8 times as likely to have stomach cancer, and twice as likely to die from it. Women are 2.4 times as likely to have and die from liver and IBD cancer and 40% more likely to have kidney cancer.	Adults are 2.3 times as likely to have diabetes and twice as likely to die from it.	Adults are 1.2 times as likely to have heart disease and 1.3 times as likely to have high blood pressure.	Adults have 40% higher HIV rates.	Infant mortality is 1.4 times higher; babies are twice as likely to die from SIDS. Mothers are 3.7 times as likely to not receive prenatal care or not begin to receive it until the third trimester.	Adults are 60% more likely to have a stroke.

TABLE 5-1 Health Disparities (2007–2008) Office of Minority Health, U.S. Department of Health and Human Services
(continued)

Racial/ Ethnic Group	Income	Insurance Coverage	Education	% of Population	Cancer	Diabetes	Heart Disease	HIV/AIDS	Infant Mortality	Stroke
Asian Americans	Median income is $15,600 higher than the national average. 10% of Asians live at the poverty level and 2.2% receive public assistance.	84% have insurance coverage, although rates of private insurance vary from 76% for Vietnamese to 84% for Chinese. Public insurance rates vary from 3.8% for Chinese to 11% for Vietnamese.	86% have a high school diploma, which is equivalent to the overall U.S. rate. 50% of Asians, compared to 28% of the United States' overall population, have earned a bachelor's degree.	5%	Men are less likely to have prostate cancer than Whites. Adults have 3 times the incidence of liver and IBD cancer. Men are twice as likely and women are 2.6 times as likely to die from stomach cancer. Vietnamese females have the highest mortality rates for cervical cancer.	Asians are 30% less likely than Whites to die from diabetes.	Asians are less likely than Whites to get and to die from heart disease and are less likely to have high blood pressure.	HIV rates are increasing for Asians; however, they still have lower HIV/AIDS rates than Whites.	SIDS is the 4th leading cause of death among Asian infants.	Asians are less likely to die from stroke than are Whites.

(continues)

TABLE 5-1 Health Disparities (2007–2008) Office of Minority Health, U.S. Department of Health and Human Services
(continued)

Racial/Ethnic Group	Income	Insurance Coverage	Education	% of Population	Cancer	Diabetes	Heart Disease	HIV/AIDS	Infant Mortality	Stroke
Native Hawaiians/ Pacific Islanders	Median household income is $50,992	Not collected.	84% have high school diplomas, 10% have bachelor's degrees, and 4% have graduate degrees.	0.1%	Men are 40% less likely to have prostate cancer, and women are 30% less likely to have breast cancer. Adults have 3 times the incidence of liver and IBD cancer. Men are twice as likely and women are 2.6 times as likely to die from stomach cancer.	Native Hawaiians have twice the rate of diabetes as White individuals.	Hawaiians are 30% more likely to have high blood pressure, but less likely to have or die from heart disease, than Whites.	The AIDS case rate for HIV is twice that of Whites.	SIDS is the 4th leading cause of infant mortality.	The risk of stroke is less than in White populations.

TABLE 5-1 Health Disparities (2007–2008) Office of Minority Health, U.S. Department of Health and Human Services *(continued)*

Racial/ Ethnic Group	Income	Insurance Coverage	Education	% of Population	Cancer	Diabetes	Heart Disease	HIV/AIDS	Infant Mortality	Stroke
Hispanic/ Latino	55% of Hispanic house-holds earn $35,000 or more. 21.5% of Hispanics live at the poverty level.	Hispanics have the highest rates of uninsured individu-als (32%). Private insur-ance cover-age varies from 58% for Cubans to 29% for Mexicans.	61% have a high school diploma and 12.5% have a bachelor's degree.	15%. Hispanics are the fastest growing group in terms of population.	Hispanic men are less likely to have prostate cancer and women are less likely to have breast cancer. Hispanic adults have a higher incidence and mortality rate for stomach and liver cancer. Women are twice as likely to have cervical cancer.	Adults are twice as likely to have diabetes, 1.5 times as likely to have end stage renal disease, and 1.6 times as likely to die from diabetes.	Hispanics are less likely to have heart disease than Whites.	Males have 3 times the AIDS rate as White males. Females have 5 times the AIDS rate as White women. Both women and men are more likely to die from AIDS than are Whites.	Puerto Rican infants are twice as likely to die from low birth weight as White children. Mexican American mothers are 2.5 times more likely to not receive prenatal care or to not receive it until the third trimester.	Hispanic adults are less likely to die of a stroke than White adults.

Selecting a Reference Group for Evaluating Disparities

The federal government considered three options in establishing a baseline from which to monitor progress in promoting health equity. First, they considered comparing a given group to the entire population. Second, they considered comparing a given group to the best performing group within the population. Finally, they considered comparing a given group with the largest fixed group. The option of a comparison to the largest fixed group was selected so that a stable baseline value could be chosen and each subsequent year's values would be measured against the same group. When the largest group is used, standard errors are the smallest. In addition, "unlike comparisons with the total population, groups are independent" when this largest group measured is used (AHRQ, 2003, p. 30). At the time of selection of this comparison group, non-Hispanic Whites, individuals at 400% or more of the federal poverty level, and college graduates were the largest fixed groups. "This choice of a comparison group was not meant to suggest that Whites or persons with high income or college education are superior or that disparities are an issue for racial and ethnic minorities or less affluent persons only. In fact, Whites and persons with high income or college education are not the best performing group in many instances" (AHRQ, 2003, p. 30).

Other Disparities in Prevalence

There are a variety of other disparities not mentioned in the earlier grid. Asthma morbidity and mortality rates are also "disproportionately high among ethnic minorities including African Americans . . . The striking ethnic disparities in asthma prevalence cannot be explained entirely by environmental, social, cultural or economic factors." Genetic factors are thought to play a role in asthma-related health disparities (Mathias, et al., 2009, p. 337).

Gay males are more likely than heterosexual males to experience depression, anxiety, and suicidal ideation. Lesbian, gay, and bisexual youth are more likely to have substance abuse issues, to attempt suicide, and to be at risk of being a victim of violence (Lewis, 2009). Hispanic injection drug users have a greater prevalence of hepatitis C than other groups (National Institute on Drug Abuse [NIDA], 2011). There are a greater number of Hispanic/Latino gang members (49%) compared to Black gang members (35%) or White gang members (9%), making Hispanic teens more likely to be at risk for homicide, which is a leading cause of death among 10 to 24 year olds.

Disparities in Quality of Care

Quality of care measures such as safety (avoiding harming patients by use of care that is intended to help them), effectiveness (provision of care based on scientific standards to all patients who might benefit but not those unlikely to benefit), patient-centeredness (care that is individualized, respectful, and responsive to values and preferences), and timeliness of care (reduced waiting times and delays in receipt of care) were identified by the Agency for Healthcare Research and Quality and the Institute of Medicine (IOM) as being critical in promoting health equity. They are also factors that illustrate disparities in the quality of health care among groups (AHRQ, 2003, p. 38). However, some have argued that it may be necessary to develop new measures of quality that are even more responsive to the needs of ethnic and minority populations (AHRQ, 2003), rather than using existing measures of quality that are applicable to the entire population.

There are multiple examples of disparities in quality of care. Hispanics and Blacks are more likely than other groups to suffer from diabetes and diabetes-related complications such as retinopathy, neuropathy, and leg amputations (AHRQ, 2003; Tirado, 2011). Twenty-nine percent of Blacks who smoke receive smoking cessation counseling while hospitalized, compared to 40% of Whites; this is in spite of the fact that smoking is the single most preventable cause of mortality. In another example, "[c]ompared to White adults (86%), Black adults achieve adequate hemodialysis less often (82%)" (AHRQ, 2003, p. 45). Hispanics who are hospitalized for acute myocardial infarction are less likely to receive optimal care (AHRQ, 2003). Twelve percent of Hispanics, 12% of Asians, and 8% of Whites are restrained in long-term care. Ten percent of Blacks and 8% of Whites in long-term care get pressure sores. Postoperative respiratory failure is higher in poor areas than near-poor areas and middle-income areas compared to high-income areas. Post-operative septicemia is higher among Blacks, Hispanics, and Asians compared with Whites.

When compared with Whites, Blacks are less likely to receive expensive or innovative treatments for cancer (Shavers & Brown, 2002). Blacks are also less likely to receive treatment for lung cancer and, when they do get treatment, less likely to get surgery (Shavers & Brown, 2002). Black, Asian, and Hispanic women "are more likely to be diagnosed at an advanced stage of breast cancer and have worse stage-for-stage survival than do White women" (Han et al., 2009, p. 247).

It is important to consider not only incidence rates and mortality rates for varied diseases, but also differences in treatments that are provided based on ethnic/racial background, income, and geographic location. It is also critical to consider when varied ethnic and racial groups access care and what barriers contribute to accessing care.

Disparities in Access to Care, Use of Care, and Cost of Care

Access issues include the ability to gain entry into the healthcare system, transportation barriers, the ability to schedule convenient appointments, feasible wait times, and the ability to obtain preventive and acute care. Issues of access to care also encompass the ability of providers to communicate effectively with patients by being culturally sensitive, attending to their language needs, and modifying teaching based on patient's health literacy needs.

Insurance coverage is a major factor that impacts access. Racial and ethnic minorities are less likely to have health insurance. Twenty percent of Blacks, 33% of American Indians, and 23% of Hispanics, compared to 12% of Whites, have public insurance. Individuals who are uninsured receive less preventive care, are diagnosed with more advanced disease stages, and have poorer health status. Individuals with lower incomes and less education as well as Blacks and Hispanics are less likely to receive routine health care and are more likely to receive acute care treatment. Hospitalizations for conditions that could have been treated in ambulatory care such as hypertension, angina, chronic obstructive pulmonary disease, and bacterial pneumonia are higher among Blacks and individuals of lower income (AHRQ, 2003).

Thirty-one percent of Hispanics, 26% of Blacks, and 20% of Whites have trouble receiving referrals to specialists. Twenty-nine percent of the poor, 26% of the near-poor, and 18% of those with higher incomes have trouble getting specialty referrals. Black, Asian, and American Indian women over 40 are less likely to receive mammography than non-Hispanic White women; lower income women are also less likely to get mammograms. Thirty-four percent of Asian women report not having a Pap smear, compared to 23% of Hispanic women, 18% of White women, and 16% of Black women. Ten percent of Blacks, 20% of Asian Pacific Islanders, and 17% of Hispanics receive a kidney transplant within 3 years of renal failure, compared to 26% of Whites. Sixty-three percent of the poor, 64% of the near-poor, 61% of middle-income patients, and 74% of high-income individuals with diabetes receive an annual retinal eye examination. Fifty-nine percent of Hispanics, 58% of American Indians, and 67% of Whites have had their cholesterol checked within the last 5 years. Fifty-six percent of the poor, 60% of the near poor, 67% of middle income, and 75% of high income persons have had their cholesterol checked, while 58% of individuals with less than a high school education, 69% of high school graduates, and 78% of those with a college education had their cholesterol checked. Hispanics and low income individuals are "more likely to experience difficulties or delays due to financial or insurance reasons or forego health care because their family needs money" (AHRQ, 2003, p. 75).

In general, ethnic and racial minorities are more likely to refuse treatment and to have longer periods from an initial abnormal screening to treatment initiation, both of which make them more likely to suffer from a variety of health disparities (Shavers & Brown, 2002). For example, a systematic review of ethnic differences in use of dementia care and provision of treatment showed that individuals from ethnic and racially diverse groups "accessed diagnostic services later in their illness and once they received a diagnosis, were less likely to access anti-dementia medication, research trials, and 24-hour care" (Cooper, Tandy, Balamurali, & Livingston, 2010, p. 193). Ethnic minorities were also more cognitively impaired and had a longer duration of memory loss at the time of diagnosis. They did not or were not able to access care at the same rate as White individuals with dementia (Cooper et al., 2010).

Language Fluency and Health Literacy

When considering health disparities it is vital to consider language fluency and how that can impact health literacy. Comparing people above the age of 5, 62% of Vietnamese, 50% of Chinese, 24% of Filipinos, 23% of Asian Indians, 42% of Native Hawaiians/Pacific Islanders, and 12% of Latino individuals living in the United States are not fluent in English. Fluency has a marked effect on communication between healthcare providers and patients as well as on health literacy, the ability to understand and follow a treatment plan, and health screening prac-

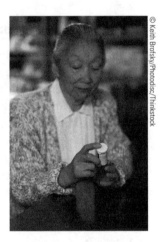

tices. For example, "non-English speaking Asians and Pacific Islander women living in the [United States] tend to have the lowest rates of Pap tests relative to women in other racial categories," a reality that is thought to be related to both health literacy and access barriers (Yu, Chou, Johnson, & Ward, 2010, p. 451).

Overall, 75% of individuals with physical or mental health problems have trouble understanding their doctor's recommendations. Fifty-eight percent of Asians and 54% of Hispanics, compared with 40% of non-Hispanic Whites, report having trouble comprehending health information; broken down by education level, 60% of those with less than a high school education, 47% of high school graduates, and 36% of college graduates report having trouble understanding health information. There are also major sources of miscommunication, in that not all individuals believe that pathogens cause disease or that visions and communicating with dead ancestors are unusual. It is important to keep in mind that Western and Eastern healing philosophies differ greatly (AHRQ, 2003).

The Immigrant Paradox

Acculturation (adopting American norms and health behaviors) has a negative effect on blood pressure, cardiovascular risk, and mental health (Egan, Tannahill, Petticrew, & Thomas, 2008). Certain groups of immigrant women have better pregnancy outcomes than first-generation women born in the United States. The term "immigrant paradox" was coined to describe the fact that immigrant populations often have better health than U.S.-born individuals of the same racial and ethnic background. As years of living in the United States increase, health disparities also increase. "Adaptation to U.S. behavioral norms can lead to the adoption of nutritional, physical, and substance use behaviors that in turn lead to increased risk of common chronic diseases" (Williams & Mohammed, 2008, p. 157). In addition, discrimination and chronic stress associated with life in an industrialized society contributes to poor health (Williams & Mohammed, 2008).

One theory used to explain the immigrant paradox was that only the "healthiest" immigrants were physically, socially, and economically able to migrate (Gallo et al., 2009); however, that has been shown to not be the case. The concept of immigrant paradox highlights the importance of understanding protective social and cultural factors that contribute to resiliency and health in addition to simply focusing on cultural and ethnic differences that undermine health (National Institute of Child Health and Human Development, 2003).

Gender, Age, and Disability-Related Disparities

Women suffer higher morbidity rates than males even though they live an average of 6 years longer. Women are more likely to need long-term care, are at greater risk for Alzheimer's disease, more likely to experience depression, and are more often uninsured. In addition, lack of health care during pregnancy has long-term consequences for both the mother and the child. Childhood is a critical developmental stage and children are dependent on adults for access to care. Many children live in poverty; black and lower income children are less likely than White and more affluent children to receive childhood immunizations, and "[o]ver 1 out of 5 children spends some time being uninsured" (AHRQ, 2003, p. 167).

The percentages of poor (6.8%), near-poor (7.3%), and middle-income (2.8%) elderly who delay seeking care are higher than in high-income elderly groups (1.2%). Elderly individuals are more likely to have trouble obtaining specialty referrals than younger individuals and are also more likely to have trouble understanding health-related information (AHRQ, 2003).

Persons with disabilities, those who utilize long-term care, and individuals at the end of life face special challenges related to access to health care. Poor persons (11%), the near-poor (9%) and middle-income individuals (7%) who are disabled report greater challenges in getting to a healthcare provider than do higher income persons (4%) (AHRQ, 2003, p. 207). Nationally, 70% of Americans say they wish to die at home, although only 25% of deaths actually occur at home. End-of-life care provided in a hospital is costly: Up to "one-quarter of Medicare dollars are spent on 5% of beneficiaries in the last year of life" (AHRQ, 2003, p. 210).

Rural Populations

Access to care is limited in rural areas because there are fewer healthcare providers, transportation is more difficult in rural areas given that distances are greater and public transportation is more often lacking, and providers in rural areas are less likely to offer evening and weekend appointments. It is also more difficult to obtain referrals to specialists in rural areas. Many rural hospitals have closed or have experienced significant financial difficulties (AHRQ, 2003). Rural gang membership is greater than in urban areas: 17% of rural White teens belong to gangs as compared to 8% of those in cities (Egley & O'Donnell, 2009). White women living in Appalachia have a higher risk of developing cervical cancer (CRCHD, 2011b). In general, rural populations are less likely to engage in preventive health care and health screenings (Paskett et al., 2008).

FACTORS CONTRIBUTING TO HEALTH DISPARITIES

Numerous, complex, intertwined factors within and outside the healthcare delivery system contribute to health disparities. Factors associated with the healthcare delivery system that contribute to disparities include: (1) lack of insurance coverage, (2) the quality of health insurance and how consistently the patient has had insurance, (3) the availability of trained healthcare providers and healthcare facilities within one's geographic area, (4) ineffective provider–patient communication, (5) the degree of fragmentation within the healthcare system and lack of follow-up care, and (6) language and cultural barriers between providers and patients. Lack of insurance following loss of a job even, when it is followed by gaining access to insurance, can result in needing to locate a new care provider and cause disruptions in care during a critical period in terms of a person's health. High co-pays and deductibles can prompt individuals not to seek care. Lifetime coverage limits that are exceeded during a period of a major illness can also leave a person without access to care (CRCHD, 2004). Even in systems such as the Veterans Health Administration System and the Medicare program, where health care is provided to everyone, health disparities based on racial and ethnic background persist (Williams & Rucker, 2000).

Factors outside the healthcare delivery system that influence health disparities include age, gender, education level, socioeconomic status (SES), race and ethnicity, transportation barriers, problems taking time off from work for health care, childcare issues, lack of knowledge of appropriate health care, cultural beliefs that interfere with seeking health care, and lack of trust for healthcare providers and systems (CRCHD, 2004; Shavers & Brown, 2002). Issues such as access to good loans, the opportunity to earn a living wage, and fair hiring practices are also factors that affect health equity (CRCHD, 2004).

Socioeconomic Status and Stress

One of the strongest predictors of having a greater disease burden (or a health disparity) is socioeconomic status (SES). Income has an effect on access to education, occupation, health insurance, and living conditions (including exposure to toxins and violence), all of which contribute to health disparities. Socioeconomic status also has an impact on behavioral factors such as smoking, physical inactivity, obesity, and alcohol and drug use. It affects whether one can afford healthy, nutritious food or access a healthy place to exercise. Lower-income people have less access to preventive care, lower-intensity hospital care when hospitalized, and worse outcomes from cardiac and vascular procedures. They also receive lower quality ambulatory care. Disparities based on SES persist "across the life cycle and across varied measures of health, including health status, morbidity, and mortality" (Fiscella & Williams, 2004, p. 1139). Hahn and colleagues (1995) described the effect of poverty as being equivalent to the risk of cigarette smoking in terms of health. It is interesting that whether one measures SES based on income, occupational status, or wealth, the effect on health continues to be significant (Williams & Mohammed, 2008).

Stress, which is prevalent in lower SES environments, has a negative influence on health in that it increases allostatic load (Fiscella & Williams, 2004). Exposure to racial/ethnic discrimination also contributes to stress and poorer health outcomes (Egan et al., 2008). As much as 30% of the population has experienced bias and 60% of those who report experiencing bias report chronic, everyday discrimination (Kessler, Mickelson, & Williams, 1999). Factors such as social networks (friends, family, participation in organized groups, having a sense of belonging in the larger society), a sense of control at home or work, a balance between effort and reward, and security and autonomy also contribute to health or to stress (Egan et al., 2008). "Socioeconomic position is associated with the types and levels of stressors to which the individual is exposed, the availability of resources to cope with stress, and the patterned responses and strategies developed over time to manage environmental challenges" (Williams & Mohammed, 2008, p. 136).

When health disparities begin early in life they often have a lasting impact. The health of mothers and fetuses and their SES are closely linked. Fetal exposure to smoking and drug use have been linked to behavioral disorders in children. Exposure to less cognitive stimulation, family conflict, childhood abuse, and environmental toxins that can be experienced in low-income communities contribute to health disparities. Children of low SES are at greater risk of "death from infectious disease, sudden infant death, accidents and child abuse and . . . they have higher rates of asthma, developmental delay, learning disabilities, and conduct disorders (Fiscella & Williams, 2004, p. 1140). Research shows that preschool and school-age interventions programs can reduce health disparities that derive from low SES.

Low SES among adolescents is linked to higher rates of pregnancy, sexually transmitted disease, depression, obesity, abuse, dropping out of school, and suicide. Adults from low SES are likely to live 6 years less than someone with a college education. Elderly individuals with low SES experience "greater physical disability, greater limitations in activities of daily living, and more rapid cognitive decline" (Fiscella & Williams, 2004, p. 1141).

Income differences between low and high-income people constitute more than three times the difference in health between Black and White individuals and more than four times the difference in health between Whites and Hispanics. This reality highlights the importance that income plays in shaping health and explains why interventions such as providing free lunches for low-income children, food stamps, rental assistance, and other programs have been implemented (Williams & Mohammed, 2008; Pamuk et al., 1998).

INTERVENTIONS FOR MINIMIZING HEALTH DISPARITIES

When educating populations who experience significant health disparities, it is crucial to rely on the cultural expertise of members of the target group in designing educational materials. Nicholson and colleagues (2008) found that articles that report about progress in eliminating disparities about colon cancer are more likely to have a positive effect on health behaviors than articles that presented the reality that Blacks are doing worse than Whites or that Black outcomes are improving but at a slower rate than seen in White populations. The negative emotions reported in response to the ads that described Blacks as being more at-risk created resistance to the message and had a negative impact on health screening behaviors. The researchers reported that "the greater the amount of negative affective response, the less likely an individual was to want to be screened" (p. 2951). This was explained by the authors as such: "People tend not to believe, or view as prejudiced, information that threatens their self-concept or a favorable image of their referent group" (p. 2947).

Previous experience with discrimination has been associated with delays in seeking health care. Because of this, education should emphasize progress that is being made rather than highlighting the stark nature of disparities that exist. However, by emphasizing progress alone, attempts to obtain legislative action and programmatic funding may be hurt. Another approach is "impact framing," which involves describing the ways that a health disparity influences a patient, a family, and a given community. Impact framing makes the given disparity personal and illustrates why it makes a difference in the lives of the affected group (Nicholson et al., 2008).

Authors have also advocated for using information technology to enhance access to care and increase people's involvement in their care as a way to manage health disparities. Options include renewing one's prescription online, emailing a physician or nurse practitioner with a question, checking lab test results online, obtaining appointment reminders, receiving medication reminders, and using the Internet to obtain health-related information. The Internet has now surpassed physicians as the most popular health education resource (Gibbons, 2011). However, a study conducted at Kaiser found discrepancies among use of online options, in that 42% of Whites registered to use online services while only 30% of Blacks did so (Roblin et al., 2009). Diverse populations are more likely to be handheld wireless Internet users than are Whites, but it is unclear how to successfully promote information technology for the purpose of managing health in these populations (Gibbons, 2011).

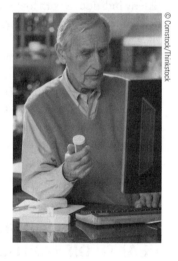

Fewer diverse healthcare providers have adopted electronic health records as part of their practice. The same is true for providers who primarily serve Hispanic patients, rural patients, the uninsured, or those on Medicaid. Electronic medical records allow for the monitoring of vital clinical parameters among groups who experience health disparities. Smart technologies that monitor glucose levels, weight, and vital signs can be connected to the electronic medical record so that a physician or nurse practitioner is notified of abnormal results from in-home monitoring. Such technology has the potential to narrow the health disparities gap by allowing for careful monitoring of disease progression. A barrier that needs to be addressed involves making sure that the health literacy needs of the given population are given adequate attention. Another question that needs to be resolved is whether lack of trust or a history of discrimination influences the acceptability of smart technologies among populations who experience health disparities (Gibbons, 2011).

Because disparities are often associated with diagnosis at an advanced disease state, increasing access to screening and prevention activities has been a priority (Shavers & Brown, 2002). On-time mammography, for example, is low among Hispanic and

Asian women. Interventions that involve community members who educate about the importance of health screening have been more successful in decreasing health disparities than has providing culturally specific and sensitive educational materials. The use of promotoras, or lay health advisors, has increased health-screening behaviors, and making low or no-cost mammography available via mobile vans or vouchers has also been effective (Han, et al., 2009).

It is crucial to tailor prevention and treatment approaches to the needs of specific cultural groups rather than to believe that improving the quality of the overall healthcare delivery system will reduce disparities. Policies that are aimed at increasing funding for prevention, screening, and access to health care are effective in minimizing health disparities. Bringing care to the communities, schools, and churches where people live is another viable option—for example, school-based primary health clinics have been effective in improving rates of immunization, providing health education, making mental health services accessible, and offering basic health screening in a nonthreatening environment. Scheduling difficulties, transportation barriers, and lack of trust toward health providers are minimized when care is provided in a familiar and comfortable setting. One limitation associated with offering care within community settings that needs to be modified is that many private and some public funding sources do not reimburse for care provided in these locations (Federico et al., 2010).

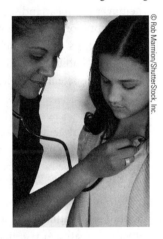

Increasing the diversity of the workforce is an excellent way to reduce health disparities. Training all providers to offer patient-centered, holistic care is also a priority. Starfield (1992) suggested there are four vital components to consider when providing care to underserved populations: (1) providing first contact access to needed services (thus avoiding complicated referral policies), (2) ensuring continuity of care, (3) providing effective care coordination, and (4) offering comprehensive care that includes holistic interventions for needed physical, mental, and social issues. One way to accomplish these goals is to encourage the use of a medical home where the patient and provider are familiar with one another and a spectrum of services are provided at one location.

Cultural Competence and Patient-Centered Interventions

To minimize health disparities, nurses need to attempt to understand the people they work with (both patients and other healthcare providers) from the frame of reference of that person's culture. It is important to understand the values, traditions, religious views, likes, dislikes, rituals, behaviors, and beliefs that guide decision making in order to help improve a person's health. It is also necessary to have knowledge of prevention and incidence rates and treatment outcomes for varied diagnoses and populations. Being sensitive to different belief systems about disease causation and exploring whether the person relies on folk healers or herbal medicines allows a nurse to obtain a comprehensive history and select an intervention that is consistent with patient values. It is also critical to honor attitudes toward family involvement in care while navigating legal guidelines about respecting patient privacy and information sharing (Leninger & McFarland, 2002). Cultural competency has been defined as "a design, implementation, and evaluation process that accounts for special issues of select population groups (ethnic, racial, and linguistic) as well as differing educational levels and physical abilities" (AHRQ, 2003, p. 124). There are demonstrable links between cultural competence, quality of care, and elimination of racial and ethnic disparities (AHRQ, 2003).

Closely associated with the concept of cultural competence is the quality measure of patient centeredness mentioned by the IOM. Providers need to develop a partnership with patients and their families to make sure that a patient's needs and preferences drive healthcare decisions, that individualized care is provided, and that education is understood. Adequate patient–provider communication "increases awareness of risky behaviors, helps patients make complex choices . . . such as selecting the best treatment, . . . and increases the likelihood that patients understand and adhere to treatment regimens" (AHRQ, 2003, p. 120). It has been documented that American Indians/Alaska Natives (44%), Blacks (23%), Hispanics (33%), low-income populations (31% of poor, 25% of near poor, 17% of middle income and 13% of higher income individuals), and the less educated (30% of those without a high school education and 17% of those with some college) report poor communication with providers (AHRQ, 2003). "Compared to Whites (22%), Blacks (27%), Hispanics (34%), and Asians (41%), report being under-involved in healthcare decision making" (AHRQ, 2003, p. 122). Likewise, 30% of the poor, 26% of the near poor, 24% of middle-income patients, and 20% of high-income patients report feeling disenfranchised. Asians (55% of Chinese and 39% of Filipinos) are more likely to report that their doctor does not understand their background and values as compared to 40% of Whites (AHRQ, 2003).

A good first step in developing cultural competence is to understand one's own background, biases, beliefs, and traditions. This is actually more difficult than it appears to be. Articulating what one grew up with and what one just came to know is a bit like describing the wind. As Edward T. Hall (Hall & Hall, 1990) commented, culture hides more than it reveals. What it hides it hides most effectively from those who were raised in and live by certain cultural norms. Individuals who grow up from an early age in a given culture just learn what a given gesture, facial expression, or tone of voice means. It is hard to describe how close one should stand to another person in a professional setting but it is something that one learns by growing up in a given culture. Likewise, the role of women or elders or children often differs from culture to culture.

As challenging as it can be to identify one's own world view, begin by reflecting on the religious beliefs, kinship and social relationships, gender roles, economic factors, attitudes toward education, health rituals, traditional remedies, food preferences, personal space rules, and communication patterns that you were raised to believe in as a child. Did your family value being on time and see that cultural value as a sign of respect or did they focus instead on being fully present and attentive to whatever activity or person they were engaged with at the moment? How did your family care for you when you were sick as a child? Did your parents prepare special foods when you were sick? Think about patients whom you have cared for who were raised with different norms, different health beliefs, and different health practices than your own. To provide culturally competent care, a nurse must understand his or her own perspective and be able to bridge cultural differences.

CULTURAL COMPETENCE CASE STUDY

Review the following case study, based on incidents that occurred during a student's public health rotation. Consider what you would have done differently and the ways the student demonstrated cultural competence during her visits with her assigned patient.

> Nadiya, a 21-year-old Asian Indian woman of Punjabi descent who was in an arranged marriage, was referred to the public health department after giving birth to her second child. I called and set up a home visit. A thin, long-haired, pale-looking woman carrying an infant came to the door. Nadiya willingly answered my questions, but she would look at her sister-in-law before answering me. Did Nadiya look to her sister-in-law because she wanted to seek her sister-in-law's approval or was it because she was looking to see if she was paying attention to our conversation? The children's immunizations were up-to-date. Nadiya told me that she was tired due to waking up to breastfeed her baby. She was interested in birth control, specifically Depo-Provera, as she did not want to have any more children. Nadiya lived in the house with four generations of her husband's extended family: a paternal

great-grandfather; two grandparents, one brother, his wife, and their son; a sister and the 3-year old who was her son; and another unmarried sister—13 people in all.

I observed that Chandra, Nadiya's newborn daughter, had stopped breastfeeding and was lying in her mother's arms. I looked at her general appearance; she was resting quietly and staring out. I tried to get her attention; she did not look at me. The body language between this mother–daughter dyad seemed off. I had the uneasy feeling that something was not right. I made a mental note to make more assessments at the next home visit. I recapped the visit by mentioning the date and time that I would visit next week. When I rang their doorbell at 10:30 a.m. the following Tuesday, Nadiya was the one who opened the door to welcome me. With Nadiya's help, I took her children's head circumferences, lengths, and weights. The measurements appeared to be within normal limits. Nadiya repeated during this visit that she really wanted to use a birth control method. She emphasized that she did not want to have any more children. I asked her what her husband thought about this; she shrugged. Her reported height was 5 feet 1 inch and her weight was 96 pounds. Her plan was to breastfeed for only six months, just as she did with her first child. "It takes too much time; she gets hungry too soon," she reasoned. I looked at how Chandra was feeding at her mother's breast. She turned her face to her mother's breast and her body faced upward. I demonstrated how Nadiya could hold Chandra close, with her baby's tummy and most of her body facing Nadiya. "This will help prevent nipple pulling and soreness. It will also promote closeness with your baby," I softly told her. Nadiya had told me earlier that she liked to sing but she did not do it anymore. I encouraged her to talk and sing to Chandra while looking at her and making eye contact, with the explanation that it was important for language and speech development.

I was a tumble of emotions with each response Nadiya provided to my queries. Sadness, frustration, and anger were just some feelings that welled up inside me. Before her arranged marriage more than 2 years ago, she was a college sophomore taking Commerce in India. Nadiya came to the United States to follow her parent's wishes. I asked her if she had made new friends in this country. She shook her head. She did not know how to drive and relied on those in the household to drive her. She reported that she did not have a bank account and that she simply received a monthly allowance from her husband to spend for herself and her children. She did not know how much her husband earned. Neither did she know his level of education. Hearing this, I had to keep my emotions in check and not let these cloud my judgment.

When we reached the question about her plans for the future, Nadiya hesitated for a moment. "Any plans of going back to school? There's a community college nearby," I prompted her. She said that she wanted to improve her English by attending "English as a Second Language" classes. From there she wanted to continue her education and learn employable skills. Her husband, Kali, had told her that she had to stay at home to care for their children until they were a little older. She added that she also wanted to learn how to drive. "Being able to drive your children to school and help them with their homework is a good reason to tell your husband so that you can achieve your plans later on," I encouraged her. "I did not think of that; thank you for the suggestion," she replied. The next question on the list I asked her was, "Do you ever feel helpless or hopeless?" Nadiya hesitated before she nodded, "I sometimes feel lonely and down." I asked her if her husband or anyone else ever physically hurt her. She answered, "No, my husband does not physically hurt me." She pointed to her heart and her forehead and said, "Here; I'm sometimes affected here."

We scheduled our last visit for the following week. I was surprised when an older man opened the door for us. I introduced myself and he called Nadiya. After that, he promptly went upstairs. I found out that he was Nadiya's father-in-law. I completed a Denver II on Nadiya's older child, Amara. At 1 year, 3 months, and 12 days old on assessment, Amara's Denver II interpretation was "Suspect" with four cautions noted. She had failed to play ball with the examiner, drink from a cup, scribble, and walk backwards. Nadiya was not perturbed that Amara could not drink from a cup. She told me that she fed Amara herself because she did not want to clean up the mess. I encouraged her to allow self-feeding, with the suggestion that she place plastic or newspapers under the child when she was eating for easier clean-up.

I learned that all the adult males (her husband, his father, and brother), except the great-grandfather, took turns and came home only once or twice a week. They stayed and slept at their place of business (a gasoline station). Her mother-in-law would go to work daily and returned to sleep at the home. Nadiya did not get along with her mother-in-law. Her eyes widened as she complained, "She woke me up at 5:30 this morning because she was mad that I did something she did not like! I don't get enough sleep as it is!" It was the first time I saw Nadiya fired-up and angry. Her voice quivered as she said, "I won't be able to take it anymore if she slaps or hurts me. I am going to leave this house if that happens." I let her settle down a bit before commenting, "Yes, you should not let anyone hurt you. Would you like me to mail you information on resources to call or to go to if you feel unsafe or if someone has hurt you?" She agreed.

I had read that the impact of cultural assimilation into U.S. society and the practice of arranged marriages, the high regard for male infants (especially first-born), and a postpartum tradition of confinement can contribute to the development of postpartum depression in new mothers like Nadiya (Goyal, Murphy, & Cohen, 2006). I had to ask Nadiya sensitive questions to assess for this risk. "Are you under pressure to bear a son? How do the members of this family look at your daughters?" Nadiya nodded her head and bemoaned, "Yes, my husband wants me to bear him a son. What happens if I give birth to another girl? I do not want to take the risk. That is why I want birth control. " I touched her arm as she continued, "My husband's family plays with my daughters; but, my mother-in-law sometimes jokingly asks the girls why they were not boys." I could not help but clench my jaw. Nadiya added that her husband was more caring and approachable when they were newly married. "But now, when I talk to him about my situation with my mother-in-law, he just says that it's between me and her."

Almost everything I heard from Nadiya saddened and concerned me. Having found out that her husband was the eldest son in the family, I thought it would be very unlikely that she could suggest that they move into a place of their own. I did not even broach the subject with her. I simply provided guidance and teaching on various topics like her need to follow up with her provider regarding birth control options, the benefits of "tummy time" for Chandra, car seat safety, the importance of getting the seasonal and H1N1 flu shots, and how to make the home child-safe. As we were wrapping up, I happened to shake the bell (from the Denver II kit) behind baby Chandra's head, near her ear; there was no reaction. I tried again, to no avail. I placed her on her abdomen to see how high she could hold her head up. She could not raise her head up by 45 degrees. This was a gross motor milestone for a 2-month infant. When Nadiya placed Chandra on her lap facing us, I rang the bell again. This time, I could see a sharp spark of realization dawn on Nadiya as she herself flinched from the sound of the bell, "That hurts my ears; but she does not even react." She did not need pushing to know that she had to talk to the doctor about scheduling a hearing test. It was a good thing that she had changed her appointment to Thursday. She was worried. As I prepared her for the end of our working relationship, she said "I am so alone and sometimes I do not know what to do anymore." When I returned to the office, I emphasized that a public health nurse needed to continue providing services to this family (Personal communication, Mary Anne Sandoval, May 13, 2010).

How did this student demonstrate cultural competency or the lack thereof when working with Nadiya? Was there anything you would have done differently? What cultural norms influenced the treatment plan for Nadiya and her family? How did the short duration of the visits impact outcomes? What other priorities needed to be addressed?

Culturally and Linguistically Appropriate Standards for Health Care

There are national standards developed by the Office of Minority Health for cultur- ally and linguistically appropriate healthcare services (CLAS); these were created from relevant laws along with input from healthcare providers, accreditation/credentialing agencies, and the public. The standards were developed to improve access to care, qual- ity of care, and health outcomes and were issued by the U.S. Department of Health and Human Services in 2000 as a way of correcting current health-related inequities. The standards are focused on healthcare organizations and are required to be adhered to if federal funds are received. The standards are also used by legislators in develop- ing laws, by agencies such as the Joint Commission on Accreditation of Healthcare Organizations, by the American Nurses Association to develop professional standards, and by educators to ensure their curricula are culturally competent.

According to the U.S. Department of Health and Human Services (2001), "cultural and linguistic competence is a set of congruent behaviors, attitudes, and policies that come together in a system, agency, or among professionals that enables effective work in cross-cultural situations" (p. 2). Competence implies the ability to consider cultural beliefs, needs, and behaviors of patients when providing health care.

There are 14 CLAS standards. The first CLAS standard emphasizes the ability to provide understandable, respectful care that is compatible with the patient's cultural health beliefs, practices, and preferred language. This standard requires being famil- iar with traditional healing systems and, when appropriate, integrating them into treatment plans. Standard 2 requires healthcare organizations to recruit, retain, and promote diverse staff members that are representative of the service area. This stan- dard covers the hospital leadership, governing boards, clinicians, and subcontractors.

Standard 3 requires that staff at all levels receive ongoing training about cultural and linguistic competence. This standard covers effective communication, techniques for conflict resolution, effects of cultural difference on health promotion, and the impact of poverty on health outcomes. Standard 4 requires that bilingual staff and interpreters be provided at no cost during all hours of operation to patients with limited English proficiency. Standard 5 requires that organizations post signs and make it known that language-assistance services are available. Standard 6 requires that translators demonstrate language competence and have 40 hours of training in cross-cultural issues. This standard discourages use of family members as interpreters and specifically states minor children should not function as interpreters. Standard 7 requires that patient-related materials (consent forms, handouts) and signs reflect the languages spoken in the service area. Standard 8 requires organizations to have a strategic plan and oversight mechanisms to ensure culturally competent care is provided. Standard 9 states that organizations should conduct ongoing self-assessments to determine that cultural and linguistic competence measures are included in performance improvement programs, patient satisfaction assessments, and outcomes-based evaluations. This self-assessment is to focus on capacities, strengths, and needed areas of improvement (U.S. Department of Health and Human Services, 2001).

Standard 10 requires that data on race, ethnicity, and spoken and written language be collected from patients to ensure an equitable quality of care is provided. This standard mandates that information collected at registration is based on patient self-identification, not visual or observational categorizations. Standard 11 states that healthcare organizations should maintain an epidemiological profile of the community so they can plan to provide care that matches the needs of their service area. Standard 12 requires that healthcare organizations facilitate community and consumer involvement in implementing CLAS-related activities. Standard 13 states that conflict and grievance resolution processes must be culturally and linguistically sensitive. Standard 14 requires that the public be notified of progress the organization is making in implementing the CLAS standards. This can occur via newsletters, conference presentations, newspaper articles, television or radio presentations. or Web site postings (U.S. Department of Health and Human Services, 2001).

THE ROLE OF THE GOVERNMENT AND OTHER ENTITIES IN DECREASING HEALTH DISPARITIES

There is justifiable debate about "the appropriate division of responsibility between the individual, the public sector, and the private sector" in terms of minimizing health disparities (AHRQ, 2003, p. 2). Historically the federal government has played a key role in initiating dialogue about health disparities and in designing programs to minimize disparities. Anti-discrimination and access to care laws passed by the federal government, including the 1964 Civil Rights Act, the 1986 Emergency Medical Treatment and Active Labor Act, and the 2007 Antidumping legislation applicable to Medicare and Medicaid, as well as recent laws about the necessity of interpreters, are examples of how the government has intervened in a way that minimizes health-related disparities.

In 1999, the NIH identified health disparities as a research priority and in 2000 established the National Center on Minority Health and Health Disparities. This center has funded studies that examine how the role of genetics, daily living conditions, income, and education contribute to health disparities (Dankwa-Mullan et al., 2010). Each year the Agency for Healthcare Research and Quality publishes an annual disparities report covering disparities in access and quality of care (Chin et al., 2007). Affirmative action programs that are responsible for training diverse physicians, nurse practitioners, and nurses were mandated and funded by the government and have been responsible for producing 40% of diverse healthcare providers (Williams & Rucker, 2000). The Health Professional Shortage Areas and Medically Underserved designations identified by the Health Resources and Services Administration were designed primarily to minimize health disparities and increase the numbers of diverse practitioners (Chin et al., 2007). Healthy People 2010 and 2020 include goals that focus on the elimination of health disparities (AHRQ, 2003).

In 2003, the Institute of Medicine identified "equity as one of the six fundamental domains of high quality healthcare" (Chin et al., 2007, p. 8S). The IOM defined equity as the provision of healthcare of equal quality based solely on need and clinical factors. They published a landmark book titled *Unequal Treatment: Confronting Racial and Ethnic Disparities in Healthcare,* which helped raise awareness about the sources of and solutions for health disparities. "Disparities at the patient, clinical encounter, and system levels" were discussed (Chin et al., 2007, p. 8S). The IOM report concluded that "to the extent that minority beneficiaries of publicly funded health programs are less likely to receive high quality care, these beneficiaries—as well as taxpayers that support public health programs—may face higher future healthcare costs" (U.S. Department of Health and Human Services, 2002, p. 116).

In 2005, the Robert Wood Johnson Foundation (RWJ), a private foundation, funded an initiative called the "Finding Answers: Disparities Research for Change," a program designed to identify, evaluate, and eliminate disparities associated with diabetes, depression, and cardiovascular disease. The RWJ Foundation sponsored research in these areas and studies that analyzed the effect of pay-for-performance and public reporting measures in decreasing health disparities. They created a searchable database (http://www.solvingdisparities.org) to describe the studies they funded. A summary of their funded studies concluded that culturally tailored interventions are more effective in reducing health disparities than are programs designed to be applicable to all groups of individuals. This body of research also supported studying diverse populations under everyday, nonexperimental situations that mirror real-world conditions rather than directing funding to randomized, controlled trials that may not mirror actual challenges that contribute to health disparities (Chin et al., 2007).

Why did the government—rather than researchers, professional organizations, private foundations, or community advocates—take the lead role in bringing health disparities to the forefront of dialogue and action in 1999? Why has this discussion about health disparities only recently become a priority when, in reality, health disparities have been present long before 1999? Is the government the most appropriate entity to assume a lead role in minimizing health disparities? What other entities need to be involved? Provide rationale for your answers to these questions.

RESEARCH AND EPIDEMIOLOGY: WHY DIVERSE POPULATIONS NEED TO BE COUNTED

Reliable and representative data on health disparities are a necessity if ethnic variations in access, treatment, and treatment response are to be understood. Adequate data are necessary if we are to identify areas of the greatest need, including "disparities that are responsive to improvements in health care," monitor trends over time, and discern which programs are successful in promoting equity (AHRQ, 2003, p. 2). Having sufficient data is especially important since there is a push toward evidence-based medicine, as well as reimbursement and allocation of resources that are tied to research evidence.

Without adequate numbers of individuals from varied groups participating in research or epidemiological surveys, sufficient statistical power cannot be achieved. In addition, it is difficult to detect and account for health disparities and to make a case for needed programs. Many studies and epidemiological databases have only included small samples of non-White populations, the elderly, the disabled, Asian/Pacific Islander individuals, and American Indian/Alaska Natives. In a number of large databases that are used to track health disparities, there are multiple entries where data on race and ethnicity is missing. The lack of consistency in reporting racial and ethnic categories and not allowing mixed race individuals to select a category such as "more than one race" significantly limits the information that is available for analysis.

"In addition, most private payer administrative data sources do not include race as a category" (CRCHD, 2004, p. 25).

After 2003, consistent federal standards for collection of race and ethnicity data were developed. Ethnic categories included Hispanic/Latino, non-Hispanic White, and non-Hispanic Black. Racial categories included White; Black; Asian; Native Hawaiian or Other Pacific Islander; American Indian/Alaska Native; and more than one race. The CLAS standards suggest one cannot "guess" an individual's background during admission to a healthcare facility. However, it continues to be the case that in a number of studies and registries, admission clerks record race and ethnicity data without asking the person to self-identify or provide their birth location, which is also a valuable data element. As one example of the magnitude of missing data, it has been estimated that one-third of American Indian and Alaska Native children are misidentified or not identified correctly, resulting in inaccurate death statistics (Epstein, 1997).

Socioeconomic status and level of education are not consistently collected, making it difficult to analyze the complex interactions that lead to health disparities. The National Healthcare Disparities Report (2003) recommended collecting SES data for (1) poor individuals below 100% of federal poverty level, (2) near-poor individuals whose income is 100 to 199% of federal poverty level, (3) individuals with middle incomes at 200 to 399% of federal poverty level, and (4) high incomes, which are 400% or more of the federal poverty level. These categories were suggested because differences between middle and high income people are significant in terms of health disparities (AHRQ, 2003).

Having an accurate baseline from which to gauge progress is vital. Many interventions and surveys have focused on Black and Latino populations, while other groups who experience disparities—such as pediatric and geriatric populations—are less frequently studied (Chin, 2007). At present it is not clear why disparities exist and which of the multiple contributing factors is most important. The complicated interrelationships between race, ethnicity, income, and education make analysis difficult. Data limitations have hindered efforts at minimizing health disparities (AHRQ, 2003), so it is vital to collect data on rural and urban areas and to track underutilization of services and high utilization of care, both of which can indicate poor healthcare quality. Given that different populations have different needs for service and different values, many have argued that measures are needed that capture the needs of specific racial, ethnic, age, gender, disability-related, and location-specific priorities (AHRQ, 2003).

It is necessary to recruit adequate numbers of diverse participants into large clinical trials to increase study generalizability and to reduce health disparities. However, it is difficult to recruit diverse participants because of a lack of trust regarding medical research, long questionnaires that impose high subject burdens and are not pertinent from the point of view of participants, extended follow-up periods that require long-term commitment, narrowly defined eligibility criteria for research participation, and a shortage of minority researchers who are skilled at recruiting diverse patients. Study recruitment is often not a priority for physicians and staff of busy clinics. Space for confidential interviewing is yet another barrier, as is obtaining a human subject's approval from multiple institutions if the study is a collaborative effort (Paskett et al., 2008).

Advantages for diverse populations participating in clinical trials include increased access to the newest treatments and technologies and having adequate data for the legislature to use when creating funding agendas and priorities. Solutions that have been suggested include use of a community advisory board, recruiting and explaining the study in a group format, using multiple recruitment sites, offering incentives for participation, establishing a toll-free number for participants to contact researchers, and creating personalized and culturally appropriate recruitment materials (Paskett et al., 2008).

Options for Monitoring and Simultaneously Minimizing Health Disparities

Several methods of monitoring and evaluating health disparities are also ways of minimizing disparities. The Surveillance Epidemiology and End Results (SEER) software is available on the National Cancer Institute Website. By using this calculator it is possible to explore cross-sectional and trend data (cancer rates, survival, stage at diagnosis) according to geographic area, SES, and/or race and ethnicity. Four absolute and seven relative summary measures of disparity can be calculated. It is a valuable online resource for designing research, intervening, and monitoring progress in eliminating cancer-related health disparities (SEER, 2010).

Another solution for minimizing health disparities involves increased funding for community based participatory research (CBPR). CBPR is a collaborative approach that begins with a research topic of importance to the community and adds academic knowledge "with a goal of promoting social change, improving community health, and reducing disparities" (Dankwa-Mullan et al., 2010, p. S 23). Rather than being a method, CBPR is an orientation that relies on equitable engagement of all partners throughout the research process from problem definition through data collection and analysis, to the dissemination and use of findings to help effect change" (Dankwa-Mullan, et al., 2010, p. S23).

FUTURE TRENDS AND ASSOCIATED COSTS

Although significant disparities exist, improvement is possible and necessary in order to contain healthcare costs and provide equitable care to the entire U.S. population. As Braveman and colleagues (2010) commented, "the health of the most socially advantaged group in a society indicates a level of health that should be possible for everyone" (p. S194). Many of the factors that contribute to health disparities are modifiable if, as a society, we adopt policies to promote equity and health.

However, "demographic trends indicate that the numbers of Americans who are vulnerable to suffering the effects of healthcare disparities will rise over the next half century . . . Some racial and ethnic minorities are growing at a much more rapid pace than the White population. Nearly 1 in 2 Americans will be a member of a racial or ethnic minority by the year 2050" (AHRQ, 2003, p. 1). In addition, the baby boomer population is aging and will place significant demands on the healthcare system. Beyond the human costs of health disparities, there are substantial financial costs that are borne by taxpayers associated with delayed and increasingly expensive treatment, costs that result in higher healthcare insurance premiums, and malpractice costs, as well as costs from months and years of lost productivity. Elimination of health disparities needs to be a top public policy priority (AHRQ, 2003).

HEALTH POLICY OPTIONS FOR REDUCING HEALTH DISPARITIES

If policies to reduce health disparities are not adopted, existing disparities will increase and quality of life for everyone will be impacted. Evidence indicates that disparities in access to, use of, and quality of care result in significant medical, social, and economic consequences (Schnittker & McLeod, 2005). A variety of health policy recommendations have been proposed for reducing health disparities, including:

1. expanding healthcare insurance coverage;
2. funding community-level interventions (community-based participatory research and education) specifically designed to reduce geographic differences in health;
3. empowering patients and family members to become more active partners in their health care;
4. facilitating coordination of care between care providers and systems of care by integrating health, social, and supportive services;

5. supporting pay-for-performance and public reporting of health outcomes;
6. funding more primary prevention activities;
7. conducting economic analyses to determine which interventions provide the highest level of benefit for the resources expended;
8. beginning by targeting the most preventable/curable diseases and diseases with the highest economic burden;
9. targeting groups with the highest need and amount of health disparity;
10. recruiting diverse providers and educating all providers to understand the culture and language of the communities that they serve;
11. using patient navigators, case managers, and promotoras
12. focusing on demand and supply level impediments (such as limitations on cigarette company advertisements);
13. reimbursing for evidence-based interventions known to be effective with given conditions;
14. providing reimbursement for care delivered via mobile health using information technology; and
15. activating shared cultural norms and practices when motivating behavioral change (Chin et al., 2007; CRCHD, 2004).

For example, the term cultural leverage, which is a focused strategy for improving the health of ethnic communities by incorporating their cultural practices and products into interventions, is commonly used. Values, rituals, music, and communication practices of varied racial and ethnic groups are taught to staff and incorporated into programs designed to foster behavioral change. It is thought that culturally tailored approaches work because they are the sine qua non of individualized care (Chin et al., 2007).

Whichever health policy approach is selected, it is well known that multi-factored interventions are most effective. Whatever option is selected, nurses should be involved because they are cost-effective providers, are able to spend time with patients, and know how to tailor interventions to match the specific needs of an individual who has a health disparity. Nurses are trained to work in teams, have been educated to be patient-centered, and have learned about cultural differences during their undergraduate education (Chin et al., 2007).

DISCUSSION QUESTIONS

1. Discuss one factor or one healthcare policy within the United States that contributes to a specific health disparity.
2. What should the role of government be in decreasing health disparities?
3. What should the role of community and church groups be in decreasing health disparities?
4. Why should groups who experience health disparities be involved in helping to minimize health disparities?
5. Talk about one positive way the quality of care provided in the clinical setting where you are working this semester minimizes a specific health disparity. Talk about one way in which the quality of care in that facility needs to be improved to further minimize a specific health disparity.
6. Discuss an example of a gender-related, an age-related, and a language-related health disparity.
7. Why should the United States develop health policies designed to minimize health disparities? What are the most important reasons for doing this?
8. How do patient navigator programs (in which recovered patients help newly diagnosed patients understand where to get help and how to deal with the healthcare system) help to minimize health disparities?
9. How could the burden of a disease be greater in one group than another? Give an example that explains your answer.
10. What factors might influence an individual to refuse or delay treatment?
11. How are language fluency and health disparities related?
12. What is the immigrant paradox and why is it important to consider?
13. Why do health disparities exist in systems like Medicare and the Veteran's Administration, where everyone in that system can theoretically access care?
14. Which national laws, policies, and standards influence how health disparities are defined or treated?
15. What are the differences between prevalence and incidence rates?
16. Talk about several of the healthcare disparities that are the most costly to treat.
17. Why is increasing first contact access to services important?
18. Should disease incidences and mortality rates be compared to a White population, the population with the best health in a given category, or the total U.S. population? Explain your answer.

CHECK YOUR UNDERSTANDING

Rank order the following health policy options (1 to 15) in terms of their cost. Offer a rationale for why the policy should or should not be adopted, and who should pay for the policy change.

The health policy options you are to rank are:

1. Expanding healthcare insurance coverage

2. Funding community-level interventions (community-based participatory research and education) specifically designed to reduce geographic differences in health

3. Empowering patients and family members to become more active partners in their health care

4. Facilitating coordination of care between care providers and systems of care by integrating health, social, and supportive services

5. Supporting pay-for-performance and public reporting of health outcomes

6. Funding more primary prevention activities

7. Conducting economic analyses to determine which interventions provide the highest level of benefit for the resources expended

8. Beginning by targeting the most preventable/curable diseases and diseases with the highest economic burden

9. Targeting groups with the highest need and most health disparity

10. Recruiting diverse providers and educating all providers to understand the culture and language of the communities that they serve

11. Using patient navigators, case managers, and promotoras

12. Focusing on demand and supply level impediments (such as limitations on cigarette company advertisements)

13. Reimbursing for evidence-based interventions known to be effective with given conditions

14. Providing reimbursement for care delivered via mobile health using information technology

15. Activating shared cultural norms and practices when motivating behavioral change (Chin et al., 2007; CRCHD, 2004).

Please complete the following table and you proceed with this assignment.

Rank Order	Health Policy Option	Rationale for Why the Health Policy Should or Should Not Be Adopted	Who Should Pay for Implementing the Policy? Provide a Rationale for Your Answer.
1. (Most Costly)			
2.			
3.			
4.			
5.			
6.			
7.			
8.			
9.			
10.			
11.			
12.			
13.			
14.			
15. (Least Costly)			

WHAT DO YOU THINK?

1. Which health disparities are most common in the clinical setting where you are placed this semester?
2. What are the largest barriers to health and health care you or someone in your family has faced? How did you or your family member navigate around those barriers?
3. What did being sick mean in your family? How did that meaning differ compared to another family you knew? Who cared for you when you were sick as a child?
4. How would you improve the measurement or monitoring of health disparities in the United States?

5. Should federal funding be allocated to reduce health disparities based on location (such as a rural area or inner city where there are fewer healthcare providers)?

6. Are disabled individuals at greater risk for health disparities? Explain your answer.

7. Does everyone have a right to equal quality health care? Why or why not?

8. Are there dangers associated with requiring physicians to use evidence-based data when prescribing medical treatments? Explain your answer.

9. Do you agree or disagree with the statement that the health of the healthiest group in a society shows what everyone should be able to achieve in terms of health? Explain your answer.

10. Should translators be available 24 hours a day in healthcare facilities or should English as the official language of the United States as a policy be followed? Explain your answer.

11. Have you or anyone in your family ever had trouble receiving a referral to a specialist? Describe what factors influenced that slow referral.

12. Have you neglected any yearly recommended health screenings since being in nursing school? What factors motivated you to neglect those screenings or to schedule them in a timely fashion?

13. Has it ever been hard for you to ask a patient what their ethnic or racial background was? How did you handle that?

14. Have you ever forgotten or had trouble understanding what a healthcare provider was recommending that you do to improve your health? Discuss that situation.

15. Should free school lunch programs be continued or discontinued? Explain your answer.

16. Should limits be placed on the amount of healthcare dollars expended on individuals over the age of 95? Explain why that would or would not be a good idea.

REFERENCES

Agency for Healthcare Research and Quality [AHRQ]. (2003). *National healthcare disparities report.* Rockville, MD: U.S. Department of Health and Human Services.

Braveman, P. A., Cubbin, C., Egeter, S., Williams, D. R., & Pamuk, E. (2010). Socioeconomic disparities in health in the United States: What the patterns tell us. *American Journal of Public Health, 100*(S1), S186–S196.

Center to Reduce Cancer Health Disparities [CRCHD]. (2004). *Economic costs of cancer health disparities: Summary of meeting proceedings.* Bethesda, MD: U.S. Department of Health and Human Services.

Center to Reduce Cancer Health Disparities [CRCHD]. (Dec 6–7, 2004). *Summary of meeting proceedings: Economic costs of cancer health disparities.* Bethesda, MD: National Cancer Institute.

Center to Reduce Cancer Health Disparities [CRCHD]. (2011a). *Health disparities defined.* Retrieved from http://crchd.cancer.gov/disparities/defined.html

Center to Reduce Cancer Health Disparities [CRCHD]. (2011b). *Cancer health disparities*. Retrieved from http://www.cancer.gov/cancertopics/factsheet/cancer-health-disparities

Chin, M. H., Walters, A. E., Cook, S. C., & Huang, E. S. (2007). Interventions to reduce racial and ethnic disparities in healthcare. *Medical Care Research and Review, 64*, 7S–28S.

Cooper, C., Tandy, A. R., Balamurali, T., & Livingston, G. (2010). A systematic review and meta-analysis of ethnic differences in use of dementia treatment, care, and research. *American Journal of Geriatric Psychiatry, 18*(3), 193–203.

Dankwa-Mullan, I., Rhee, K. B., Staff, D. M., Pohlhaus, J. R., Sy, F., Stinson, N., & Riffin, J. (2010). Moving toward paradigm-shifting research in health disparities through translational, transformational, and transdisciplinary approaches. *American Journal of Public Health, 100*(S1), S19–S24.

Egan, M., Tannahill, C., Petticrew, M., & Thomas, S. (2008). Psychosocial risk factors in home and community settings and their associations with population health and health inequalities: A systematic meta-review. *BMC Public Health, 8*, 239. Doi:10.1186/1471-2458-8-239.

Egley, A., & O'Donnell, C. E. (2009). *OJJDP Fact Sheet: Highlights of the 2007 National Youth Gang Survey*, Washington, DC: USDOJ, Office of Justice Programs, Office of Juvenile Justice and Delinquency Prevention. Retrieved from http://www.ncjrs.gov/pdffiles1/ojjdp/225185.pdf

Epstein, M., Moreno, R., & Bacchetti, P. (1997). The underreporting of deaths of American Indian children in California, 1979 through 1993. *American Journal of Public Health, 87*(8), 1363–1366.

Federico, S. G., Abrams, L., Everhart, R. M., Melinkovich, P., & Hambidge, S. J. (2010). Addressing adolescent immunization disparities: A retrospective analysis of school-based health center immunization delivery. *American Journal of Public Health, 100*(9), 1630–1634.

Fiscella, K., & Williams, D. R. (2004). Health disparities based on socioeconomic inequities: Implications for urban healthcare *Academic Medicine, 79*(12), 1139–1147.

Gallo, L. C., de los Monteros, K. E., Allison, M., Roux, A. D., Polak, J. F., Watson, K. E., & Morales, L. S. (2009). Do socioeconomic gradients in subclinical atherosclerosis vary according to acculturation level? Analyses of Mexican-Americans in the multi-ethnic study of atherosclerosis. *Psychosomatic Medicine, 71*(7), 756–762.

Gibbons, M.C. (2011). Use of health information technology among racial and ethnic underserved communities. *Perspectives in Health Information Management*, 1–13.

Goyal, D., Murphy, S. O. & Cohen, J. (2006). Immigrant Asian Indian women and postpartum depression. *Journal of Obstetrical and Gynecological Neonatal Nursing, 35*(1), 98–104.

Hahn, R. A., Eaker, E., Barker, N. D., Teutsch, S. M., Sosniak, W., & Krieger, N. (1995). Poverty and death in the United States. *Epidemiology, 6*(5), 490–497.

Hall, E. T. & Hall, M. R. (1990). *Understanding cultural differences*. Yarmouth, ME: Intercultural Press.

Han, H., Lee, J., Kim, J., Hedlin, H., Song, H., & Kim, M. (2009). A meta-analysis of interventions to promote mammography among ethnic minority women. *Nursing Research, 58*(4), 246–254. Doi: 10.1097/NNR.Obo13c3181acOf7f.

Kessler, R. C., Mickelson, K. D., & Williams, D. R. (1999). The prevalence, distribution, and mental health correlates of perceived discrimination in the United States. *Journal of Health and Social Behavior, 40*(3), 208–230.

La Veist, T. A., Gaskin, D. J., & Richard, P. (2009). *The economic burden of health inequalities in the United States*. Washington, DC: Joint Center for Political and Economic Studies.

Leninger, M., & McFarland, M. (2002). *Transcultural nursing: Concepts, theory, research, and practice*. (3rd ed.), New York, NY: McGraw-Hill Professional.

Lewis, N. M. (2009). Mental health in sexual minorities: Recent indicators, trends, and their relationships to place in North America and Europe. *Health and Place, 15*, 1029–1045.

Mathias, R. A., Grant, A. V., Rafaels, N., Hand, T., Gao, L., Vergara, C., . . . Barnes, K. C. (2009). A genome-wide association study on African ancestry populations for asthma. *Journal of Allergy and Clinical Immunology, 125*(2), 336–347.

National Institute of Child Health and Human Development (2003). *Health disparities: Bridging the gap.* Bethesda, MD: U.S. Department of Health and Human Services.

National Institute on Drug Abuse [NIDA]. (2011). *Health disparities news: Recent findings.* Retrieved from http://www.drugabuse.gov/about/organization/healthdisparities/news/index.html.

Nicholson, R. A., Kreuter, M. W., & Lapka, C., Wellborn, R., Clark, E. M., Sanderes-Thompson, V., . . . Casey, C. (2008). Unintended effects of emphasizing disparities in cancer communication to African-Americans. *Cancer Epidemiology, Biomarkers & Prevention, 17,* 2946–2953.

Pamuk, E. R., Makuk, D. M., Heck, K. E., Reuben, C., & Lochner, K. (1998). *Health, United States, 1998, with socioeconomic status and health chartbook.* Hyattsville, MD: National Center for Health Statistics.

Paskett, E. D., Reeves, K. W., McLaughlin, J. M., Katz, M. L., McAlearney, A. S., Ruffin, M. T., . . . Gehlert, S. (2008). Recruitment of minority and underserved populations in the United States: The Centers for Population Health and Health Disparities experience. *Contemporary Clinical Trials, 29*(6), 847–861.

Roblin, D. W., Houston, T. K., Allison, J. J., Joski, P. J., & Becker, E. R. (2009). Disparities in use of a personal health record in a managed care organization. *Journal of the American Medical Informatics Association, 16*(5), 683–689. DOI: 10.1197/jamia.M3169 PMCID: PMC2744719.

Shavers, V. L. & Brown, M. L. (2002). Racial and ethnic disparities in the receipt of cancer treatment. *Journal of the National Cancer Institute, 94*(5), 334–357.

Schnittker, J. & McLeod, J. D. (2005). The social psychology of health disparities. *Annual Review of Sociology, 31,* 75–103.

Starfield, B. (1992). *Primary care: Concept, evaluation, and policy.* New York, NY: Oxford University Press.

Surveillance Epidemiology and End Results [SEER]. (2010). Health disparities calculator. Retrieved from http://seer.cancer.gov/hdcalc

Tirado, M. (2011). Role of mobile health in the care of culturally and linguistically diverse U.S. populations. *Perspective in Health Information Management,* 1–7.

U.S. Department of Health and Human Services (2001). *National standards for culturally and linguistically appropriate services in healthcare: Executive Summary.* Washington, DC: Office of Minority Health.

U.S. Department of Health and Human Services. (2002). *Health, United States, 2002: With chart book on trends in the health of Americans.* Hyattsville, MD: National Center for Health Statistics. Table 28, Life expectancy at birth, at 65 years of age, and at 75 years of age, according to race and sex: United States, selected years 1900–99, p. 116.

Yu, T., Chou, C., Johnson, P. J., & Ward, A. (2010). Persistent disparities in Pap test use: Assessments and predictions for Asian women in the US, 1982-2010. *Journal of Immigrant Minority Health, 12,* 445-453.

Williams, D. R., & Mohammed, S. A. (2008). Poverty, migration, and health. In A. Lin and D. Harris (Eds.), *The colors of poverty* (pp. 135–169). New York, NY: Russell Sage Foundation.

Williams, D. R., & Rucker, T. D. (2000). Understanding and addressing racial disparities in healthcare *Healthcare Financing Review, 21*(4), 75–90

For a full suite of assignments and additional learning activities, see the access code at the front of your book.

CHAPTER 6

Health Literacy

Bonnie Raingruber

OBJECTIVES

At the conclusion of this chapter, students will be able to:

- Articulate why there is a need to address health literacy.
- Explain how types of health literacy differ.
- Compare and contrast definitions of health literacy.
- Critique health literacy screening tools.
- Describe health literacy challenges typically encountered when working with children and adolescents.
- Identify effective strategies for improving health literacy.

INTRODUCTION

Since 1990, health literacy has become a popular topic within the health promotion literature and a major concern of governmental and healthcare agencies. Health literacy is one of four top priorities in public health in the United States (Clement et al., 2009). Improving health literacy is an objective listed in both Healthy People 2010 and 2020 (Speros, 2005). In 2004, the Institute of Medicine issued a report that explained health literacy as a function of both social and individual factors, reframing the issue as one of shared responsibility (Baur, 2010). The Joint Commission on Accreditation of Hospitals includes a standard of accreditation that patients must receive oral and written information about their care that is understandable to them. To be understandable, information must be tailored to a patient's health literacy needs. In addition, the Joint Commission's national patient safety goals require that patients be active participants in their care, a reality that is difficult for individuals with low health literacy (Murphy-Knoll, 2007). In 2010, the National Institutes of Health (NIH), the Agency for Health Care Research and Quality (AHRQ), and the Centers for Disease Control and Prevention (CDC) introduced funding opportunities that focused on improving health literacy. Also in 2010, the Office of the Surgeon General sponsored a workshop and a number of town halls to identify best practices to improve health literacy. A national action plan derived from that effort and released by the U.S. Department of Health and Human Services emphasized the importance of coordinating healthcare services, public health programs, and educational efforts (Baur, 2010). Earlier, in 2007, the World Health Organization (WHO) had already identified health literacy as "having a central role in determining inequities in health in both rich and poor countries" (Nutbeam, 2008, p. 2073).

Lower health literacy has been linked to higher healthcare costs, longer hospitalizations, infrequent use of preventative health care, delays in seeking care, higher levels of chronic disease, and more frequent and inefficient use of costly services (Hinojosa, et al., 2010; Paasche-Orlow & Wolf, 2007). Individuals with lower health literacy put off health care, enter the system in poorer health, and are often hospitalized for reasons that could have been prevented (Hinojosa, Hinojosa, Nelson, & Delgado, 2010).

Health literacy is a risk factor that is mediated by access to and utilization of health care, patient–provider communication, social support, and self-care abilities (von Wagner, Steptoe, Wolf, & Wardle, 2009). When patients are unfamiliar with their disease, they are less likely to ask questions of a provider and less likely to share in decision making about their health (Peerson & Saunders, 2009). Oftentimes, providers are unaware of their patient's limited literacy, and as a result they fail to tailor teaching and treatment recommendations to ensure understanding. Providers may become frustrated that patients with lower health literacy use unscientific descriptions of their medical problems or are not accurate in presenting their medical history (Paasche-Orlow & Wolf, 2007). Lower health literacy results in individuals misunderstanding healthcare instructions, which can lead to not adhering to prescribed treatments or not taking an active role in self-care. Individuals with lower health literacy are more likely to make medication errors and not understand when to seek care for adverse side effects; they are also frequently not familiar with the health benefits associated with setting self-care goals and as a result are not motivated to do so. These individuals are not equipped to select the best insurance policy for their needs, locate a provider that is a good fit for their condition, or draft a letter explaining an error on a healthcare bill (Paasche-Orlow & Wolf, 2007; Rothman et al., 2010).

Health literacy has been described as predicting health status and health outcomes to a greater degree than economic status, age, or ethnic/racial background

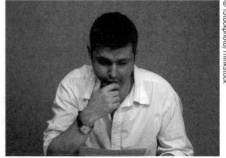

© iStockphoto/Thinkstock

(Speros, 2005). Individuals with inadequate health literacy are more than twice as likely to be hospitalized compared to those with adequate health literacy (Baker, Parker, Williams, & Clark, 1998). These individuals also experience shame and worry that their limited literacy will be exposed. "Distrust of providers, pessimism about treatment, and lower satisfaction with care" are common among those with low health literacy (Paasche-Orlow & Wolf, 2007, p. S20).

As the healthcare system becomes more fragmented and complex, it becomes even more difficult for individuals with poor health literacy to navigate the healthcare system (Speros, 2005). As von Wagner and colleagues (2009) commented, "Medical decisions often involve technical terms, complex ideas, multiple options, and the need to differentially weigh the relative value of unfamiliar choices" (p. 869). Low health literacy makes it difficult to navigate complex medical systems and participate as an active partner in shared decision making. Individuals with lower health literacy are more likely to rely on emotional or experiential knowledge rather than analytical information processing to make healthcare decisions, even though analysis is needed in weighing benefits and risks of varied health treatments.

Navigation skills are broad in that they include the ability to locate an office in a large medical center, use the Internet to obtain health information, schedule and obtain coverage for needed health conditions, ask relevant questions during brief appointments, choose between complex healthcare options, understand where to obtain help if needed, and how to select a provider that meets one's needs. Many interventions have been directed toward improving the health literacy of individuals, although efforts to reform the healthcare delivery system to make it more user friendly and understandable to all is also needed (von Wagner et al., 2009).

The National Adult Literacy Survey (NALS) documented that 25% of the United States population is functionally illiterate and a slightly higher number have marginal literacy skills (Speros, 2005). The United States ranked 12th among 20 high-income nations in terms of literacy (Perlow, 2010). Individuals over the age of 65, immigrants, those from lower socioeconomic backgrounds, those with less education, people who are experiencing poor health, and African American and Hispanic individuals are the most likely to suffer from poor health literacy (Baur, 2010; Cutilli & Bennett, 2009; Paasche-Orlow et al., 2005). Forty-six percent of this at-risk population has more than one disability. Thirty-five percent did not speak English before they began their formal education (Cutilli & Bennett, 2009). Among respondents with Medicare or Medicaid, 27% and 30%, respectively, had below-basic health literacy (Perlow, 2010). In fact, individuals who have the greatest need to understand healthcare information are least likely to be able to do so (Speros, 2005).

Low health literacy "affects 39% of adult Americans, more than obesity, diabetes, HIV/AIDS, and breast cancer combined" (Fetter, 2009, p. 798). Health literacy will continue to be a major challenge because elderly and minority populations are growing, numbers of Americans with limited English proficiency are increasing, more medications are being prescribed, hospital stays are shorter, and treatment is shifting to home-based and community-based settings.

To understand health literacy, healthcare professionals must assess cognitive skills, knowledge of relevant facts, age-related cognitive decline in working memory, learning and communication disorders, mental disabilities, reading and mathematical ability, verbal skills, English language fluency, and any visual and hearing deficits experienced by their patients (Baur, 2010; von Wagner et al., 2009). For patients to be fully participating partners in their health care, they must have the necessary attention, memory, and decision-making skills needed to engage in healthy behaviors.

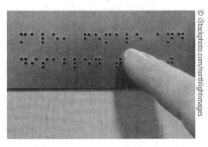

Required health literacy skills include the ability to locate and evaluate information, follow healthcare directives, and analyze information to select the best course of action from among choices. Having accurate and disease-specific knowledge, as well as familiarity with treatment options, has been shown to be a prerequisite to goal setting and motivation in order to engage in behavioral change (von Wagner et al., 2009). As for ambulatory care and community-based settings where patients, not healthcare personnel, are responsible for carrying out treatments, health literacy issues can be even more pronounced than in hospital settings (Hasnain-Wynia & Wolf, 2010).

Health literacy is important because of its relationship to health status, health disparities, medical costs, and active patient participation in decision making (Mancuso, 2009). Adequate health literacy helps patients "understand the problem, seek information from various sources, [and] make informed and shared decisions that lead to better treatment adherence and subsequent self-management" (Ishikawa & Yano, 2008, p. 118).

TYPES OF HEALTH LITERACY

Nutbeam (1999) described three types of health literacy:

Level 1: Functional health literacy, or the ability to read, write, and understand factual information regarding health risks.

Level 2: Interactive health literacy, or the ability to optimize prevention and self-management of disease via problem solving, communication, and decision making while applying new information to changing circumstances.

Level 3: Critical health literacy, or the ability to analyze information and participate in navigating health-related barriers while taking action at both the individual and community level by influencing social norms (Peerson & Saunders, 2009).

Interactive health literacy includes the concepts of motivation or inclination to act in health promoting ways, personal empowerment, and behavioral change (Nutbeam, 2000, 2008).

In 2003, the National Assessment of Health Literacy (NAAL), the largest survey focused on health literacy, was conducted by the U.S. Department of Education. Three types of literacy, including prose, document, and quantitative, were evaluated. Prose literacy required that the participant read several paragraphs and search, comprehend, and use the health information presented in formats similar to those seen in brochures and instructional handouts. Document literacy measured the ability to use information from noncontinuous texts such as applications and food labels. Quantitative literacy required that individuals use numbers to calculate medication doses and complete other computations. Individuals were ranked as having below-basic, basic, intermediate and proficient health literacy. Below-basic literacy is less than what is needed to function in a healthcare setting. Individuals with basic literacy can read and understand simple information and complete one-step mathematical calculations, while having an intermediate level of literacy allows one to summarize health-related

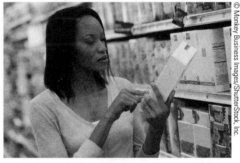

content and develop inferences. Proficiency implies individuals can understand lengthy and complex written material and synthesize the information to arrive at conclusions (Cutilli & Bennett, 2009).

The NAAL found that 12% of individuals had proficient health literacy, 53% had an intermediate level of health literacy, 22% had basic health literacy, and 14% had below-basic health literacy. White and Asian/Pacific Islander adults had higher health literacy than Black and Hispanic adults. Individuals who spoke Spanish before starting school had below-basic health literacy; adults over 65 had the lowest average health literacy. Women overall scored six points higher on health literacy measures than men. Individuals with less than a high school diploma and those living at or below poverty levels reported lower health literacy (Cutilli & Bennett, 2009). More than 50% of the adult population in the United States has difficulty understanding health insurance, Medicare forms, and pre- or postoperative instruction (Fetter, 2009).

DEFINITIONS OF HEALTH LITERACY

Health literacy has to do with whether individuals are able to comprehend health and self-care information and whether healthcare institutions are able to provide education that is accessible to everyone. Health literacy involves "assessing, understanding, and using information to make health decisions" (Peerson & Saunders, 2009, p. 285). The ability to read and comprehend, to manage numerical calculations, and to use information in healthcare decision making are all aspects of health literacy. Health literacy includes the ability to read and understand prescription labels, over-the-counter medication labels, appointment slips, health instructions, directions to appointments, admission forms, insurance forms, and consent forms. It also involves recognizing the value of health prevention activities such as physical exams, mammograms, immunizations, and Papanicolaou (PAP) smears. Being informed about healthy menu choices and exercise options are also important components of health literacy. Clues that a person has difficulty with health literacy include not being able to name medications or dosages, trouble with remembering one's health history, or frequently making comments about leaving one's glasses at home when being asked to read over healthcare instructions in an office or hospital setting (Speros, 2005).

Numerous different definitions have been used for health literacy, including:

1. "The ability to perform health-related tasks requiring reading and computational skills." This definition resulted from the TOFHLA research sponsored by the Robert Wood Johnson Foundation (Speros, 2005, p. 635).
2. "A constellation of skills, including the ability to perform basic reading and numerical tasks required to function in the healthcare environment" (American Medical Association Ad Hoc Committee on Health Literacy for the Council on Scientific Affairs, 1999, p. 553).
3. "The degree to which individuals have the capacity to obtain, process, and understand basic health information and services needed to make appropriate health decisions" (U.S. Department of Health and Human Services, 2000, pp. 11–12). This definition is used in the Healthy People initiatives and by the National Institutes of Health. It is not limited to individuals in healthcare settings, but also applies to community settings. Inherent in the definition within the "capacity to obtain" phrase is that health care is accessible (affordable and tailored to various needs—e.g., vision, hearing, and mobility needs) (Perlow, 2010).
4. "The cognitive and social skills which determine the motivation, and ability of individuals to gain access to, understand, and use information in ways that promote and maintain good health" (WHO, 1998, p. 10). This definition

includes the knowledge and confidence to take action by changing personal lifestyles and improving the health of communities (Nutbeam, 2008).

5. "The ability to make sound health decisions in the context of everyday life at home, in the community, at the workplace, in the healthcare system, the marketplace, and the political arena enabling people to exert control over their health, seek out information and assume responsibility for their health" (Kickbusch, Wait, & Maag, 2005, p. 8).

6. "A wide range of skills and competencies that people develop to seek out, comprehend, evaluate, and use health information and concepts to make informed choices, reduce health risks, and increase quality of life" (Zarcadoolas, Pleasant, & Greer, 2005, pp. 196–197).

7. "The knowledge and skills required to understand and use information relating to health issues such as drugs and alcohol, disease prevention and treatment, safety and accident prevention, first aid, emergencies, and staying healthy (Australian Bureau of Statistics, 2006, p 4.)

8. "The ability of U.S. adults to use printed and written health-related information to function in society, to achieve one's goals, and to develop one's knowledge and potential" (White, 2008, p. viii). This definition was used in the National Assessment of Adult Literacy in 2003.

9. "The ability to find, understand, appraise, and communicate information to promote health across the life-course" (Rootman & El-Bihbety, 2008, p. 11). This definition came from a Canadian expert panel on literacy.

Authors have stressed that attributes of the healthcare system must be mentioned in definitions of health literacy, not just individual, patient-level characteristics. Healthcare system attributes include things such as rules governing what health plans cover, changing formulary coverage, and physicians who leave the network. Other healthcare system issues include shortened timeframes for patient–provider communication, more emphasis on factual/scientific explanation, and an increase in specialized/fragmented care (Paasche-Orlow & Wolf, 2007).

TOOLS FOR MEASURING HEALTH LITERACY

A variety of standardized patient screening forms for evaluating health literacy have been published. Screening tools are not routinely used in clinical practice in spite of the fact that the literacy needs of many patients go undetected.

In 1992, the Robert Wood Johnson Foundation funded physicians from Emory University and the University of California at Los Angeles to conduct a 2-year study on the ability to read and complete mathematical calculations needed to function in a healthcare setting. This was one of the first studies on health literacy conducted on a large scale. These researchers developed the Test of Functional Health Literacy in Adults (TOFHLA), which has come to be the gold standard of health literacy screening. The TOFHLA measures reading and numeracy skills as well as comprehension. Both English and Spanish versions of the TOFHLA exist, as well as a 14-point font format for those with impaired vision. A score of 0–59 indicates inadequate functional health literacy, scores from 60 to 74 indicate marginal functional health literacy, and scores of 75–100 indicate adequate functional health literacy. Reliability is 0.98 and criterion and content validity are good. The full-length TOFHLA takes 25 minutes to administer. Fifty items measure reading comprehension and 17 items measure numerical ability. Within the reading comprehension section are instructions for preparing for an upper gastrointestinal series, a patient rights and responsibilities section of a Medicaid application and a consent form. The numerical section asks individuals to comprehend instructions on prescription bottles, directions for monitoring blood glucose levels, keeping clinic appointments, and applying for financial assistance (Baker, Parker, Williams, & Clark, 1998; Speros, 2005).

A brief TOFHLA contains 2 reading passages and 4 numerical items, and it takes 12 minutes to administer. Reliability for the reading section is good (0.97) but questionable for the numerical items (0.68). A short TOFHLA, which takes 7 minutes to administer, has good reliability and validity. However, with the short TOFHLA only reading comprehension is measured, not health literacy. The Spanish versions of the TOFHLA have no reported reliability or validity data (Baker, Parker, Williams & Clark, 1998; Mancuso, 2010).

The National Assessment of Adult Literacy was developed in 2004 by the National Center for Education Statistics in the U.S. Department of Education. The NAAL consists of 28 health tasks in each of three literacy categories. Scores are below-basic, basic, intermediate, and proficient. The NAAL demonstrated 37% of Americans had basic or below-basic health literacy, which could make it difficult to locate health information in complex documents or could create challenges when making simple inferences regarding health conditions. The NAAL documented that lower health literacy predicted health disparities, poor access to information, and limited health insurance coverage (Bankson, 2009; von Wagner et al., 2009).

Between the administration of the National Adult Literacy Survey in 1992 and the NAAL in 2003, quantitative literacy scores in the United States improved to some degree but prose and document literacy did not. In a world where medical terminology and treatment options are becoming increasingly complex, less than half the adult population has adequate health literacy. Tasks such as identifying drinks permitted before a medical test or calculating dosages of over-the-counter medications are beyond the capabilities of individuals with marginal healthcare literacy (Nath, 2007).

The Health Activity Literacy Scale (HALS) evaluates health promotion, health protection, disease prevention, health care and maintenance, and navigation skills, including a focus on oral communication. It takes up to 1 hour to administer. Reliability and validity are still being evaluated (Nutbeam, 2008).

The Adult Literacy and Life Skills Survey (ALLS) includes subscales of literacy, document literacy, numeracy, problem-solving, and health literacy. It covers health promotion, health protection, disease prevention, health care, disease management, and navigation. Included are activities such as reading newspapers, comprehending bus schedules, calculating time of medication administration, locating health facilities, providing consent, planning an exercise regime, or avoiding the use of certain products that interfere with health (Peerson & Saunders, 2009).

The Wide Range Achievement Test (WRAT) evaluates reading, word recognition, and arithmetic but is not based on scenarios from healthcare settings. The WRAT is a standardized reading test with good reliability and validity that is used to determine grade level reading ability. The test takes 20–30 minutes to administer. One level is designed for children age 5 to 11, while another is for ages 12–64. The MART was developed from the WRAT. The MART has good reliability and validity with an administration time of 3 to 5 minutes. It only measures word recognition, not understanding, and it has not been researched in studies other than the original publication, which is a major limitation (Mancuso, 2010).

The Rapid Estimate of Adult Literacy in Medicine (REALM) only takes 5 minutes to administer and is therefore considered to be a practical option for use in busy healthcare practices, including primary care and public health settings. It is a word recognition test based on 125 health-related words. Patients are asked to read the words aloud and are scored based on correct pronunciation. Test–retest reliability is 0.98 and validity is good. A shortened version of the REALM relies on 66 words which can be administered in 3 minutes. Validity (0.96) and reliability (0.99) of the shortened version remain excellent. Yet another shorter version contains 11 words and can be administered in 2 minutes; here, reliability (0.91) continues to be good but the validity is questionable (0.64). All three forms of the REALM are available in English and only measure reading and pronunciation, not understanding (Mancuso, 2009; von Wagner et al., 2009).

The Short Assessment of Health Literacy for Spanish-speaking Adults (SAHLSA) was developed from the REALM. It is a word recognition test in which each term must be associated with a similar word to demonstrate comprehension. There is no numerical section. Reliability (0.92) is excellent but validity is questionable (0.65). Scoring takes 3–6 minutes. The SAHLSA was tested on a small sample of females and needs to be evaluated with additional populations (Mancuso, 2009).

The Newest Vital Sign (NVS) assessment allows for quick (3 minutes or less) clinical screening. It requires that individuals read and evaluate an ice cream nutrition label accompanied by six questions that test reading and quantitative skills. It has been shown to be sensitive in assessing marginal rates of health literacy. It is available in English and Spanish and is free and downloadable off the Internet (http://www.pfizerhealthliteracy .com). The NVS requires further testing because, although the English version has acceptable reliability (0.76), the Spanish version does not (0.69) (Fetter, 2009; Mancuso, 2009; von Wagner et al., 2009). Why do you think the authors of the Newest Vital Sign tool selected the name for their test that they did?

Chew and colleagues (2004) proposed using brief screening questions, including: 1) How often do you have someone help you read hospital materials?; 2) How confident are you filling out medical forms by yourself?; and 3) How often do you have problems learning about your medical condition because of difficulty understanding written information? Their research was conducted on primarily male Caucasian veterans, and the questions did not do a good job identifying individuals with marginal health literacy (Mancuso, 2009).

The Spoken Knowledge in Low Literacy Patients with Diabetes (SKILLD) scale focuses specifically on diabetes knowledge. Scores on this instrument correlate with Hemoglobin HbA_{1C} results. The Literacy Assessment for Diabetes (LAD) is a word recognition test measuring the ability to pronounce words and can be administered in 3 minutes. The vocabulary is at a 4th, 6th or 16th grade reading level. It will be interesting to see if the trend toward use of disease-specific health literacy scales continues (Nath, 2007).

When individual assessment is not possible, the Prevalence Calculator can be used to give a rough percentage of individuals within a given geographic area that could be expected to have inadequate health literacy. It is available without charge at www.pfizer healthliteracy.com/physicians-providers/prevalence-calculator.html (Nath, 2007).

According to Nutbeam (2008), any instrument that is used to evaluate health literacy needs to gauge the ability of an individual to access information from a variety of sources, evaluate that information, personalize that information to their situation, and use it to gain benefit. The instrument also has to have adequate reliability and validity and be easily administered in busy healthcare and community-based settings.

Mancuso (2009) suggested that health literacy instruments need to minimize the potential of embarrassment by being given in a private setting where the rationale for the screening is explained. In addition, unless the screening will be used to tailor health communications or education to the health literacy need of the specific patient, then the test serves no purpose. Mancuso also stressed that health literacy measures need to be developed for languages other than English and Spanish.

According to Paasche-Orlow and Wolf (2007), current instruments do not adequately evaluate listening, verbal fluency, memory span, and navigation skills, all of which are important components of health literacy. Rather, existing instruments primarily measure reading and mathematical skills. In addition, they have been designed to measure functional health literacy rather than interactive or critical health literacy (Ishikawa & Yano, 2008). Other critiques point out that existing instruments do not consider age, gender, language, cultural, contextual, and setting-specific factors (Peerson & Saunders, 2009).

HEALTH LITERACY NEEDS WITHIN IMMIGRANT POPULATIONS

Heart attacks, cancer, diabetes, strokes, and HIV/AIDS are among the health disparities that disproportionately affect immigrant populations. Significant language and health literacy challenges interfere with immigrants obtaining adequate care for these disparities. Health education for immigrant populations needs to incorporate cultural beliefs and values, culturally sensitive images, and common healing practices. If providers are discussing the statistical risk of getting an illness or the probability that treatment will be effective, narrative descriptions and visual presentations should be used to reinforce mathematical meanings. Providing education in the primary language of the individual receiving care is also critical, as is exploring whether other family members should be involved in the patient's care. When possible, representatives from the target audience should be involved in design of web-based, videotaped, and print materials to ensure that all phrases and references are understandable and culturally appropriate (Kreps & Sparks, 2008; Nath, 2007).

HEALTH LITERACY ISSUES INVOLVING CHILDREN

Health literacy education is being included in preschools, day-care centers, kindergarten, and K–12 education as a way of empowering young people and promoting health equity. Initially, familiar safety symbols such as crosswalk signs and poison symbols are introduced, which are then followed by more sophisticated health promotion education as the child matures. By introducing health-related content early, and by repetition of content, young people learn to process, integrate, and act on health information gathered from a variety of sources (Mogford, Gould, & Devought, 2010).

Health attitudes and behaviors formed during childhood have a direct effect on adult health habits (Borzekowski, 2010; Mogford, Gould, & Devought, 2010). As Sanders and colleagues (2010) commented, each of the 10 leading health indicators—physical activity, obesity, tobacco use, substance use, responsible sexual behavior, mental health, injury prevention, environmental quality, immunizations, and access to care—are shaped by childhood experiences. Some schools are recommending health literacy be a graduation competency. All schools use the National Health Education Standards (NHES) as guidelines for creating and presenting health-education curricula from kindergarten through high school (Sanders et al., 2009).

However effective it may be to teach children and young adolescents to take an active role in their own health, they also rely on parents and guardians. It is necessary to assess what a child or adolescent can do on his or her own and what they can do when helped by adults. With this assessment, healthcare providers can offer health education that meshes with the developmental abilities and needs of young people (Borzekowksi, 2010). Researchers have reported that one-half of parents studied could not accurately interpret a medication dosing table for acetaminophen (Rothman et al., 2010). Other authors have reported that 36% of parents are unable to follow an immunization schedule, interpret a growth chart, understand food labels, identify portion sizes, or mix formula correctly (Sanders et al., 2009). Illustrated medication schedules have been helpful with parents whose healthcare literacy is insufficient to manage their child's care (Rothman et al., 2010). Frequently, education needs to be targeted to both the young person and their parent or guardian.

WAYS OF IMPROVING HEALTH LITERACY

An Institute of Medicine report (Nielsen-Bohlman et al., 2004) (Nielsen-Bohlman, Panzer & Kindig, 2004) concluded that most healthcare providers do not have an adequate understanding of the barriers created by inadequate health literacy. It may be that their years of training and exposure to the healthcare field have created a sense of comfort and familiarity with terms and treatments, and this familiarity may make it hard to comprehend how a patient could be confused by prevention or treatment recommendations. When beginning to tailor healthcare communications to the literacy needs of patients, it is important to ask the individual if they prefer verbal instructions, computer-based education, videos, or written material (Nath, 2007). It is also important to assess the health literacy of each patient.

Often, healthcare providers rely almost exclusively on written information in the form of pamphlets and handouts to reinforce or teach self-care in spite of the fact that individuals with poor health literacy cannot adequately comprehend written materials (von Wagner et al., 2009). This trend needs to be reversed. How many times in the previous month have you given a patient or family member health-related written information without thinking about their health literacy level?

Health education that is designed to increase health literacy makes use of lay language, audiovisual, and pictorial materials to clarify concepts, and concrete examples or stories. Content is delivered in a shame free environment while targeting only a few key points per session, emphasizing patient concerns, speaking slowly, avoiding medical jargon, being sensitive to cultural issues, and limiting the amount of information covered in one session. When written information is given out, shorter words should be used, sentence structure must be simplified, active voice needs to be used, and the overall length of the handout minimized so that only key content is included. Prior to beginning health teaching, it is important to assess patient readiness, to tailor the type of education to patient preference, and to provide contact information should the patient think of questions at a later date (Seligman et al., 2007).

Any written information that is provided must be translated into the person's primary language (Clement et al., 2009; Speros, 2005). Oftentimes it is helpful to involve more literate family members in healthcare decisions and treatments if the individual with lower literacy agrees (von Wagner et al., 2009). It is useful to confirm important health history with others and reinforce the importance of action items with family members (Paasche-Orlow & Wolf, 2007).

In general, it is necessary to make education interactive so that patients can ask questions and take a more active role in their own self-care (Nath, 2007). It is effective to ask individuals to repeat back what has been taught to assess comprehension. One technique, called "Show me" or "Teach back," involves having the patient explain what has just been taught to the healthcare provider to ensure that the information was understood (von Wagner et al., 2009). Another similar technique is called teach-to-goal, in which "a learner is asked to exhibit comprehension and gets repeated rounds of focused teaching until mastery is exhibited" (Paasche-Orlow & Wolf, 2007, p. S22). A simple but effective statement and question is, "We don't always do a good job of explaining things. Can you tell me in your own words what your care plan is and what you are going to do to improve your health?"

It is necessary to use nonjudgmental questions and avoid conveying frustration, anger, or contempt for individuals who have trouble completing medical forms, following signs, or complying with treatments they do not understand. Years of familiarity with medical jargon and procedures make understanding the medical system seem like second nature to nurses. It is important to remember even simple terms and directions can seem confusing to individuals with low literacy (von Wagner et al., 2009). For example, a medication label that reads "Take 1 tablet every 12 hours" has been shown to be more understandable to individuals with low literacy than one that reads "Take one tablet twice a day." Finally, it is important to enhance patient's self-efficacy by acknowledging success and efforts at behavioral change (Nath, 2007).

Nurses must assess and document the literacy needs of patients (Murphy-Knoll, 2007). Nurses should also become involved in committees that redesign enrollment and consent documents to ensure that third- to sixth-grade language is used and phrases that are included are clear (Speros, 2005). For example, medication instruction handouts can be presented using pictures of the prescribed medication, pictures of daily activities, and clocks to help improve medication adherence for individuals aged 65 and over and/or people with poor health literacy (Hussey, 1994).

Educational materials designed for individuals with low health literacy need to include content that focuses on benefits that derive from behavior change; emphasize conditions that will facilitate change; and encourage setting short-term, measurable goals and action plans (Seligman et al., 2007). For example, discussing how a diabetic patient would feel better after taking insulin shots for uncontrolled blood sugar values helps to motivate the person to agree to use injections when they might have otherwise been reluctant to do so. Involving patients in creating personalized action plans enhances motivation and increases the likelihood of success. One example of an action plan is, "I will walk around the block before I sit down to watch television three times during the next week" (Seligman et al., 2007, p. S71).

A variety of innovative approaches designed to improve health literacy have been described in the literature. Songs, plays, street theater, and computer games have been used to engage individuals with low health literacy in the health education content being presented (Silk et al., 2008). Games that require participation and engagement can be used to teach nutrition education and cardiovascular risk prevention (Lyons et al., 1997). Fotonovelas, a type of suspenseful story, have been used among Latinas with low literacy. Fotonovelas are especially effective when the Latina community participates in developing the story board and taking photographs or creating drawings that illustrate the selected health condition. Fotonovelas have been used to provide information on nutritional education, HIV prevention, and a variety of other health-related topics (Hinojosa et al., 2010).

Interestingly, Silk and colleagues (2008) found that use of video games was less effective in conveying nutrition information than websites designed with simple wording and healthy recipes. The authors hypothesized that the intense focus and concentration required in a video game and the availability of game consoles in low-income households would make use of video game instruction highly effective. However, results indicated that individuals play video games for completion rather than for learning. Even though the computer game was designed to use points to measure retention of content, participants preferred to use a website with similar content than the video game. The relatively small sample size (n = 155) prompted researchers to suggest that larger studies need to be conducted.

Another group of researchers examined the effectiveness of a computer interface, the Embodied Conversational Agent (ECA), to provide health education. One randomized study focused on hospital discharge instructions while another targeted the value of walking for older adults. An animated character that used hand gestures, head nods, and raised eyebrows to emphasize significant content interacted with patients who were using a touch screen attached to a wheeled computer kiosk. Use of computers allowed for providing health information in a consistent manner and in a self-paced, low-key environment. Participants with lower health literacy were more satisfied with the ECA than were those with adequate health literacy. Patients commented that the ECA allowed them to take as much time as they needed to understand, while their healthcare provider was always rushed and in a hurry (Bickmore et al., 2010).

The use of consistent personnel and the concept of a patient-centered medical home in which the needs of the patient are known to providers and the patient is comfortable have also been mentioned as ways to address health literacy needs (Rothman et al., 2010). Waiting times prior to medical appointments can be well spent if health education videos or electronic kiosks outfitted with headphones and health information are available for use (Sanders et al., 2009).

A number of web-based resources and toolkits are available for use in healthcare settings to manage health literacy issues. The American Medical Association Foundation published a toolkit for medical practitioners titled "Health Literacy: A Manual for Clinicians" (Bankson, 2009). In April of 2010, AHRQ released a health literacy toolkit to address the needs of healthcare systems (Hasnain-Wynia & Wolf, 2010). The Diabetes Literacy and Numeracy Education Toolkit (DLNET) uses color-coded measuring devices and portion sizes to convey diabetes education (Wolff et al., 2009). The Living with Diabetes Guide is a low-literacy guide that was developed by the American College of Physicians to motivate self-care (Seligman et al., 2007).

A personal health record that is culturally and linguistically competent uses simple forms to record visits with healthcare providers, medications, and questions. Since it is small enough to fit in a back pocket, it is a convenient way to store reliable healthcare data and questions an individual wishes to raise with a healthcare provider (Kupchunas, 2007). Look up each of these toolkits to determine which ones might be helpful in your practice.

Motivational Interviewing

Motivational interviewing was developed by William Miller in 1983 and has been used to decrease alcohol and substance abuse, HIV risk behavior, and obesity as well as increase physical activity and participation in diabetic care. Motivational interviewing takes 10 to 15 minutes and relies on nondirective questioning about what health behavior the patient wants to change, how they wish to begin, and what they believe a reasonable goal would be. The purpose of motivational interviewing is to increase the self-esteem and self-efficacy of the patient by reflective listening, active engagement, and open-ended dialogue. Healthcare providers adopt the stance of partner, expressing empathy for the patient's point of view, recognizing that reluctance to change is normal, acknowledging everyone experiences discrepancies between their behavior and goals, and creating confidence that the patient can achieve the goals that they establish. Motivational interviewing requires that a nurse listens without interrupting to provide advice or instruction. Because the approach is at odds with the patriarchal stance many healthcare practitioners are socialized into, it requires patience and focused concentration. It also requires engaging patients who are reluctant to or uncomfortable with setting their own healthcare goals (Soderlund, Nilsen, & Kristensson, 2008).

Theme Parks and Health Museums

Health museums, exhibits, and theme parks are being used as innovative ways of increasing health-related knowledge and understanding. Although not exclusively designed for individuals with low health literacy, this approach would certainly be an effective way to increase health literacy. Tourist, cultural, entertainment, and health sector personnel are collaborating to create educational experiences in which participants learn about the human body (Seymour, Ashton, & Edwards, 1986).

One such proposed museum, the Body, Mind, City Museum in Liverpool, is a mixture of a science Exploratorium and a Walt Disney-type theme park. Hands-on exhibits, interactive videos, computer games, rides that take a person through a large blood vessel, and a walk-through-the-brain exhibit are used to create a sense of wonder and fun. Planned exhibits test a visitor's stamina, flexibility, coordination, and balance. A dark tactile maze is proposed to provide insight regarding how a blind person experiences the world. An IMAX theatre is also planned (Seymour, Ashton, & Edwards, 1986).

The Deutsches Hygiene Museum in Dresden, founded in 1911, includes exhibits on human anatomy and physiology, health, and disease. The California Museum of Science and Industry in Los Angeles has exhibits about human anatomy and physiology. One such exhibit, The Dynamic Kidney, shows how nephrons work. Another exhibit features a 6-foot-tall tooth and teaches principles of corrective dentistry. A 16-foot human heart walkthrough is also available. The Cleveland Health Education Museum, founded in 1936, includes exhibits of the brain, nervous system, birth process, blood vessels, and microbes. Satellite health education is transmitted from the museum to elder centers, business locations, and health fairs. The Don Harrington Discovery Centre in Amarillo, Texas and the Health Adventure in Asheville, North Carolina offer educational programs to children and the community. Trips to hospitals, traveling health shows, and summer camps are used. Other health museums include the Mayo Medical Museum in Minnesota and the Fort Crawford Medical Museum in Wisconsin (Seymour, Ashton, & Edwards, 1986).

The participatory nature of these health adventures help people to retain what they have seen and experienced. Each visitor has a unique experience that builds on their own informational base. An advantage is that affordable education is provided to a large number of people. The wonder of the human body is presented by combining artistic presentations, multimedia exhibits, and life-sized models (Seymour, Ashton, & Edwards, 1986).

Universal Design

Universal design is a concept that ensures all products, communications, and environments will be usable by all people regardless of their health literacy, age, or access needs. It is a cost-effective approach because, from the beginning phases of design, the product, communication, and/or environment is created to be usable without the need for adaptation, thus saving time and money (Perlow, 2010). In 2004, the federal government mandated that all health records and data linkages be universal by the year 2014 (Fetter, 2009).

Textbooks are designed using multiple formats (written, audio, Braille, etc.) so that individuals with varied literacy needs can use them. Online systems are designed using the Digital Accessible Information System (DAISY) standard so that talking books and print-format documents can be readily adapted to varied learning styles. Information is tailored to various experience, literacy, and physical ability levels. Audio components are captioned. Font size and style can be adapted. Text-to-speech software is used, sign language translation is included, variable reading speed is enabled, and dictionaries are linked with online sites (Perlow, 2010).

Building design is created to be accessible to individuals with mobility, vision, hearing, and literacy needs. Each of these design features ensures that content is accessible to a broad spectrum of individuals. The goal is to reach the largest number of individuals and to make health information and services usable, available, and accessible (Perlow, 2010).

Health-Related Websites

Eighty percent of individuals with basic health literacy do not use the Internet to seek out health-related information (Cutilli & Bennett, 2009). This is not due to lack of access, as it has been estimated that Internet connections and computers are available in many low-income households (Silk et al., 2008). One factor may be that the quality of health information found on the Internet varies greatly. Ninety percent of diet and nutrition information has been found to be unreliable, if not conflicting, while only 5% of cancer content was deemed to be unreliable. Higher quality education tends to be found on government, professional, and charitable organization sites. In addition, the existence of editorial boards, publication of conflict of interest statements, and evidence-based criteria or references are indications of quality content. However, it is often the case that credible websites lack engaging design features. Furthermore, downloading content is often a slow and frustrating experience for consumers with low levels of literacy (Reavley & Jorm, 2010). Even websites created by the U.S. Food and Drug Administration have been evaluated as presenting content at 10th grade level or higher, making them inaccessible to individuals with low levels of health literacy (Rothman et al., 2010). It is helpful for healthcare providers to hand out a list of relevant and respected health education websites that is tailored to the specific health literacy needs of the patient (Reavley & Jorm, 2010).

CASE STUDIES

Think back over the last 6 months of patients you have observed being cared for in a hospital, community-health, or primary care clinic. Which patients might have had health literacy issues? What could have been done to do a better job of addressing their health literacy needs? As you read through the following case studies, consider which health literacy needs were influencing the behaviors of the patients described below. Suggest alternative ways of meeting their health literacy needs.

> Mr. Roberts is a 77-year-old, retired, African American schoolteacher who was hospitalized for right-sided flank pain. It was determined he had a large kidney stone blocking his right ureter, which required surgery. Although he was an avid reader and well educated, he refused to sign the consent because he did not understand the risks associated with the surgery described in the consent or a number of terms that were used in the document. What should the nurse caring for Mr. Roberts do? Should his wife be included in discussions with the physician? Should the nurse bring a medical dictionary to the bedside so Mr. Roberts could look up terms in the consent he did not understand? Why is it important for him to have surgery? How might Mr. Roberts's pain level and/or age be influencing his decision?

> Mrs. Johns, a 95-year-old woman, was taken by ambulance to the emergency room for a nosebleed that she could not stop. Her son was concerned because she was on Coumadin. She had missed a scheduled blood level test to monitor her Coumadin level. At the emergency room she could not remember her birthday when asked by the ward clerk who was admitting her. Mrs. Johns's nosebleed stopped when the nurse

instructed her to lower her head below her knees and packed her nose. Her Coumadin level was barely elevated, so no medications to counteract the effect of Coumadin were needed. A urinalysis indicated she was not dehydrated. The nurse instructed her to stop blowing her nose, a habit that she exhibited several times in the emergency room. After approximately 30 minutes, she was discharged home. What does this case study have to do with health literacy? How might the emergency room visit have been prevented?

Mrs. Ambrose lived in a rural mountain town with her husband, who smoked four packs of cigarettes a day, and her 4-year-old son. The son had severe asthma. Mrs. Ambrose was soft-spoken and had a 3rd-grade education. On leaving the emergency room following her son's asthma attack, the nurse gave Mrs. Ambrose a brochure explaining the importance of not smoking in the home and describing how to use the peak flow meter and nebulizer. The following day Mrs. Ambrose returned to the emergency room when her son experienced another asthma attack. When the nurse asked if she used the nebulizer, Mrs. Ambrose explained she could not get it to work. She could not demonstrate to the nurse how to use the peak flow meter and just stared at the nurse when asked if her husband had been smoking outside. How should the nurse proceed in tailoring health education to Mrs. Ambrose's health literacy needs?

Ms. Smith was an 85-year-old woman who had a small stage I cancerous tumor removed from her right breast. When the nurse explained the need for getting a mammogram twice yearly to follow up, Ms. Smith balked at the idea, saying it was hard for her to get to the clinic, that mammograms hurt her, and her insurance only paid for one mammogram a year. In addition, she said that she felt the radiation she would be exposed to during the mammogram was dangerous. How should the nurse tailor education to fit Ms. Smith's needs? Which aspects of health literacy were influencing Ms. Smith's attitude?

Ms. Talbun was attempting to fill out a State Children's Health Insurance Program (SCHIP) form but was unable to answer all of the questions. She lived in one of the 26 states where the SCHIP form was written at 10th grade level, but Ms. Talbun had only completed 5th grade before she dropped out of school. She was embarrassed to tell anyone she could not understand the questions on the SCHIP form. What should she do? Who might she ask for help (Sanders et al., 2009)?

Ms. Robinson had gained 60 pounds over a 2-year period and was having difficulty losing weight. Her nurse practitioner prescribed Phenlramine HCL after asking her if she had heart or lung problems. Ms. Robinson answered that she did not and wondered why the nurse practitioner would ask that question, since she had been seeing her for the last 7 years. Ms. Robinson took one-half of a pill and experienced multiple side effects. She was so anxious she felt like eating more, not less. She could not concentrate at work and started crying at home after her husband made a brief comment about something inconsequential. That night she could not sleep so she looked up the side effects and counter-indications of Phenlramine on the Internet. She found that anyone with a history of pulmonary hypertension should not take Phenlramine and that it was an amphetamine. Ms. Robinson remembered that one doctor 10 years ago had told her she might have pulmonary hypertension when a chest X-ray had shown infiltrates throughout her lung fields. Since those had gone away with antibiotics, Ms. Robinson assumed she actually had pneumonia. In addition, she did not realize a possible diagnosis of pulmonary hypertension was a "lung problem" that she should mention when her nurse practitioner questioned her about her medical history. Ms. Robinson returned to her nurse practitioner and explained she could not tolerate taking the Phenlramine and was actually afraid to do so. Which health literacy issues and healthcare system issues influenced Ms. Robinson's treatment in this situation?

DISCUSSION QUESTIONS

1. Why has health literacy only recently become a priority topic? Why is it a priority?
2. Does health literacy play a central role in shaping health disparities? Explain your answer.
3. Talk about a time you observed a patient not having sufficient time to explain their health concerns to a provider.

4. Which health screening tool would be the best choice for the clinical setting where you are currently assigned?

5. Should health screening tools be generic or disease-specific? Provide a rationale for your answer.

6. Why is it important for health screening tools to measure more than reading and mathematical ability?

7. Should health literacy be a high school graduation competency? Why or why not?

8. What are the advantages of teach-to-a-goal and teach-back methods of providing health education?

9. How might a patient misunderstand a medication label that reads "Take one tablet three times a day?"

10. Why have fotonovelas been effective? In which population have they primarily been used?

11. Which populations might not respond to education provided by an embodied conversational agent?

12. What are the advantages of motivational interviewing? How might you incorporate motivational interviewing into your nursing practice within the next 2 weeks?

13. What are the advantages of and challenges associated with requiring that all healthcare data systems be universal by 2014?

CHECK YOUR UNDERSTANDING: EXERCISE ONE

Using the definitions of health literacy included in this chapter and listed here, describe which definitions are: (1) practical and applicable to the healthcare settings in which your clinical experiences have occurred, (2) highlight individual responsibility for health, (3) focus on both hospitals and community-based settings, (4) encompass only reading and mathematical skills rather than comprehension and analysis, (5) include social influences that shape health, and (6) include aspects of the healthcare system.

CHECK YOUR UNDERSTANDING: EXERCISE TWO

Match the definitions of health literacy with the description that follow that is most clearly evident in the definition. Although several of the descriptions apply to more than one definition, please select the one description that can only apply to one definition (only one description should be matched to any one definition).

Definitions of Health Literacy

A. WHO definition of health literacy
B. Healthy People definition of health literacy
C. American Medical Association definition of health literacy
D. TOFHLA definition of health literacy
E. Zarcadoolas and colleagues definition of health literacy
F. Kickbusch and colleagues definition of health literacy
G. The Australian Bureau of Statistics definition of health literacy
H. The NAAL definition of health literacy
I. The Canadian expert panel definition of health literacy

Definition Descriptions

1. Definition includes the social determinants of health
2. Definition emphasizes individual responsibility for health literacy
3. Definition applies primarily to adults in the United States
4. Definition includes access issues
5. Definition includes a focus on quality of life
6. Definition specifically mentions political factors
7. Definition applies across the lifespan and includes communication as a skill
8. Definition is limited to healthcare settings, not community-based environments
9. Definition makes note of disease and accident prevention

CHECK YOUR UNDERSTANDING: EXERCISE THREE

Mrs. Tom is a 94-year-old woman. She has a history of atrial fibrillation, high blood pressure, hearing loss, repeated urinary tract infections, chronic obstructive pulmonary disorder, and advanced Alzheimer's disease. A nurse practitioner Mrs. Tom was seeing was confused about what brought Mrs. Tom to the clinic and when Mrs. Tom began taking Pradaxil. Each time the nurse practitioner asked for clarification on these topics, Mrs. Tom would become increasingly agitated. What should the nurse practitioner do to obtain an accurate history? Review the following interventions and select the intervention(s) that you would use in this instance. Explain your choice or choices.

1. Establishing a timeline of events
2. Seeking clarification from a family member or caretaker
3. Repeating back and summarizing what Mrs. Tom had said
4. Asking for additional specific information
5. Consulting her previous healthcare provider
6. Using motivational interviewing

WHAT DO YOU THINK?

1. Would you evaluate your own health literacy as being at the level of functional, interactive, or critical? Provide an illustration and rationale for your answer.
2. If you were designing a health museum or theme park, what exhibits and activities would you include? Who would your target audience be?
3. Should health literacy be one of the top four public health priorities within the United States? Explain your answer.
4. Have you ever received health information that wasn't understandable? Have you ever been reluctant to question your healthcare provider about a medical issue? What factors contributed to those situations?
5. Have you ever worked with a patient who did not understand their healthcare education? How should that situation have been handled differently to achieve a better outcome?
6. Have you or anyone in your family ever struggled to select healthcare insurance or to dispute a denied claim? Describe what that was like.
7. Which of the health literacy definitions described in this chapter do you prefer? Explain your rationale.
8. Should health literacy screening tools be used with all patients in all settings? Why or why not?
9. What sort of health literacy evaluations or health education interventions do you think would work with nonemergent patients waiting in an emergency room?
10. If you were a senator and wanted to sponsor a piece of legislation to increase health literacy within the U.S, what interventions would you propose for inclusion in that legislation?

REFERENCES

American Medical Association Ad Hoc Committee on Health Literacy for the Council on Scientific Affairs (1999). Health literacy: Report of the council on scientific affairs. *Journal of the American Medical Association, 281*, 552–557.

Australian Bureau of Statistics (2008). *Health literacy, Australia.* Catalogue No. 4233.0 Retrieved from http ://www.abs.gov.au

Baker, D. W., Parker, R. M., Williams, M. V., & Clark, W. S. (1998). Health literacy and the risk of hospital admission. *Journal of General Internal Medicine, 13*, 791–798.

Bankson, H. L. (2009). Health literacy: An exploratory bibliometric analysis, 1997–2007. *Journal of the Medical Library Association, 97*(2), 148–150.

Baur, C. (2010). New directions in research on public health and health literacy. *Journal of Health Communication, 15*(1), 42–50.

Bickmore, T. W., Pfeifer, L. M., Dyron, D., Forsythe, S., Henault, L. E., Jack, B. W., Silliman, R., & Paasche-Orlow, M. K. (2010). Usability of conversational agents by patients with inadequate health literacy: Evidence from two clinical trials. *Journal of Health Communication, 15*, 197–210.

Borzekowksi, D. L. (2010). Considering children and health literacy: A theoretical approach. *Pediatrics, 124*, S282–S288.

Chew, L. D., Bradley, K. A., & Boyko, E. J. (2004). Brief questions to identify patients with inadequate health literacy. *Family Medicine, 36*, 588–594.

Clement, S., Ibrahim, S., Crichton, N., Wolf, M., & Rowlands, G. (2009). Complex interventions to improve the health of people with limited literacy: A systematic review. *Patient Education and Counseling, 75*, 340–351.

Cutilli, C. C., & Bennett, I. M. (2009). Understanding the health literacy of America: Results of the National Assessment of Adult Literacy. *Orthopedic Nursing, 28*(1), 27–34.

Fetter, M. S. (2009). Promoting health literacy with vulnerable behavioral health clients. *Issues in Mental Health Nursing, 30*, 798–802.

Hasnain-Wynia, R., & Wolf, M. S. (2010). Promoting health care equity: Is health literacy a missing link? *Health Services Research*, 897–903.

Hinojosa, M. S., Hinojosa, R., Nelson, D. A., & Delgado, A. (2010). Salud de la Mujer Using Fotonovelas to increase health literacy among Latinas. *Progress in Community Health Partnerships: Research, Education and Action, 4*(1), 25–30.

Hussey, L. C. (1994). Minimizing effects of low literacy on medication knowledge and compliance among the elderly. *Clinical Nursing Research, 3*, 132–145.

Ishikawa, H. & Yano, E. (2008). Patient health literacy and participation in the health-care process. *Health Expectations, 11*, 113–122.

Kickbusch, I., Wait, S., & Maag, D. (2005). *Navigating health: The role of health literacy.* Retrieved from www .emhf.org/resource_images/NavigatingHealth_FINAL.pdf

Kreps, G. L., & Sparks, L. (2008). Meeting the health literacy needs of immigrant populations. *Patient Education and Counseling, 71*, 328–332.

Kupchunas, W. (2007). Personal health record: New opportunity for patient education. *Orthopedic Nursing, 26*(3), 185–193.

Lyons, G. K., Woodruff, S. I., Candelaria, J., Rupp, J. W., & Elder, J. P. (1997). Effect of a nutrition intervention on macronutrient intake in a low English-proficient Hispanic sample. *American Journal of Health Promotion, 11*, 371–374.

Mancuso, J. M. (2009). Assessment and measurement of health literacy: An integrative review of the literature. *Nursing and Health Sciences, 11*, 77–89.

Mancuso, J. M. (2010). Impact of health literacy and patient trust on glycemic control in an urban USA population. *Nursing and Health Sciences, 12*, 94–104.

Mogford, E., Gould, L., & Devoght, A. (2010). Teaching critical health literacy as a means to action on the social determinants of health. *Health Promotion International, 26*(1), 4–13.

Murphy-Knoll, L. (2007). Low health literacy puts patients at risk: The Joint Commission proposes solutions to a national problem. *Journal of Nursing Care Quality, 22*(3), 205–209.

Nath, C. (2007). Literacy and diabetes self-management. *American Journal of Nursing, 107*(6), 43–49.

Nielsen-Bohlman, L., Panzer, A. M., & Kindig, D. A. (2004). Health literacy: A prescription to end confusion. Committee on Health Literacy, Board on Neuroscience and Behavioral Health, Institute of Medicine. Washington, D.C. National Academies Press.

Nutbeam, D. (1999). Literacies across the lifespan: Health literacy. *Literacy and Numeracy Studies, 9*, 47–55.

Nutbeam, D. (2000). Health literacy as a public health goal: A challenge for contemporary health education and communication strategies into the 21st century. *Health Promotion International, 15*, 259–267.

Nutbeam, D. (2008). The evolving concept of literacy. *Social Science and Medicine, 67*, 2072–2078.

Paasche-Orlow, M. K., Parker, R. M., Gazmararian, J. A., Nielsen-Bohlman, L. T., & Rudd, R. R. (2005). The prevalence of limited health literacy. *Journal of General Internal Medicine, 20*, 175–184.

Paasche-Orlow, M. K., & Wolf, M. S. (2007). The causal pathways linking health literacy to health outcomes. *American Journal of Health Behavior, 31*(Suppl 1), S19–S26.

Peerson, A., & Saunders, M. (2009). Health literacy revisited: What do we mean and why does it matter? *Health Promotion International, 24*(3), 285–296.

Perlow, E. (2010). Accessibility: Global gateway to health literacy. *Health Promotion Practice, 11*(1), 123–131.

Reavley, N. J., & Jorm, A .F. (2010). The quality of mental disorder information websites: A review. *Patient Education and Counseling*. Doi: 10.1016/j.pec.2010.10.015.

Rootman, I., & El-Bihbety, D. G. A. (2008). *Vision for a health literate Canada: Report of the expert panel on health literacy*. Ottawa, ON: Canadian Public Health Association.

Rothman, R. L., Yin, H. S., Mulvaney, S., Patrick, J., Homer, C. & Lannon, C. (2010). Health literacy and quality: Focus on chronic illness care and patient safety. *Pediatrics, 124*, S315–S326.

Sanders, L. E., Shaw, J. S., Guez, G., Baur, C., & Rudd, R. (2009). Health literacy and child health promotion: Implications for research, clinical care and public policy. *Pediatrics, 124*, S306–S314.

Seligman, H. K., Wallace, A. S., De Walt, D. A., Schillinger, D., Arnold, C. A., Bryant-Shilliday, B., . . . Davis, T. C. (2007). Facilitating behavior change with low-literacy patient education materials. *American Journal of Health Behavior, 31*(suppl 1), S69–S78.

Seymour, H., Ashton, J., & Edwards, P. (1986). Health museums or theme parks: A new approach to intersectoral collaboration. *Health Promotion, 1*(3), 311–317.

Silk, K. J., Sherry, J., Winn, B., Keesecker, N., Horodynski, M. A., & Sayir, A. (2008). Increasing nutrition literacy: Testing the effectiveness of print, web-site, and game modalities. *Journal Nutrition and Educational Behavior, 40*, 3–10.

Soderlund, L. L., Nilsen, P., & Kristensson, M. (2008). Learning motivational interviewing: Exploring primary health care nurses' training and counseling experiences. *Health Education Journal, 67*(2), 102–109.

Speros, C. (2005). Health literacy: Concept analysis. *Journal of Advanced Nursing, 50*(6), 633–640.

U.S. Department of Health and Human Services (2000). *Healthy People 2010 (2nd ed.), With understanding and improving health and objectives for improving health*. (2 vols.) Washington, DC: U.S. Government Printing Office.

von Wagner, C., Steptoe, A., Wolf, M .S., & Wardle, J. (2009). Health literacy and health actions: A review and framework from health psychology. *Health Education Behavior, 36*(5), 860–877.

White, S. (2008). *Assessing the nation's health literacy: Key concepts and findings from the National Assessment of Adult Literacy (NAAL)*. Chicago, IL: American Medical Association Foundation.

World Health Organization [WHO]. (1998). Division of health promotion, education and communications. Health education and health promotion unit. *Health Promotion Glossary*. Geneva, Switzerland: Author.

Wolff, K., Cavanaugh, K., Malone, R., Hawk, V., Gregory, B. P., David, D, . . . Rothman, R. L. (2009). The diabetes literacy and numeracy education toolkit (DLNET): Materials to facilitate diabetes education and management. *Diabetes Education, 35*(2), 233–236, 238–241, 244–245.

Zarcadoolas, C., Pleasant, A. & Greer, D. S. (2005). Understanding health literacy: An expanded model. *Health Promotion International, 20*, 195–203.

For a full suite of assignments and additional learning activities, see the access code at the front of your book.

CHAPTER 7

Artistic, Creative, and Aesthetic Approaches to Health Promotion

Bonnie Raingruber

OBJECTIVES

At the conclusion of this chapter, students will be able to:

- Define "aesthetic" and discuss why aesthetic approaches are valuable additions to health promotion practice.
- Describe how poetry, literature, narrative stories, music, photo-voice, art, soap operas, cartoons, dance, and theater can be used to promote health.
- Discuss why creative and aesthetic approaches to health promotion are effective.
- Identify which populations respond most effectively to creative and artistic approaches to health promotion.
- Describe how aesthetic approaches have been used to educate healthcare providers.
- Discuss how aesthetic components of healthcare environments influence healing.
- Define aesthetic knowledge and explain its role within the nursing profession.

INTRODUCTION

The word aesthetics comes from the Latin term *aesthetica*, which is translated as "perception, sense, feeling, awareness, knowledge of the fine arts, and the standards used to understand the arts" (Caspari, Eriksson, & Naden, 2006, p. 852). Aesthetic influences shape both physical and psychological feelings. "Art captures and expresses humanity . . . Art is life's spirit" (Caspari, Erickson, & Naden, 2006, p. 852).

Art is a process, a way of approaching life as well as an outcome. Pictures and drawing, stories and storytelling, poems and poetry writing, music and listening to music, dance and dancing, plays and dramatic performances are all art. Art requires technical capability and an inner capacity to know how to bring elements together into a unified whole (Chinn & Kramer, 2004; Leight, 2002). "Art is important for it commemorates the seasons of the soul, or a special or tragic event in the soul's journey. Art is not just for oneself, not just a marker of one's own understanding. It is also a map for those who follow after us" (Estes, 1995, p 13). The arts and humanities help us make sense of the human condition by exploring emotion, ambiguity, complexity, and uncertainty (Fox, 2009). Art has been described as a conversation with multiple meanings, interpretations, and points of view (Kester, 2004). As Milligan and Woodley (2009) commented, the humanities "provide a platform from which we can articulate what it means to be human" (p. 135).

A clear link between creativity and healing has been documented. When a person engages in creative work, the parasympathetic system slows the heart rate, decreases blood pressure, slows breathing, diverts blood to the intestines, and produces relaxation. The hypothalamus is also stimulated and hormone levels are balanced. Endorphins and other neurotransmitters that strengthen the immune system and relieve pain are stimulated (Lane, 2005). By engaging in or watching artistic activities, one's mood is improved. "Throughout history, people have used pictures, stories, dances, and chants as healing rituals" (Stuckey & Nobel, 2010, p. 255). Holistic approaches to health promotion that include aesthetic interventions help to create and sustain health.

EDUCATING HEALTHCARE PRACTITIONERS

Education that incorporates the study of artistic and aesthetic approaches has been used to train dietitians, physicians, nurses, and other healthcare providers to help them develop an attitude of contextual understanding and relational involvement rather than a stance of detached observation (Milligan & Woodley, 2009). Aesthetic approaches have included reading assigned literature that focused on issues relating to health promotion, then presenting the perspective of the protagonist; creating a class poem in which each student adds one line (Milligan & Woodley, 2009); or visiting an art gallery and dialoguing about the health conditions and symptoms illustrated in paintings (Pardue, 2005). Milligan and Woodley (2009) concluded that although it is not clear that "any of us can teach compassion, we can through narrative, conserve the compassion our students already have and pave a softer path through the hard environment trodden by healthcare students and professionals" (p. 137).

Leffers and Martins (2004) listed 22 books and described how literature can be used with nursing students to develop compassion for the struggles experienced by the poor, homeless, immigrants, and victims of violence. Students presented creative summaries about the books they were assigned. Presentations included: (1) a model graveyard and a description of the stories and struggles of families who were buried there, (2) a clothesline project that displayed stories and tattered clothing of abused children, (3) a monologue describing the life experience of the main characters from the assigned book, (4) a truth-or-consequences game to dialogue about assumptions regarding those who live in poverty, and (5) a presentation of scenes from a popular movie to illustrate how a child who is afraid of gangs feels. How might this same approach be incorporated into a book club in a wealthy community to help residents develop an understanding of the perspectives and priorities of individuals from a low-income section of town?

A type of creative writing called 55-word stories has been used to help family medicine fellows to gain insight into key moments from their training. Each story includes a setting, characters, conflict, and an outcome or resolution. Fifteen minutes is devoted to writing, followed by time for editing. At first fellows are encouraged to write down everything they can remember, to write without editing, take time to edit the story to 55 words, and then share it with others to get their reaction and feedback (Fogarty, 2010). Common instructions for writing, whether it be journaling or writing a 55-word short story, include not stopping or editing for the 15 minutes you should be writing (Stuckey & Nobel, 2010).

NARRATIVE STRATEGIES AND STORYTELLING

People both "understand stories and are shaped by the narratives of their lives . . . The reality of a story comes to be known by living it and allowing it to live in us through hearing or telling" (Leight, 2002, p. 109). As Estes (1995) suggests, "stories are medicine, they do not require us to do, be or act, we need only listen" (p. 14). Some stories are "observations, some are fragments, some are little pieces of pine pitch for fastening feathers to trees to show the way back to our psychic home" (Estes, 1995, p. 18). Self-knowledge begins with self-revelation. In the telling of our story we emphasize what is important, we organize and classify information, and we describe the context that makes a difference. Stories include strengths and abilities as well as challenges. They inform and heal. The role of a nurse is to engage patients in sharing their stories, interpreting their meaning, and "looking beyond the situation to focus on what might be" (Leight, 2002, p. 113).

Reading stories is as effective as sharing one's own story. The plots of stories and the development of characters within a narrative allow the reader to develop an awareness of other people and their motives. Imbedded in stories are complex past events, current struggles, and future hopes that influence the characters (Smith, 2005). Stories have a goal-oriented theme and dialogue that expresses feelings, thoughts, and actions (Matto, 2003). Stories portray how a given health problem or lifestyle choice disrupts the lives of involved characters. Even when stories are similar to our own life, they portray events and struggles as happening to another person; therefore, they allow a patient to develop a once-removed understanding of events, to step back and reflect, and to distinguish the person involved from the given health problem. Consequently, stories minimize resistance to the overall theme being emphasized. Published novels and short stories can be used or patients can be encouraged to make up their own story about a given health condition (Smith, 2005).

In one example, a book titled *Lake Rescue* from the Beacon Street Girls series was given to a group of 9 to 13-year-old girls with an elevated body mass index (BMI). *Lake Rescue* is about an overweight girl who has a poor self-esteem who becomes more active, loses weight, and feels happier. Another group of girls were given a control book and still another group received no intervention. Those girls who were assigned the intervention book had a greater decrease in BMI than girls who were given the control book or those who received no intervention (Bravender, Russell, Chung, & Armstrong, 2011). Why would a nurse need to carefully read any short story or novel that was being used to illustrate a healthcare goal or topic? Which age groups might benefit from reading a novel or short story?

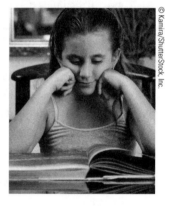

© Kamira/ShutterStock, Inc.

Sakalys (2003) suggested that narration of an illness episode is an excellent way to identify meaning, re-establish a sense of coherence in one's life, and "reclaim the illness experience from the medical meta-narrative" (p. 228). She claimed that "the assault of illness on our sense of self is compounded by the medical perspective, which often frames the illness experience in objective, depersonalized terms" (p. 230). A person can feel like a spectator in their own drama and lose themselves and their capacity for choice, and it is easy to become more focused on lab results than on how you feel.

Narrative thinking differs from analytic thinking, in that narrative approaches help identify how people make sense of things and find meaning. In narratives there is a temporal ordering of events. "Stories link past, present, and future in a way that tells us where we have been, where we are, and where we could be going." (Taylor, 2001). Action and plot transform into meaning. "Stories are the single best way humans have for accounting for our experience. They help us to see how choices and events are tied together, why things are, and how they could have been" (p. 2).

Stories need an audience. As Taylor (2001) commented, stories say "You come too . . . Join me in my experience. Let's go through this together" (p. 16). Smyth and

Pennebaker (1999) suggested that sharing is a factor that accounts for a good portion of healing associated with storytelling. The goal of the nurse is to understand what the story means to the patient's life—how their history, values, meanings, relationships, expectations, and commitments constituted their narrative (Sakalys, 2003). Asking open-ended questions, listening for meaning rather than facts, rarely interrupting, and giving control of the dialogue to the patient are priorities. The nurse can begin by asking, "Tell me about your illness. How did it begin? What did you think was causing it? What did you do? What is it like for you now? What do you imagine for the future?" (Sakalys, 2003, p. 237). The nurse should ask him or herself, "Am I listening to understand what it feels like to be this person in this situation, or am I beginning to fill in the gaps in his or her story with my assumptions?" (Freedman & Combs, 1996, p. 40–41).

When stories are made up, the person creating the story is able to give voice to their own experiences and feelings. A story about uncontrolled pain that is made up by the patient allows the nurse to see if the patient sees him or herself as a hero, a villain, or a bit-part character who is unable to influence their pain level (Carter, 2004). When a nurse is listening to a patient story, the main goals are to "give primacy to the patient's voice and to provide a relationship enabling the evolution of the patient's story" (Sakalys, 2003, p. 228).

Use of metaphors that illustrate feelings is common within stories. For example, a diagnosis of Lupus can be described as a black cloud that hangs over a family and disrupts daily life in an unpredictable way. One narrative reframing technique used in storytelling involves having a family share a metaphor that illustrates a common pattern in their life. For example, one family described a common pattern of tantrums and arguments as "The Grouchies." By renaming this negative pattern, they gained control over a situation that had previously felt overwhelming. The reframing allowed them to be creative about coming up with solutions. Family members discussed all options for taming The Grouchies. This playful approach moved the family climate away from criticizing and labeling individual family members as 'bad' to involving everyone in preventing a visit by The Grouchies (Tuyn, 2003).

One technique, life narrative interviewing, is used to encourage patients to reminisce and recall positive aspects of their life, their strengths, and resources. It is done to affirm the storyteller's sense of self and to activate positive coping strategies. Narrative life interviewing also serves the purpose of finding meaning and a sense of continuity between one's past and the present (Rybarcyk & Bellg, 1997). The nurse begins life narrative interviewing by using open-ended questions and prompts such as:

1. What is the biggest health challenge you have overcome? How did you do that?
2. Tell me about an accomplishment you are most proud of in your life.

3. What is one thing you would do differently to maintain your health if you could live your life over?
4. Tell me about a health-related goal you have been working on.

Letter writing is another form of narrative that often has an enduring impact. Letters can be sent to a patient by a primary nurse after discharge to summarize patient strengths and future health goals. Letters can also be sent following a death to highlight the person's enduring qualities or memorable moments from their life. Family members keep letters and reread them in difficult periods (Tuyn, 2003).

Sandtray: A Pictorial Type Of Storytelling

A sandtray (3 × 16 × 24 inch waterproof tray filled with sand) and small figurines can be used for a type of storytelling called mutual storytelling. A benefit of mutual storytelling is that it externalizes conflict, provides psychological safety, and allows for expressing complex meanings with multidimensional symbols (figurines). When a series of stories are shared, the method allows for desensitization and mastery of unconscious conflict over time.

In this method the patient searches through a collection of small figurines and uses them to make up a story. Sometimes a broad theme, such as "Tell me a story about something you hope for" is used to introduce the storytelling activity. Oftentimes a camera is used to take a picture of scenes from the story. As the story is told, the nurse listens for maladaptive themes, considers the overall atmosphere or tone of the story, and asks questions to learn what the figurines that were used mean to the patient. For example, the nurse can ask "What made the wolf so angry?" or "What sort of a house is that?"

In the mutual storytelling phase, the nurse creates a similar story using the same characters in a similar setting but introduces healthier adaptations and resolutions of the conflicts exhibited in the initial story. The purpose of this phase is to provide more alternatives and resolutions that the patient did not previously consider. It is helpful to ask the patient what the moral of the retold story is to see if the retold story was understood.

As an example, let's consider a story told by a 50-year-old woman who had been diagnosed with stage III breast cancer and was undergoing chemotherapy. During her career she had been a reporter for a large newspaper. The nurse prompted the woman to construct a sandtray story about something she wished for and everything that was keeping her from achieving that wish. The woman selected a small child-like figure to represent herself as well as a tiny book to place in the center of the sandtray. Surrounding those items were a variety of wild animals (tigers, lions, elephants, etc.) and a collection of healthcare personnel and health-related items (a doctor, a nurse, an ambulance, a stethoscope). When the nurse asked her what the animals and health-related items represented, the woman replied "Everything that is keeping me from finishing my novel. The animals are my cancer. They are bigger than I am and threatening me all the time. The doctor, the nurse, and the ambulance are also keeping me from finishing my novel. Most days are filled with medical appointments. Most days I feel too frightened, tired or sad to work on my novel. I had started the novel before I was diagnosed with cancer. I really enjoyed writing. All I want to do is finish my novel."

The nurse said she had a similar story that she wanted to share with the woman. The nurse moved the animals and the healthcare items farther out toward the edge of the sandtray. She selected a picket fence to put between the woman and the animals and healthcare items. Inside the fence the nurse placed a bed, a Ferris wheel, and a domestic cat. She replaced the child-like figure with a female wizard sitting in front of a desk. The nurse put the book on the desk and told the following story: "A wise woman I know decided to create some space to finish her life's work, a book that contained all the gems from her long working career. Because she knew this was a daunting task, the wise woman always made sure she carved out enough time to rest (pointing to the bed), scheduled regular time for fun (pointing to the Ferris wheel), and made sure she had what she needed to comfort and sustain herself (pointing to the domestic cat). She knew she had to keep the forces that interfered with her goal at a distance (pointing to the picket fence) so she could finish her work." Next, the nurse asked the woman what a fitting moral would be for the retold story. The woman replied, "If you keep your boundaries and pace yourself, you can do what you really want to." The nurse took this response as evidence that the woman had understood her retold story. Do you agree with that conclusion?

Mutual storytelling can be used with children, adolescents, adults, and with groups. It is an enjoyable way of evaluating and intervening with psychological issues such as one would expect when a patient had been diagnosed with a serious illness, had experienced a major life event or developmental norm, or had undergone a major loss (Gardner, 1986). Mutual storytelling using a sandtray can be done in an inpatient play room or an outpatient setting. Mutual storytelling can also be done verbally without using sandtray figures. The patient merely tells the story; the nurse listens for maladaptive themes in the story, and then retells the story including a healthier adaptation to the presented conflict.

READING AND WRITING POETRY

The poet David Whyte asserts that poetry provides a way of making sense of one's experience by giving voice to feelings individuals are not easily able to articulate (Reece, 2000). Poetry is an art form that involves collecting together details and scattered particulars into a coherent whole for the purpose of accessing meaning (Carper, 1978; Holmes & Gregory, 1998). Poets "see what others ignore or cannot find the words to adequately express" (Homes & Gregory, 1998, p. 1192). Rowe (2000) suggested that the poignant, stark nature of poetry strikes the reader from the beginning and is more often remembered than are prose or scientific jargon. Poems allow one to say a lot with a relatively few words (Frampton, 1986). Some authors have claimed that the use of poetry in healing is as old as the first chants sung around tribal fires.

No two individuals interpret a poem in exactly the same way; one's background influences how meaning is understood (Akhtar, 2000). Poetry is "dialogical: it seeks in the listener an ally whose empathy will take the form of sharing the survivor's anguish and struggle" (Kaminsky, 1998, p. 408). Poetry allows one to share a residue of another's experience that is like our own.

Poetry includes images of actual places and people to create a sense of realism and enhance the ability of the reader to be in the present moment that the author is describing (Hunter, 2002). The literal and the metaphorical are woven throughout each poem so that we can relate to the story, connect with the narrator, and understand the themes expressed. Collections of literal examples and metaphors within poetry "provide us with the opportunity to look at something from different perspectives" (Hunter, 2002, p. 143). Details, vivid examples, and particular descriptions within the poem bring the reader's awareness to the moment by drawing the reader into the world of the poem. Connelly (1999) explained that "the power of poetry is to insist on immediacy" and engage us with the particular (p. 420). The detailed complexity within poetry mirrors the ambiguity of everyday life and creates feelings of "real" and "believable."

When nurses encourage patients to write a poem about their feelings or experiences, it helps revive a sense of self-worth or creativity that had been lost as a result of a major illness (Frampton, 1986). Patients can be reminded that writing poetry allows them to listen to a part of themselves that knows what is true during a period of crisis (Remen, 1995). Also, simply reading poetry to a patient allows a nurse to be with the patient. Dialogue about the poem following the reading enables the nurse to get a sense of the patient's emotional state.

Poetry about a given topic such as pain, sudden loss, or death and dying can be used to help individuals cope with a new diagnosis or adjust to their current state of health. In Canada, a group of nurses from public health, a clinic, acute care, a detoxification center, and a university offered a series of art activities for female substance abusers to help them make sense of their world, to build on their strengths, and to involve them in a health-promoting activity. Art activities included poetry writing, mask making, collages, self-portraits, and drawings. The works were so powerful that a local art gallery hosted a 2-month show of the women's creations. The artistic works were also presented at an International Conference on Drug-Related Harm and at a nursing conference. These showings "resulted in great pride for the women and permitted expression of their voices within their own community" (Paivinen & Bade, 2008, p. 217). In expressing the value of the art and poetry sessions, one woman wrote, "For me, art is like emptying your dreams and thoughts on a piece of paper. It's like a little hummingbird, we just need a little taste then we can find our wings and fly away and take one day at a time" (p. 218). How do you think the nurses found the resources to support this project? What might a nurse say if initially a woman commented, "I think art is silly—it can't help me get over my drug habit."

Another project in Los Angeles used poetry, film, and photography to develop social capital by enhancing the African American community's ability to communicate effectively about depression (Chung et al., 2006). In yet another intervention, African American women who had survived breast cancer were interviewed and verbatim words from the focus groups were used to develop 11 poems. The nurse who wrote the poems created them to share with other nurses so that culturally competent breast cancer care could be provided to African American women. The definitions of beauty, the meaning of waiting for a diagnosis and how that impacted trust in the healthcare system, the importance of scripture, and meanings associated with silence were themes conveyed in the poems (Kooken, Haase, & Russell, 2007). By using testimonies, photographs, and poetry, barriers to breast cancer screening were minimized in another African American community. These creative works were used to address barriers such as logistic concerns, lack of knowledge, and a sense of fatalism that interfered with breast cancer screening (Gibson, 2008).

Poetry has also been used to educate nursing students and to enable practicing nurses to describe and let go of powerful clinical experiences. Poetry helps develop empathy and emotional intelligence by assisting a nurse to recognize and manage his or her feelings and those of others (Goleman, 1998). Poetry invites one to broaden their perceptual and emotional horizon by experiencing a multiplicity of diverse points of view and affective states (Roberts, 2010).

ART AND ART THERAPY

Art helps people to think differently, try new behaviors, and express emotion. "Art helps people express experiences that are too difficult to put into words, such as a diagnosis of cancer" (Stuckey & Nobel, 2010, p. 256). Art can help a person explore the meaning of past and present experiences as well as future hopes, "thereby integrating cancer into their life story and giving it meaning" (p. 256). Art can be used to increase one's understanding of themselves or others, "develop a capacity for self-reflection, reduce symptoms, change behavior, alter thinking patterns, inhibit maladaptive responses, and encourage adaptive ones" (Camic, 2008, p. 295).

Art therapy uses drawings, paintings, collages, and sculpture to explore and express emotion, thoughts, and memories, as well as to allow time for reflection and to diminish stress. Many forms of art include a tactile component such as pottery, textiles, and collage-making. Artistic ability is not important; rather, the focus is on art therapy as a means of expression. Mediums such as oil paints, tempera, clay, textiles, lead pencils, and charcoal are provided and the participant is allowed to select which ones to use. Often a theme will be suggested, but the participant is encouraged to create a product that expresses their feelings without substantial direction (Sweeney, 2009). Typical prompts include "Draw your addiction/diagnosis" or "Draw where you are on your path to health/recovery" (Matto, Corcoran, & Fassler, 2003). The participant decides when the work is finished and shares whatever they wish about their product.

The art therapist or the nurse using art therapy does not interpret or analyze the artistic creation, rather only asks questions that allow the individual to express their feelings (Matto, Corcoran, & Fassler, 2003; Sweeney, 2009). One begins by asking the person to describe their overall work; suggested questions include:

1. Tell me about your picture/sculpture.
2. What would you title the picture?
3. What thoughts immediately come to mind as you look at your drawing?
4. What are the people/objects feeling?
5. What are the affirming symbols in your piece?
6. What surprised you the most about your work?
7. What is the loudest/softest part of your work saying? Who would you like to be listening?
8. What part of your drawing do you need to let go of?
9. What would a new ending to this work look like? What would need to come about/change for that ending to take place?" (Matto, Corcoran, & Fassler, 2003, p. 268–269).

Typical follow-up questions focus on the colors used, placement of objects on a page, size and the shape of various objects, and symbols used.

Just as with mutual storytelling, it is effective to ask the participant to retell or revise the work. A person can be asked to create another drawing that represents movement toward a desired state of health. Prompts can be used, such as "Imagine overnight something has changed inside of your heart without you noticing it . . . illustrate what that change would look like" (Matto, Corcoran, & Fassler, 2003, p. 271). Although these are typical questions asked by an art therapist, the same approach can be used by a nurse working in an outpatient cancer center, a mental health unit, a home health agency, or with patients who see the same nurse frequently—for example, with patients who have sickle cell disease and see a nurse for multiple visits. Several drawings from a single individual created over time can be kept in a portfolio to document changes that are occurring (Matto, Corcoran, & Fassler, 2003).

Art therapy works because the process of creating images accelerates and promotes the recall of memories, feelings, and details. The creative process facilitates a sense of detachment that allows one to obtain a more objective perspective and to identify relevant solutions. The problem or the diagnosis becomes more fluid and open to change when it is experienced as a work of art. By creating their work of art, the individual also becomes more actively engaged in behavioral change (Matto, Corcoran, & Fassler, 2003).

By reframing or introducing people to a new way of viewing the situation, art therapists and nurses using art therapy methods invite individuals to realize that every problem contains within it an inherent strength or blessing. Reframing encourages people to view the problem or situation in a new light, which generates actions or solutions that address the issue (O'Hanlon & Weiner-Davis, 1989).

Art therapy is a relatively inexpensive intervention that has been used with a variety of populations including women undergoing treatment for breast cancer (Svensk et al., 2009), with older adults (Johnson & Sullivan-Marx, 2006), with individuals who have a substance abuse problem (Matto, Corcoran, & Fassler, 2003), and with rural residents, among others (Sweeney, 2009). Art therapy in cancer care has resulted in enhanced communication, improved processing of traumatic events, reduction of symptoms, increased energy, and enhanced questioning of traditionally gendered limits and boundaries (Svensk et al., 2009).

Exhibits in which cancer survivors display their works of art and share them with the larger community have been successful (Nainis et al., 2006). In Australia and England, community-based arts initiatives have been used to raise public awareness of mental health issues, minimize isolation associated with a diagnosis, and improve understanding of multiple cultures (Kirrmann, 2010; VicHealth, 2003). Johnson and colleagues (2006) commented that, "art-making is communication that can be felt, seen, and heard. Art is an assertive act giving the patient and others a measure of control and opening up creative discovery and possibilities for change" (p.309). Art is a creative process that engenders hope. When exhibits are used, others relate to the common experiences that show within the work and a sense of emotional connection is engendered. For individuals who are exhibiting their work, "the opportunity to reminisce and to have others participate in the reminiscence honors their histories and helps patients to find meaning" in their experience (p. 310).

One example of a group art project was used with working-class Latino women. A large piece of butcher paper was mounted on the wall, on which individuals put their age, place of birth, hobbies, family celebrations, childhood memories, and a graphic description of their current life situation. They were also asked to use clay to make an abstract representation of individuals who were important to them from their child-hood and write an unspoken message that the person had given them that still influ-enced their life today. The art activity allowed women to describe their roots and how they were managing the transition to living in the United States (Ciornai, 1983).

In Canada, a health promotion research project focused on a disadvantaged area of a large city with the goal of reducing health inequities related to social determinants of health. A vibrant art facility was funded that encouraged school age children and community residents to engage in arts during evening and weekend hours. Local artists sponsored an afterschool art club that made painting, drawing, storytelling, garden art, and open studio time available to local residents. Space, art materials, and instructors were provided. The center also provided a place for social interaction and sharing. Five hundred community members attended 25 courses in the first year. Fundraising activities involving a local restaurant owner and a local butcher are contributing to the self sufficiency of the program (Carson, Chappell, & Knight, 2007). How could you use art with a child or an adult with whom you have worked in the last month of your clinical rotation?

PHOTO-VOICE

Photo-voice is a research strategy and a process by which community members "iden-tify, represent, and enhance their community" using photography (Wang & Burris, 1997, p. 369). It is used to empower community members to record and "reflect their community's strengths and concerns, to promote dialogue . . . through large and small group discussion of the photographs, and to reach policymakers" (Wang & Burris, 1997, p. 369). Community members record issues of concern and act as catalysts for change by using pictures to tell a story that illustrates health concerns. The vivid nature of the photographs that catalogue the primary issues provide evidence of needed change. This method has also been called photo-novella and foto-novella. Stryker defined this sort of documentary photography as showing "the things that need to be said in the language of pictures" (Wang & Burris, 1997, p. 371). Photo-voice is based on Paulo Freire's approach to documentary photography: using ideas that images portray, photographs are collected with the aim of influencing policymakers. Community members actively participate in collecting and analyzing images (Wang & Pies, 2004).

Photo-voice can be used with community members who are not fluent in the domi-nant language and with people who are not literate, but nevertheless have an insight into their community that an outside professional would not. Photo-voice allows disenfranchised groups such as homeless children to "shoot back" with their cameras and to capture the social conscience of a community in visual imagery. Photo-voice allows one to step inside the viewpoint of the people who live in a given community. It contributes to a sense of community and yields a richer description of the daily challenges than can typically be found using other approaches.

Two copies of most photographs are made so that one copy can be given back to neighbors and friends who allowed their picture to be taken. This allows participants "to express their appreciation, build ties, and pass along something of value made by themselves" (Wang & Burris, 1997, p. 373). Participants are taught how to approach someone to ask if it is OK to take his or her picture. They are taught about what sorts of situations should not be photographed and whether they could be in physical danger or if privacy could be lost by taking a photograph. Community members are asked to sign consent forms agreeing that their photographs and analysis can be used in research (Wang & Pies, 2004).

Photo-voice is a method that captures community needs and also assets. The first step involves choosing the photographs that most accurately reflect community needs and assets, telling stories about what the photographs mean, identifying recurring themes that emerge, and adding a caption to each selected photograph that captures its primary meanings. Photo-voice "is a participatory method not of counting up things but of drawing on the community's active lore and stories" (Wang & Burris, 1997, p. 382). Since the photographs are discussed after they are processed, they help community members to prioritize their needs and identify relevant solutions. This approach encourages community members to become advocates for their own well-being. The method is "designed to increase the individual's and the community's access to power. It involves people at the grassroots level in all aspects of defining their community's concerns, furnishing the evidence, and getting solutions enacted into programs and policies" (Wang & Burris, 1997, p. 382). The method "affirms the ingenuity and perspective of society's most vulnerable populations" and gives them a voice in creating change (Wang & Burris, 1997, p. 384).

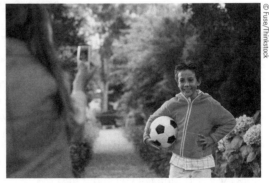

One disadvantage of the method is that photo-voice produces large numbers of photographs, which take time to discuss, digest, and analyze. The data that is generated is complex and filled with meaning. The facilitator or researcher who is familiar with local history and culture asks community members to discuss questions such as:

1. What is this photograph about?
2. What does this picture tell us?
3. What do you see here? What is really happening?
4. Why does this situation exist? How does it relate to our lives?
5. What do these photographs tell us about what should be preserved in this community? What should be changed?
6. How could those changes be brought about? What can we do? What are the barriers and resources that will get in the way of or facilitate change? (Wang & Pies, 2004, p. 98).

Photo-voice has been used to engage youth in identifying reasons for neighborhood violence. After themes had been identified that had at least four compelling photographs, youth respondents spent several minutes free writing and answering the questions here. One boy, for example, took a picture of a bus with several bullet holes. In describing the picture he wrote:

> There are two sides to every story: a person with a gun and demands and a person with fear and a wallet. As I am going to school, I can tell that the bus I ride in is always different because the bullet holes are always in different windows . . . The bullet holes are cold reminders that you never know what will happen next. This violence exists because people don't know how to deal with hardships and anger. They think it's easier to rob people for money or shoot when they are scared. But in the long run, it is much harder. We need to show people that they have special skills and help them find out what their gifts are. Once they believe they are not victims of circumstance and they can determine their destiny, they will find this strength many times more powerful than a gun. (Wang et al., 2004, p. 913)

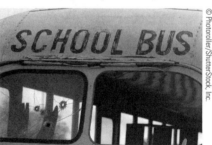

© Photoroller/ShutterStock, Inc.

How would you respond as a nurse to the boy's description of his school bus? What does the description tell you about the boy?

As part of the State Maternal and Child Health Title V federal block grant funds, photo-voice was used to help develop a 5-year plan in Contra Costa County and the San Francisco Bay area of California. One theme that emerged was the need for safe recreational areas. Pictures included a cross marking a street where children had been killed, a park sign that read "This area is not maintained by the city, enter at your own risk," and hypodermic needles sticking out of a sandbox in the park (Wang & Pies, 2004, p. 98). Another theme was neglect of property. Pictures included graffiti, trash piled on the street, a closed hospital, and a poorly maintained bathroom with filthy water sinks and toilets. This project resulted in the county reopening a city clinic that made healthcare services available to low income individuals (Wang & Pies, 2004). What other unmet needs were portrayed in the pictures described here? If you were working as a community health nurse, what would you fight for next now that the city reopened the healthcare clinic?

SOAP OPERAS

Soap operas have been used in Mexico, Turkey, Brazil, Nigeria (Hagerman, 1991), England (Howe, Owen-Smith, & Richardson, 2002; Verma, Adams, & White, 2007), the United States (Love, Mouttapa, & Tanjasiri, 2009), and Tanzania (Rogers et al., 1999) to teach health-related topics such as adult literacy, sex education, and the status of women and children. Mexico's Miguel Sabido originated the idea of using telenovelas or soap operas to offer health education and health promotion content. His first soap opera focused on adult literacy, followed by a soap opera on family planning, sex education, women's status, AIDS, and the treatment of children (Hagerman, 1991). The soap operas were designed to help people identify with and create an emotional involvement with the characters and to use realistic plots that mirrored everyday health challenges.

A soap opera titled *Coronation Street* included a central character who developed cervical cancer and experienced excessive wait times for Pap smears. The show was televised four times per week in England and had over 13 million viewers per episode. A research study compared average numbers of Pap smears taken before and after airing of the episode involving this character and found that there was a sharp increase in the number of cervical smears taken following airing of this soap opera (Howe, Owen-Smith, & Richardson, 2002).

Love and colleagues (2009) discussed the fact that an audience often views a soap opera character as a counselor, comforter, and model. This type of modeling is especially effective with low-literacy female populations. Love and colleagues (2009) did research with Thai-speaking women living in Los Angeles who learned about barriers to scheduling Pap tests in a soap opera format. The main character in the soap opera modeled desirable behavior, and this intervention was more effective than a comparison group intervention in changing attitudes about Pap smears. Sixty-five percent of women who viewed the soap opera changed their mind about talking to a physician about scheduling a Pap smear versus 48.6% in the comparison group.

A subplot on HIV/AIDS was included in the soap opera *The Bold and the Beautiful*. During the show, the AIDS and Sexually Transmitted Disease hotline numbers were displayed. Caller volume was so high the hotlines were overwhelmed (Kennedy et al., 2004). A soap opera video format was used with African American urban women living in the northeastern part of the United States and evaluated using a handheld computer. "In the video, Kayla, a young African American woman, had not heard from nor seen her partner, Steve, in 2 weeks. She was anxiously awaiting a call from him. She happened to see Steve talking to a woman whom she believed Steve was seeing. That afternoon Kayla came home to find a message from Steve on her answering machine. Steve was asking if he could come over" (Jones, 2008, p. 879). Following the video, the women are asked whether: (1) Kayla let Steve come over, (2) they had sex, and (3) they used a condom. The Women's Sex Role scale was used to evaluate perceptions to the vignette. Finally, the video required that viewers develop a realistic ending for the script. Nearly one-half of the women studied reported unprotected sex is expected to maintain a relationship and developed a story ending that involved Kayla having sex with Steve without using a condom. This study, which was funded by the National Institute of Nursing Research, highlighted a belief that put women at risk of contracting HIV/AIDS. The study resulted in future funding designed to test the effects of a series of soap opera videos on behavior change and health education knowledge (Jones, 2008).

CARTOONS

Cartoon characters facilitate children's recall because fun and fantasy are appealing. Thus, cartoon characters can and have been be used both to promote health and also to market unhealthy food choices. A study in Australia documented that cartoon characters marketing unhealthy foods created long-term brand recognition and loyalty from an early age. Similar marketing efforts in the United States have offered collectible cartoon characters along with fast food choices. Regulations that restrict the use of cartoons and collectibles to advertise non-core food choices are now being debated in both Australia and the United States (Kelly et al., 2008).

Graphic illustrations and cartoons that are included in education materials increase patient interest and attention while improving adherence. Cartoon illustrations have been used to increase compliance with emergency room discharge instructions such as suture removal, wound care, signs of infection, and ways of reducing scarring. Because the reading level of emergency room patients is often sixth grade or lower, visual representations are effective and engaging. Ninety-seven percent of patients were satisfied with cartoon-based emergency room discharge instructions compared with 66% who were satisfied with standardized discharge instructions (Delp & Jones, 1996).

Animated cartoons have been used by the United States Centers for Disease Control and Prevention to encourage mothers to take their children to get polio vaccinations. Music, movement, and dialogues were used to maintain viewer attention. Because it is easy to use voice-over technology to change the language of a cartoon, these programs are easy to export to different countries with minimal adaptation (Leiner, Handal, & Williams, 2004). The National Heart, Lung, and Blood Institute of the U.S. Department of Health and Human Services selected Garfield, the popular cat from the cartoon strip of that name, as a spokes-cat for their campaign to encourage children aged 7 to 11 to get at least 9 hours of sleep per night. Because of Garfield's popularity, he has been an effective messenger (Twery, 2006).

A participatory-based narrative approach was used in South Africa to develop eight-page cartoon booklets about two families who were dealing with HIV/AIDS in very different ways. Qualitative interviews were used to identify HIV/AIDS-associated themes such as the disempowerment of parents, poor communication between parents and children, lack of knowledge about HIV transmission, and stigmatization associated with having AIDS. These themes were then used to develop two different story lines, one of which focused on the AmaQhawe (Champion) family and the other of which that focused on the Xakekile (Unfortunate) family. The characters were developed and drawings were created by working with this rural South African community. The serialized cartoons included exercises families were to complete. An example of one fill-in-the-blank exercise required participants to respond how they would tell Themba, one of the characters, to handle being called AIDS boy. The community rated the cartoon narratives as an effective way to present AIDS-related health information (Petersen, et al., 2006).

Thirty-four cartoon characters were developed using a participatory approach involving fifth graders from five schools in the United States. The cartoon characters belonged to one of two families. "The Fitwits epitomized healthy foods and desirable lifestyle choices including physical activities and active hobbies while the Nitwits typified unhealthy food choices and undesirable lifestyle choices" (McGaffey et al., 2010, p. 1135). Character names such as Elvis Pretzley, Sunny Yolk, Fry Girls, Biggie Allbeef, Barfenstein, and the Belchers were used. The cards and game are available at http ://www.fitwits.org The activity began by having children dance to popular music. Next, a 1-minute video of the cartoon characters was used. "A portion size instruction was included using the students' own hands. Children were also taught about obesity-associated diabetes, and heart disease with a dilated, fat-encased heart" (p. 1138). Next, an activity in which students identified fat and sugar-laden foods was used followed by a trivia game to reinforce previous messages. Fifth graders increased their knowledge of portion sizes and the sugar content of various foods using this cartoon-based approach (McGaffey et al., 2010).

MUSIC

Music has been called a universal language that is effective with people from all cultural backgrounds (Olofsson & Fossum, 2009). Music has a psychological and physiological response on the human body. Even Florence Nightingale documented the value of music in promoting healing.

Attention to rhythm is an important element to consider when selecting music for therapeutic purposes. It is also important to consider melody, which has an influ-ence on emotions and moods that can lead to improved health outcomes. "Music can summon memories of past experiences and their associated emotions" (Murrock & Higgins, 2009, p. 2251). Some have argued that music serves as an audi-tory distraction that is helpful in managing pain, exertion, and other unpleasant stimuli. Listening to "calming music releases beta-endorphins, the body's natural opioid pain relievers" (Murrock & Higgins, 2009, p. 2252). Music has been shown to decrease blood pressure, heart rate, respiratory rate, and oxygen consumption. Music motivates movement and helps increase physical activity levels. The rhythm of a musi-cal piece cues the timing and cadence of physical movements.

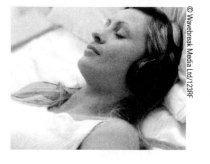

© Wavebreak Media Ltd/123RF

Music is "safe, cost-effective, non-invasive, and easy to implement in different set-tings" (Murrock & Higgins, 2009, p. 2254). It requires a minimal time investment by the nurse to yield substantial benefits. Often a duration of 20 to 40 minutes is sufficient to be effective (Liu, Chang, & Chen, 2010). The widespread availability of headphones allows patients to focus on the music while avoiding any disruption should they have a roommate. Music can be used in nursing homes, hospitals, waiting rooms, surgical centers, schools, and community settings.

Music selections should be tailored to the preferences of the listening population (Murrock & Higgins, 2009). Allowing patients to self-select music introduces a sense of familiarity in an unfamiliar environment. Patients can be encouraged to bring in their own music or family and friends can be interviewed to help determine patient preference (Sung, Chang, & Lee, 2010).

Music has been effectively used to manage pain, aid sleep, decrease anxiety associated with surgery, lower blood pressure for patients undergoing a colonoscopy, lower heart rate for ventilated patients (Chan et al., 2008), decrease labor pain, decrease stress in fibromyalgia patients (Liu, Chang, & Chen, 2010), decrease anxiety in dementia patients (Sung, Chang, & Lee, 2010), decrease side effects of chemotherapy (Olofsson, & Fossum, 2009), and increase oxytocin and relaxation levels after open-heart surgery (Nilsson, 2009). Although many healthcare settings employ music therapists, a common nursing intervention is encouraging use of music with patients to promote healing. It is important that the equipment used to play the music be of good quality and that equipment can be cleaned if shared by more than one patient (Nilsson, 2009).

DANCE

Because motivation and social support are important factors that influence whether a person continues a health-promoting activity, options such as dance, which are inherently enjoyable, are effective. Dance is a leisure activity which also has health benefits (Kreutz, 2008). It helps restore the connection between the physical body and one's emotions. Dance can be used with patients who have physical limitations as well as perceptual and communication problems (Hoban, 2000). For hospitalized individuals, scarves, paper fans, and streamers have been used so that bed-bound individuals can keep time or dance to the music (Lane, 2005).

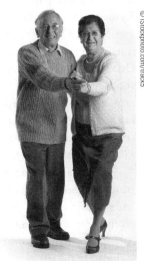

© iStockphoto.com/track5

Dance has been used to improve fitness levels of African American and Hispanic teens. Hip-hop music and high-intensity aerobic dance was evaluated as being "fun without being boring" by teens. Minimal equipment was required and everyone was able to be successful in that the routines were noncompetitive. Body mass index and resting heart rate of teens in the dance group improved compared to students enrolled in a comparison group who spent a comparable amount of time engaged in playground activities (Flores, 1995). What would a nurse want to evaluate when considering what music to use in a dance class? What are the advantages and disadvantages of letting teens select their own music choices?

Partnered tango dance classes have been used to improve the gait and balance of older individuals with Parkinson's disease. Tango was selected because it "involves frequent movement initiation and cessation, a range of speeds, and rhythmic variation" (Hackney & Earhart, 2011, p. 385). Improved balance, increases in walking distance, gait speed, and endurance were documented after 20 tango lessons.

Postmenopausal women used interactive video dance and a force-sensing pad synchronized to music to improve coordination, promote weight loss, increase endurance, improve balance, and increase flexibility. Video dance is engaging and provides rapid feedback about the accuracy of foot placement using a 3 foot x 3 foot mat. Individuals can select songs and the complexity of dance patterns so that increasing challenge is built into the dance. After each dance the dancer gets feedback on the correct number of dance steps. The total cost of the system is between $50 and $700 for professional versions (Inzitari et al., 2009). Belly dancing has also been used to tone uterine muscles prior to childbirth. It is not uncommon for women in the Middle East to practice belly dancing movements for 5 years prior to conception and to tone abdominal muscles after birth (Kananghinis, 2001).

THEATER

Live drama is a high-impact way of communicating. It is interactive and encourages audience participation while being nonconfrontational. Both those involved in a performance and the audience identify with characters in the play and the conflicts they experience. The degree of identification depends on how likable the character is, how much one wants to become like the character, and by what happens to the character. One learns through identification and modeling without having to have direct personal experience. It is easy to identify with both the characters and the decisions they face in the play or performance (Mitschke et al, 2008). In performing arts, "meaning arises in the interaction between performer, performance and spectator . . . The emphasis is on the process of the performance with the accent on pleasure and play" (Skaife & Jones, 2009, p. 203).

Theater and drama, especially street theater, has been used to disseminate health education. Semi-professional theater groups travel to locations and recruit local amateurs to join them in presenting performances that fit the cultural framework of the given community. Improvisation is used so that no two performances are similar. After performances, community health workers hold discussions to reinforce messages included in the performances (Pelto & Singh, 2010).

In one variation, actors were used to depict a realistic and undesirable health outcome. At the end of that scene, community members are invited to come on stage and act out a healthier solution to the problem being portrayed. Oftentimes, a second community member is invited on stage to act out yet another resolution to the health challenge so that multiple perspectives can be considered and the audience has an opportunity to rehearse future options (Baldwin, 2009).

In another variation, actors are given a script to read while they add emotional emphasis, gestures, and facial expressions to the dialogue. Participants are "taught [that] to create drama and tension, the character must strive to remove an obstacle that is keeping him or her from accomplishing a health-related goal" (Jackson, Mullis, & Hughes, 2010, p. 94). Street theatre as just described has been used in Nepal to present information about respiratory infections to children, in India to share information with truckers about avoiding HIV/AIDS, and in Sri Lanka to motivate children to attend school. Colorfully dressed broadcasters often walk a neighborhood singing about the upcoming performance to motivate people to attend. Often, other actors are placed in the audience to heckle the actors and stimulate interest in the performance. The language used is the language of the local people and scripts address issues of importance in the given community (Pelto & Singh, 2010). Why is it important to use the language of the local people, including slang and dialect? Why is audience involvement important?

Role-playing and improvisation in school settings have been used to develop children's social skills, imagination, and health while creating a positive attitude toward the select health-related topic. This work is based on the Confucian saying of "Tell me and I will forget. Show me and I may remember. Involve me and I will understand" (p. 128). Plays focused on HIV prevention, healthy eating, smoking, peer relations, positive self-concepts, and social skills have been taught using dramatic performances (Joronen, Rankin, & Astedt-Kurkip, 2008). "By entering the fictional world created in drama, students and teachers can move safely into" a topic (Joronen, Rankin, & Asted-Kurkip, 2011, p. 2). Drama provides opportunity for independent thinking and a release of emotion. Follow-up activities to be done at home and post-class discussions are used to reinforce topics (Joronen, Rankin, & Asted-Kurkip, 2011).

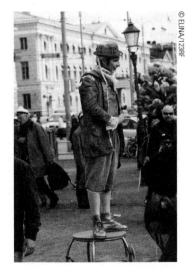

© ELINA/123RF

A variety of theatrical performances have been used to promote the health of communities and to educate groups about health-related topics. One such theatrical performance was developed by youth aged 17 to 21 who performed short skits recounting stories about HIV/AIDS risks. Sanchez-Camus (2009) began by eliciting stories from West African youth that illustrated what they considered to be a problem in terms of HIV/AIDS, what the solutions might be, and how change should be implemented. To integrate and reflect local customs, the play that youth developed was presented during a village festival and incorporated local myths regarding HIV infection and treatment. Youth decided to structure each story by having a performer representing a good conscience and healthy immune system as well as a bad conscience that was partnered with the HIV virus appear and talk to performers during key decision points. The project allowed youth to have an opportunity to express their creativity, to give to their community, and to learn about and reflect on culturally appropriate ways of avoiding HIV exposure. Why was it effective to have the HIV virus appear and talk to performers and the audience in the middle of the performance? What were the advantages of scheduling the performance during a village festival attended by individuals of many ages?

THE IMPORTANCE OF AN AESTHETIC ENVIRONMENT FOR HEALING

Healthcare facilities should be designed to promote the health of patients, staff, and visitors (Ulrich, 1991). Hospitals that include fountains, gardens, and meditation rooms for patients and staff contribute to a sense of well being. Aesthetic environments have been shown to reduce use of medications, promote sleep, improve blood pressure, and result in shorter hospital stays for patients (Ulrich, 2001).

The concept of an art cart, with posters of paintings that patients can select to hang in their hospital room, has been used along with CD players to involve patients in designing their own health-promoting environment (Lane, 2005). Other important design features are those that support family visitation, provide access to positive distractions, minimize noise and harsh lighting, and encourage patient control—as, for example, by offering ample choice in terms of the menu (Ulrich, 1991). Tidiness, décor, design, architecture, temperature, ventilation, sounds, colors, the amount of daylight, and ample personal space decrease stress and

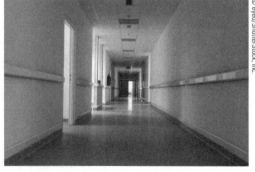

© eyed/ShutterStock, Inc.

add to a person's sense of well-being. Information kiosks, benches, and the cafeteria are also important. Beautiful environments need not be expensive. However, décor that is restful and interesting translates into higher patient satisfaction scores. "A patient who must remain on his or her back, day after day, will not be positively affected by a view of a grey ceiling" (Caspari, Eriksson, & Naden, 2006, p. 856).

Today, it is often the case that functionality is given more consideration than aesthetics when designing healthcare facilities (Caspari, Eriksson, & Naden, 2006). Consider how the Greeks used gardens, open spaces, columns, and water to create a sense of health and healing. The concepts of beauty, harmony, and balance guided all of their architecture, including in their healing centers (Caspari, Eriksson, & Naden, 2006). Now reflect on the hospital where you had your last clinical rotation. What design aspects in that environment contributed to stress reduction and well-being?

Aesthetic environments also contribute to greater job satisfaction and fewer sick calls for staff. The environment will influence patients, staff, and visitors, even if they are not consciously thinking about what surrounds them. "A person continually senses and experiences the environment as aesthetic, unaesthetic, or insignificant . . . Cognitive awareness is not necessary for aesthetics or their lack to influence health. The aesthetic sense need not convert impulses into words. It has its own language and communicates continually through all the senses to every cell of the body and the mind" (Caspari, Eriksson, & Naden, 2006, p. 852).

The Planetree model, which began in San Francisco in 1978, was built on the concept that hospitals should be warm, welcoming, and exist to care for the patient and his or her family. Physicians, nurses, and other healthcare professionals designed the first Planetree hospital by cataloguing and revising all of the influences they had found not to be healing at other hospitals where they had worked. Numerous Planetree hospitals have been developed in various countries since that time, but all emphasize that patient values must come first and that freedom and autonomy are of critical importance. The décor in Planetree hospitals, to whatever degree possible, is designed to look more like furniture and surroundings that would be found in a home rather than in a sterile hospital (Caspari, Eriksson, & Naden, 2006).

Communities as well as healthcare facilities contribute to health and well-being. Social gathering places, art projects, parks, bike lanes, and lighting are all important design aspects of healthy communities. Environments that are safe and contribute to a sense of cohesiveness are vital. "Neighborhoods that are more conducive to walking and social interactions encourage physical activity" (Semenza & Krishnasamy, 2007, p. 244). Feeling at home, recognized, welcomed, and valued as a member of a community lowers stress and facilitates health. Mental health as well as physical health is promoted by having social supports, social cohesion, and a shared sense of identity that derives from a sense of community. Local artists have been recruited to help community members plan neighborhood revitalization programs (Semenza & Krishnasamy, 2007), to create arts displays at local cafes, to offer dance or yoga lessons, to facilitate creative writing classes, or to offer pottery classes, all of which contribute to a sense of health and well-being (Stickley & Duncan, 2007).

NURSING: THE AESTHETIC ART OF KNOWING

A longstanding part of nursing's heritage is aesthetic knowing. "Aesthetic knowing in nursing practice is expressed through the actions, bearing, conduct, attitudes, narrative, and interactions of the nurse in relation to others. It is also expressed in art forms such as poetry, drawings, stories, and music that reflect and communicate symbolic meanings embedded in nursing practice" (Chinn & Kramer, 2004, p. 7).

Nursing makes use of two languages: the language of science found in quantifiable outcomes and the language of people found in observations of health and illness. Nurses must be fluent with both of these languages. Aesthetic knowing in nursing happens in the process of attending to and being with another "such that the nurse is attuned to minute differences not necessarily observable to the more casual observer" (Leight, 2002, p. 111). Aesthetic knowing relies on intuition or the ability to "gaze at the world through a thousand eyes" (Estes, 1995, p. 10). Aesthetic knowing seeks to find form in the midst of chaos; it arrives like enlightenment with a feeling of unity, clarity, and completeness (Smith, 1992). Estes (1995) reflects that nursing is "a craft of hands, a craft of stories, a craft of questions—all these are the making of something, and that something is soul. Anytime we feed soul, it guarantees increase" (p. 13). The relationships nurses create with patients are a form of aesthetic knowing. Nurses listen and help interpret or envision the future when working with patients (Leight, 2002). The "in-the-moment glimpsing of the beauty" in the nurse–patient relationship is the essence of aesthetic knowing in nursing (Leight, 2002; Smith, 1992).

Since all of the aesthetic and creative interventions described in this chapter rely on a playful approach, the nurse–patient relationship must be a trusting, open one that includes a healthy dose of enthusiasm and fun. Fortunately, aesthetic approaches are enjoyable for both the nurse and the patient.

DISCUSSION QUESTIONS

1. Which populations do you think would benefit the most from creative and artistic approaches? Explain your answer.
2. How can one work of art convey multiple meanings and interpretations?
3. What physiological responses are associated with creativity?
4. How do narrative and analytical thinking differ?
5. What benefits and challenges are associated with narrative life interviewing?

6. Why is it that no two individuals interpret a poem in exactly the same way?
7. What is the value of helping a patient understand the meanings they associate with a critical diagnosis?
8. Can photo-voice be used with individuals rather than a community? Describe how that modification might occur.
9. Why is it important to allow the "artist" to interpret their own work rather than having a professional do that?
10. How could you use an art portfolio with a patient you have worked with who had a chronic disease?
11. Why are soap operas an effective way of disseminating healthcare information?
12. What physiological effects does calming music have on the body?
13. How has dance therapy been used in health care? What populations have benefited from dance therapy?
14. What is aesthetic knowing in nursing?

CHECK YOUR UNDERSTANDING: EXERCISE ONE

A home health nurse was working with a 76-year-old male hospice patient who was alert and oriented. The nurse asked the man to tell her about his greatest successes and happiest moments. The man had been "down" and expressing the feeling that he could not handle dying of cancer for several weeks. The nurse hoped to remind the man about previous coping strategies and strengths that were a part of his life experience. The nurse was using which aesthetic technique?

A. Mutual story telling
B. Narrative reframing
C. Narrative life interviewing
D. Sandtray
E. Photo-voice

CHECK YOUR UNDERSTANDING: EXERCISE TWO

A critical aspect of nursing is connecting with patients and identifying which particular intervention would work best for a given person. Recognizing that you do not have a specific case study to base your answer on, complete the following grid to summarize which general populations you think would or would not respond to artistic and creative interventions designed to promote health. Provide a rationale for your answers.

Intervention	Populations for Which the Intervention Would Likely Work	Populations That Would Be Unlikely to Respond to This Intervention	Rationale for Your Answer
Storytelling			
Sandtray			
Poetry			
Art			
Photo-voice			
Soap operas			
Cartoons			
Music			
Dance			
Theater/Drama			

Which of the listed interventions have you seen nurses use with their patients? Which interventions would you be comfortable facilitating? Which would you not be comfortable facilitating? Please discuss your answers and outline a plan for how you will increase your own sense of aesthetic knowing in your nursing practice over the next 5 years.

WHAT DO YOU THINK?

1. Of the aesthetic and creative approaches described in this chapter, which are you most likely to use in your nursing practice?
2. Do you agree that stories are medicine? Why or why not?
3. Describe how you could use narrative reframing in your practice. Provide a specific example.
4. Which of the interventions described in this chapter could you use or modify for use in an inpatient setting?
5. What soap opera plot would you use if you were designing a health education program?
6. How would you introduce a dance program to wheelchair-bound patients?
7. How would you use street theater to teach a health-related topic? Which health-related topic would you target?

8. Which aspects of the facility where you are having your clinical rotation are healing? Which aspects could be redesigned to promote a healing atmosphere for patients and staff?
9. What part of the Planetree model impressed you the most?

REFERENCES

Akhtar, S. (2000). Mental pain and the cultural ointment of poetry. *International Journal of Psychoanalysis, 81*, 229–243.

Baldwin, A. (2009). Applied theatre: Performing the future. *Australian Psychiatry, 17*, S133–S136.

Bravender, T., Russell, A., Chung, R. J., & Armstrong, S. C. (2010). A novel intervention: A pilot study of children's literature and healthy lifestyles. *Pediatrics, 125*(3), 513–517.

Camic, P. M. (2008). Playing in the mud: Health psychology, the arts and creative approaches to healthcare. *Journal of Health Psychology, 13*, 287–298.

Carson, A. J., Chappell, N. L., & Knight, C. J. (2007). Promoting health and innovative health promotion practice through a community arts centre. *Health Promotion Practice, 8*(40), 366–374.

Carper, B. (1978). Fundamental patterns of knowing in nursing. *Advances in Nursing Science, 1*(1), 13–23.

Carter, B. (2004). Pain narratives and narrative practitioners: A way of working in relation with children experiencing pain. *Journal of Nursing Management, 12*, 210–216.

Caspari, S., Eriksson, K., & Naden, D. (2006). The aesthetic dimension in hospitals: An investigation into strategic plans. *International Journal of Nursing Studies, 43*, 851–859.

Chan, M. F., Chung, Y. F., Chung, S. W., & Lee, O. K. (2008). Investigating the physiological responses of patients listening to music in the intensive care unit. *Journal of Clinical Nursing, 118*, 1250–1257.

Chinn, P. L. & Kramer, M. K. (2004*). Integrated knowledge development in nursing* (6th ed.). St. Louis, MO: Mosby.

Chung, B., Corbett, C. E., Boulet, B., Cummings, J. R., Paxton, K., McDaniel, S., . . . Gilk, D. (2006). Talking wellness: A description of a community-academic partnered project to engage an African-American community around depression through the use of poetry, film, and photography. *Ethnic Disparities, 16* (1 Suppl 1), S67–S78.

Ciornai, S. (1983). Art therapy with working class Latino women. *The Arts in Psychotherapy, 10*, 63–76.

Connelly, J. (1999). Being in the present moment: Developing the capacity for mindfulness in medicine. *Academic Medicine, 74*, 420–424.

Delp, C. & Jones, J. (1996). Communicating information to patients: The use of cartoon illustrations to improve comprehension of instructions. *Academic Emergency Medicine, 3*(3), 264–270.

Estes, C. (1995). *Women who run with the wolves: Myths and stories of the wild woman archetype.* New York, NY: Ballantine Books.

Flores, R. (1995). Dance for health: Improving fitness in African-American and Hispanic adolescents. *Public Health Reports, 110*(2), 189–193.

Fogarty, C. T. (2010). Fifty-five word stories: Small jewels for personal reflection and teaching. *Family Medicine, 42*(6), 400–402.

Fox, A.L. (2009). Evaluation of a pilot arts and health module in a graduate community nutrition program. *Canadian Journal of Dietetic Practice and Research, 70*(2), 83–86.

Frampton, D.R. (1986). Creativity and dying patients. *British Medical Journal, 293*, 1593–1595.

Freedman, J., & Combs, G. (1996). *Narrative therapy: The social construction of preferred realities.* New York, NY: Norton.

Gardner, R. (1986). *The psychotherapeutic techniques of Richard Gardner.* Cresskill, NJ: Creative Therapeutics.

Gibson, L. M. (2008). Teaching strategies to facilitate breast cancer screening by African-American women. *Journal of the National Black Nurses Association, 19*(2), 42–49.

Goleman, D. (1998). *Working with emotional intelligence*. London, UK: Bloomsbury.

Hackney, M. E. & Earhart, G. M. (2009). Effects of dance on gait and balance in Parkinson's disease: A comparison of partnered and non-partnered dance movement. *Neurorehabilitation and Neural Repair, 24*(4), 384–392.

Hagerman, E. (1991). As the Third World turns. *World Watch, 4*(5), 5–7.

Hoban, S. (2000). Motion and emotion: The dance/movement therapy experience. *Nursing Homes Long Term Care Management*, 33–34.

Holmes, V., & Gregory, D. (1998). Writing poetry: A way of knowing nursing. *Journal of Advanced Nursing, 28*(6), 1191–1194.

Howe, A., Owen-Smith, V., & Richardson, J. (2002). The impact of a television soap opera on the NHS Cervical Screening Programme in the North West of England. *Journal of Public Health Medicine, 24*(4), 299–304.

Hunter, L. P. (2002). Poetry as an aesthetic expression for nursing: A review. *Journal of Advanced Nursing, 40*(2), 141–148.

Inzitari, M., Greenlee, A., Hess, R., Perera, S. & Studentski, S. A. (2009). Attitudes of postmenopausal women toward interactive video dance for exercise. *Journal of Women's Health, 18*(8), 1239–1243.

Jackson, C. J., Mullis, R. M., & Hughes, M. (2010). Development of a theater-based nutrition and physical activity intervention for low-income, urban, African-American adolescents. *Progress in Community Health Partnerships: Research, Education, and Action, 4*(2), 89–98.

Johnson, C. M., & Sullivan-Marx, E. M. (2006). Art therapy: Using the creative process for healing and hope among African-American older adults. *Geriatric Nursing, 27*(5), 309–316.

Jones, R. (2008). Soap opera video on handheld computers to reduce young urban women's HIV sex risk. *AIDS behavior, 12*, 876–884.

Joronen, K., Konu, A., Rankin, S., & Astedt-Kurki, P. (2012). An evaluation of a drama program to enhance social relationships and anti-bullying at elementary school: A controlled study. *Health Promotion International, 27*(1), 5–14. DOI: 10.1093/heapro/dar012.

Joronen, K., Rankin, S., & Astedt-Kurki, P. (2008). School-based drama interventions in health promotion for children and adolescents: Systematic review. *Journal of Advanced Nursing, 63*(2), 116–131.

Kaminsky, M. (1998). Voicing voicelessness. On the poetics of faith. *American Journal of Psychoanalysis, 58*, 405–416.

Kananghinis, A. (2001). Belly dancing makes birth better. *Australian Nursing Journal, 9*(2), 37.

Kelly, B., Hattersley, L., King, L., & Flood, V. (2008). Persuasive food marketing to children: Use of cartoons and competitions in Australian commercial television advertisements. *Health Promotion International, 23*(4), 337–344.

Kennedy, M. G., O'Leary, A., Beck, V., Pollard, K., & Simpson, P. (2004). Increases in calls to the CDC and National STD and AIDS hotline following AIDS-related episodes in a soap opera. *Journal of Communication, 54*(2), 287–301.

Kester, G. H. (2004). *Conversation pieces: Community + communication in modern art*. Berkeley: University of California Press.

Kirrmann, K. (2010). CoolTan arts: Enhancing well-being through the power of creativity. *Mental Health and Social Inclusion, 14*(20, 12–16.

Kooken, W. C., Haase, J. E., & Russell, K. M. (2007). I've been through something: Poetic explorations of African-American Women's Cancer Survivorship. *Western Journal of Nursing Research, 29*, 896–919.

Kreutz, G. (2008). "Does partnered dance promote health" The case of tango Argentiono. *Journal of Recreational and Social Promotion and Health, 128*(2), 79–84.

Lane, M. R. (2005). Creativity and spirituality in nursing. *Holistic Nursing Practice, 19*(3), 122–125.

Leffers, J. & Martins, D. C. (2004). Journey to compassion: Meeting vulnerable populations in community health nursing through literature. *International Journal for Human Caring, 8*(1), 20–28.

Leight, S. B. (2002). Starry night: Using story to inform aesthetic knowing in women's health nursing. *Journal of Advanced Nursing, 37*(1), 108–114.

Leiner, M., Handal, G., & Williams, D. (2004). Patient communication: A multidisciplinary approach using animated cartoons. *Health Education Research Theory and Practice, 19*(5), 591–595.

Liu, Y., Chang, M., & Chen, C. (2010). Effects of music therapy on labour pain and anxiety in Taiwanese first-time mothers. *Journal of Clinical Nursing, 19*, 1065–1072.

Love, G. D., Mouttapa, M., & Tanjasiri, S. P. (2009). Everybody's talking: Using entertainment-education video to reduce barriers to discussion of cervical cancer screening among Thai women. *Health Education Research, 24*(5), 829–838.

Matto, H., Corcoran, J., & Fassler, A. (2003). Integrating solution-focused and art therapies for substance abuse treatment: Guidelines for practice. *The Arts In Psychotherapy, 30*, 265–272.

McGaffey, A., Hughes, K., Fidler, S. K., D'Amico, F. J., & Stalter, M. N. (2010). Can Elvis Pretzley and the Fitwits improve knowledge of obesity, nutrition, exercise, and portions in fifth graders? *International Journal of Obesity, 34*, 1134–1142.

Milligan, E. & Woodley, E. (2008). Creative expressive encounters in health ethics education: Teaching ethics as relational engagement. *Teaching and Learning in Medicine, 21*(2), 131–139.

Mitschke, D. B., Loebl, K., Tatafu, E., Matsunaga, D. S. & Cassel, K. (2010). Using drama to prevent teen smoking: Development, implementation, and evaluation of crossroads in Hawaii. *Health Promotion Practice, 11*(2), 244–248. DOI: 10.1177/1524839907309869.

Murrock, C. J. & Higgins, P. A. (2009). The theory of music, mood, and movement to improve health outcomes. *Journal of Advanced Nursing, 65*(10), 2249–2257.

Nainis, N., Paice, J. A., Ratner, J., Wirth, J. H., Lai, J. & Shott, S. (2006). Relieving symptoms in cancer: Innovative use of art therapy. *Journal of Pain and Symptom Management, 31*(2), 162–169.

Nilsson, U. (2009). Soothing music can increase oxytocin levels during bed rest after open-heart surgery: A randomized control trial. *Journal of Clinical Nursing, 18*, 2153–2161.

Ogden, T. H. (1999). The music of what happens in poetry and psychoanalysis. *International Journal of Psychoanalysis, 80*, 979–994.

O'Hanlon, W. H., & Weiner-Davis, M. (1989). *In search of solutions: A new direction in psychotherapy*. New York, NY: Norton.

Olofsson, A., & Fossum, B. (2009). Perspectives on music therapy in adult cancer care: A hermeneutic study. *Oncology Nursing Forum, 36*(4), E223–E231.

Pardue, K. T. (2005). Blending aesthetics and empirics: Teaching health assessment in an art gallery. *Journal of Nursing Education. 44*(7), 334–337.

Paivinen, H. & Bade, S. (2008). Voice: Challenging the stigma of addiction; a nursing perspective. *International Journal of Drug Policy, 19*, 214–219.

Pelto, P. J. & Singh, R. (2010). Community street theatre as a tool for interventions on alcohol use and other behaviors related to HIV risks. *AIDS Behavior, 14*, S147–S157.

Petersen, I., Mason, A., Bhana, A., Bell, C. C. & Mckay, M. (2006). Mediating social representations using a cartoon narrative in the context of HIV/AIDS. The AmaQhawe family project in South Africa. *Journal of Health Psychology, 11*, 197–208.

Reece, R. L. (2000). Preserving the soul of medicine and physicians: A talk with David Whyte. *The Physician Executive, 26*(2), 14–19.

Remen, R. (1995). Wholeness. In: B. Moyers & B. Flowers (Eds.)., *Healing and the mind* (pp. 343–363). London, UK: Harper Collins.

Roberts, M. (2010). Emotional intelligence, empathy, and the educative power of poetry: A Deleuzo-Guattarian perspective. *Journal of Psychiatric and Mental Health Nursing, 17*, 236–241.

Rogers, E. M., Vaughan, P. W., Swalehe, R. M., Rao, N., Svenkerud, P., & Sood, S. (1999). Effects of an entertainment-education radio soap opera on family planning behavior in Tanzania. *Studies in Family Planning, 30*(3), 193–211.

Rowe, R. C. (2000). Poetry and verse: An ideal medium for scientific communication. *Drug Discovery Today, 5*(10), 436–437.

Rybarczyk, B., & Bellg, A. (1997). *Listening to life stories: A new approach to stress intervention in healthcare*. New York, NY: Springer.

Sanchez-Camus, R. (2009). The problem of application: Aesthetics in creativity and health. *Health Care Analysis, 17*, 345–355.

Sakalys, J. A. (2003). Restoring the patient's voice: The therapeutics of illness narratives. *Journal of Holistic Nursing, 21*(3), 228–241.

Semenza, J. C. & Krishnasamy, P. V. (2007). Design of a health promoting neighborhood intervention. *Health Promotion Practice. 8,* 243–256.

Skaife, S. E., & Jones, K. (2009). The art therapy large group as a teaching method for the institutional and political aspects of professional training. *Learning in Health and Social Care, 8*(3), 200–209.

Smith, M. (1992). Enhancing esthetic knowledge: A teaching strategy. *Advances in Nursing Science, 14,* 52–59.

Smith, M. J. (2005). Story theory: Advancing nursing practice scholarship. *Holistic Nursing Practice, 19*(6), 272–276.

Smyth, J. M., & Pennebaker, J. W. (1999). Sharing one's story: Translating emotional experiences into words as a coping tool. In C. R. Snyder (Ed.), *Coping: The psychology of what works* (pp. 70–89). New York, NY: Oxford University Press.

Stickley, T., & Duncan, K. (2007). Art in mind: Implementation of a community arts initiative to promote mental health. *Journal of Public Mental Health, 6*(4), 24–32.

Sung, H., Chang, A. M., & Lee, W. (2010). A preferred music listening intervention to reduce anxiety in older adults with dementia in nursing homes. *Journal of Clinical Nursing, 19,* 1056–1064.

Svensk, A. C., Oster, I., Thyme, K. E., Magnusson, E., Sjodin, M., Eisemann, M., . . . Lindh, J. (2009). Art therapy improves experienced quality of life among women undergoing treatment for breast cancer: A randomized controlled study. *European Journal of Cancer Care, 18,* 69–77.

Sweeney, S. (2009). Art therapy: Promoting wellbeing in rural and remote communities. *Australasian Psychiatry, 17*(Suppl), S151–S154.

Stuckey, H. L., & Nobel, J. (2010). The connection between art, healing, and public health: A review of current literature. *American Journal of Public Health, 100*(2), 254–263.

Taylor, D. (2001). *Tell me a story: The life-shaping power of our stories.* St. Paul, MN: Bog Walk Press.

Tuyn, L. K. (2003). Metaphors, letters, and stories: Narrative strategies for family healing. *Holistic Nursing Practice, 17*(1), 22–26.

Twery, M. J. (2006). The cartoon character Garfield and the "sleep well, do well, star sleeper" campaign. *Pediatrics, 118*(3), 1259.

Ulrich, R. S. (1991). Effects of interior design on wellness: Theory and recent scientific research. *Journal of Healthcare and Interior Design, 3,* 97–109.

Verma, T., Adams, J., & White, M. (2007). Portrayal of health-related behaviours in popular UK television soap operas. *Journal of Epidemiological and Community Health, 61,* 575–577.

VicHealth (2003*). Creative connections: Promoting mental health and wellbeing through community arts participation.* Carlton, Australia: Victorian Health Promotion Foundation.

Ulrich, R. (2001). Effects of healthcare environmental design on medical outcomes. In A. Dilani (Ed.), *Art, Design, & Health.* (pp. 49–59) Stockholm, Sweden: Svensk Byggtjanst.

Wang, C. & Burris, M. A. (1997). Photo-voice: Concept, methodology, and use for participatory needs assessment. *Health Education Behavior, 24*(3), 369–387.

Wang, C .C., Morrel-Samuels, S., Hutchinson, P. M., Bell, L., & Pestronk, R. M. (2004). Flint photo-voice: Community building among youths, adults, and policymakers. *American Journal of Public Health, 94*(6), 911–913.

Wang, C. C. & Pies, C. A. (2004). Family, maternal, and child health through photo-voice. *Maternal and Child Health Journal, 8*(2), 95–102.

For a full suite of assignments and additional learning activities, see the access code at the front of your book.

CHAPTER 8

Rural Health Promotion

Alexa Colgrove Curtis

OBJECTIVES

At the conclusion of this chapter, the student will be able to:

- Define a rural community for the purpose of nursing health-promotion program development, policy analysis, and research.
- Identify critical issues affecting the health of rural communities in America.
- Discuss the epigenetic forces affecting the future of rural health in America.
- Recognize the regional, cultural, socioeconomic, and racial and ethnic diversity of rural communities in the United States.
- Articulate cultural factors that may affect the delivery of health-promotion services to rural communities in the United States.
- Examine barriers to the delivery of health-promotion services in rural communities.
- Articulate the role of nursing in the provision of health-promotion services in the rural community.
- Identify opportunities for the utilization of information technologies to improve health-promotion services in the rural community.
- Apply relevant theoretical frameworks to rural health research proposals and the development of health-promotion services in the rural community.
- Develop nursing health-promotion interventions for rural residents across the developmental spectrum corresponding with the Healthy People 2020 objectives.

THE FUTURE OF RURAL HEALTH

Nursing health promotion is critical to the vitality of rural communities in the United States. In *Quality Through Collaboration: The Future of Rural Health Care*, the Institute of Medicine (IOM) projected that the burden of chronic disease in rural communities will become enormous unless health-related behavioral risk factors are addressed

(IOM, 2005). The actualization of nursing health-promotion activities at multiple intersects within the rural community holds unrealized potential to lessen the burden of chronic disease and substantially impact the future trajectory of rural health. Public health nurses, school nurses, home health nurses, community-based advanced practice nurses, and tertiary care nurses all play an integral role in protecting the future of the rural community through innovations in nursing health promotion.

DEFINING THE RURAL COMMUNITY

Rural communities are most commonly identified using population density and geographic parameters. The U.S. Census Bureau identifies rural communities as regions that do not meet the population criteria for an urban area (50,000 people with a population density exceeding 1,000 per square mile) or an urban cluster (2,500 people) (Hart, Larson, & Lishner, 2005; U.S. Census Bureau, 2011d; U.S. Census Bureau,

FIGURE 8-1   Distribution of Metro and Non-Metro Counties in the United States

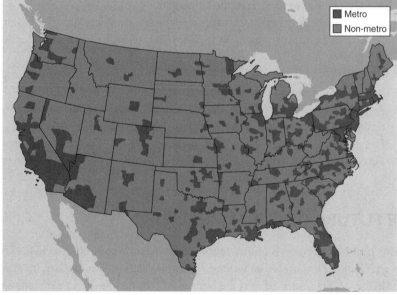

Source: United States Department of Agriculture Economic Research Service, http://maps.ers.usda .gov/new_rural/

2011a). Many reports of rural health use the United States Office of Management and Budget's (OMB) nonmetropolitan county designation (counties that do not meet the U.S. Census Bureau urban criteria) as the operational definition of a rural region (U.S. Census Bureau,

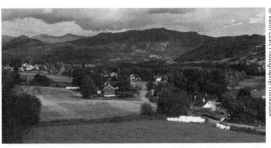

2011c). The OMB further divides nonmetropolitan counties into "micropolitan" counties with a minimum population of 10,000 residents including an urban cluster and the less dense "noncore" counties without an urban cluster (U.S. Census Bureau, 2011c). "Frontier" rural areas are sparsely populated regions situated in remote geographic locations with a population density of less than six residents per square mile (Rural Assistance Center [RAC], 2011a). The Rural Urban Commuting Area (RUCA) codes used by the Economic Research Service of the United States Department of Agriculture (USDA) and the Office of Rural Health Policy (ORHP) specify the degree of rurality through a combination of census tract statistics and geographic commuting data (Rural Health Research Center, 2011b). Calculation of the rural population will vary depending on which rural taxonomy is employed. Using the 2000 Census data and definitions, 21% of the population (59,061,367 citizens) lives in rural communities in the United States (U.S. Census Bureau, 2011b).

Rural Demographics

The socioeconomic and racial and ethnic demographics of rural communities in the United States vary considerably by region; however, trends can be identified. Overall, rural residents are older than those of suburban or urban communities as a result of the persistent migration of youth to urban centers and retired persons to rural regions (IOM, 2005). This regional age gradient is projected to widen in upcoming decades as the baby boomer generation ages. Given this trend, rural communities in the future will include an increasingly disproportionate representation of America's oldest citizens (Morton, 2004). Therefore, it is imperative that future plans for nursing health-promotion activities in rural communities carefully consider the specific needs of a rapidly expanding geriatric population.

Rural regions in the United States have been historically homogenous and predominantly White, but populations of racial and ethnic minorities in rural communities nationwide are steadily growing (IOM, 2005). Considerable regional variability exists in the distribution of racial and ethnic minorities across the United States. Rural Black populations are located predominantly in the Southeast of the United States;

the majority of the American Indian and Alaskan Native population reside west of the Mississippi in California, Oklahoma, Arizona, Texas, New Mexico, Washington, and Alaska; the rural Hispanic population is established in the Southwest; and rural Asian/ Pacific Islanders are primarily concentrated in Hawaii (Peek & Zsembik, 2004; Probst, Samuels, Jespersen, Willert, Swann, & McDuffie, 2002; Rhoades & Cravatt, 2004). Although regional distributions of rural racial and ethnic minorities exist, progressive geographic dispersion is increasing the diversity in rural communities throughout the United States, particularly in the Midwest and the Southeast regions (IOM, 2005; National Public Radio, 2011). As historically homogenous rural communities continue to diversify, close attention must be given to the development of inclusive and culturally congruent health-promotion activities that are responsive to the evolving regional demographics.

Significant socioeconomic disparities found in rural communities affect opportunities for health-promotion services. In general, rural residents have lower incomes and experience higher poverty rates than urban and suburban residents (IOM, 2005). This is in part a consequence of lower literacy rates, less postsecondary education, and fewer stable job opportunities in rural America. The lowest literacy rates in rural regions are found among the older, disabled, and racial and ethnic minority residents (IOM, 2005). Similar to urban populations, rural minority populations and female-headed single parent households are at the greatest socioeconomic disadvantage (IOM, 2005). Directly related to economic disadvantage and employment disparities, rural residents overall are less frequently covered by private health insurance and more frequently rely upon publicly funded sources of health care than urban and suburban residents (IOM, 2005).

RURAL COMMUNITY CULTURE AND HEALTH PROMOTION

The culture of rural communities in the United States is as diverse and regionally variable as the population sociodemographics. Dependent on the cultural composition of the particular community, residents of rural regions and intra-regional microsystems within rural settings may exhibit a spectrum of similar and disparate perceptions on health, illness, and normative healthcare practices, challenging the provision of culturally congruent nursing health promotion (Bushy, 2009). In rural communities where indigenous practices are more prevalent, there may be increased availability of alternative and complementary health-promotion services consistent with the cultural orientation of the local residents. Conversely, minority groups living in rural regions dominated by a culture other than their own may be geographically isolated from culturally responsive health care (Stamm, Lambert, Piland, & Speck, 2007).

Although the culture of rural communities in the United States is highly variable, common cultural propensities of small and remote communities can affect the provision of nursing health-promotion services. In general, residents of rural communities tend to be more socially and politically conservative, demonstrate greater conformity to traditional gender roles, and may be more actively involved in traditional faith-based activities than urban or suburban populations (Bushy, 2011; Leipert, 2010; Long & Weinert, 1989; Winters & Lee, 2010). Perhaps a result of extended geographic separations between residents, services, and resources, many rural residents have also retained a proud commitment to self-reliance, personal hardiness, intergenerational family support, and a strong affinity to the local community (Bales, 2010; Bushy, 2009; Leipert, 2010). These cultural proclivities can manifest both assets and challenges in the provision of nursing health-promotion services in the rural community.

Some rural religious practices, both contemporary and indigenous, may be grounded in a more philosophically fatalistic perspective on life, potentially encouraging a relatively passive approach to health and health care. An operating assumption that life events are "God's will" and that "God will provide" could reduce the impetus for some rural residents to seek out preventive healthcare services, especially when services are not easily accessible or culturally normative. On the other hand, traditional religious affiliations may also provide protection from some behavioral health risks and provide opportunities for health-promotion activities in rural and remote regions (Borders & Booth, 2007; Bushy, 2011; Nonnemaker, Mcneely, & Blum; 2003; Wong, Rew, & Slaikeu, 2006). Religious organizations frequently function as centers for socialization and collaboration in the rural community, and therefore may be productive venues for community health assessment, dissemination of health information, and the culturally congruent delivery of family-centered nursing health-promotion services (Bushy, 2011). The American Nurses Association recognizes religion-based nursing activities, historically known as "parish nursing," as a nursing sub-specialty, now identified as "Faith Community Nursing" (International Parish Nurse Resource Center, 2011). With appreciation for the importance of the religious community to the small town environment, the utilization of Faith Community Nursing practitioners may be a potentially productive mechanism to increase health-promotion activities within more traditional rural communities.

The philosophically conservative, and often faith-based, nature of the rural community may also create barriers to the delivery of healthcare services. A conservative milieu can affect the acceptability and accessibility of socially controversial health services in the isolated community. For example, school-based health centers providing confidential reproductive and mental health services for adolescents are frequently less available to youth in rural communities (Santelli et al., 2003). Similarly, abortion services are severely restricted in rural communities in the United States, limiting the accessible options for rural women experiencing unintended pregnancy (Abortion Access Project, 2009). The provision of controversial nursing health-promotion services, protected in large urban regions by a diverse political environment, can be restricted in rural communities through fiscal and regulatory control of small local governing bodies. Unfortunately, the rural residents most in need of more controversial prevention services are often the least geographically mobile, the least financially and socially empowered, and therefore the most vulnerable to health disparities and poor health outcomes.

Self-reliance, personal hardiness, and productivity are persistently valued personal traits among many rural residents (Bales, 2010; Bales, Winters, & Lee, 2010; Bigbee, 1991; Bushy, 2011; Leipert, 2010). Consequently, the underlying conceptualization of "health" in the rural community may be understood as perseverance, functionality, and the ability to work (Bushy, 2011; Lee & McDonagh, 2010; Weinert & Long, 1987). One study of rural women of childbearing and child-rearing age defined health as: (1) a lack of major health problems, (2) minimal or no use of routine medications, (3) being mentally and physically active, and (4) having the ability to perform necessary tasks without limitations or undue stress (Bales, 2010). Other research suggests that an appreciation for "functionality" among rural residents may be evolving to embody less emphasis on the work role and focus more on individual capacity to pursue personal goals (Lee & McDonagh, 2010, p. 27). Using either definition of functionality, a cultural perspective of "get it done" and "if it ain't broke, don't fix it" may impede the prioritization of preventive health-promotion activities in the daily life of rural residents. In fact, data show that rural residents engage in fewer health-promotion activities, from seat belts to mammograms, than urban or suburban populations (Bennett, Olatosi, & Probst, 2008; Dunkin, 2000; Gamm, Hutchison, Dabney, & Dorsey, 2003; IOM, 2005).

Given an appreciation for the cultural emphasis on functionality, successful integration of health-promotion activities for adults in the rural community may be most effectively oriented around the goal of increasing productivity and capacity and best provided in a manner that does not disrupt the daily work routine. For example, data suggest that rural women view health maintenance activities and the development of personal "hardiness" as essential to their functional capacity as maternal and community caretakers (Bales, 2010; Leipert, 2010). Building on this culturally embedded commitment to self-reliance and functionality, rural residents can potentially be directed into increased engagement in health promoting self-care activities from a perspective of goal-oriented enhanced capacity, productivity, and self-sufficiency.

Another facet of the self-reliant personality trait encountered in rural communities is a fiercely defended sense of independence, self-determination, and personal freedom. Research suggests that rural residents are inclined to seek health care based on a self-assessment of individual need, the availability of resources, and the perceived relative importance of the healthcare services (Bales et al., 2010; Lee & McDonagh,

2010). Health-promotion activities requiring the rural resident to submit to externally imposed dictates may encounter significant resistance. In addition, some rural residents may be less inclined to access entitlement programs if they are conceived of as "hand-outs" related to a state of perceived dependency on external resources in compliance with bureaucratic mandates. Therefore, staged risk reduction approaches to health-promotion interventions, allowing the rural participant to direct the behavioral change process and control resource utilization, may be more successful in rural communities than externally scripted interventions. One model of staged risk reduction used to direct behavior change includes: (1) recognizing and labeling behavioral risk through health education and guided self-assessment; (2) personal commitment to behavior changes incorporating considerations of self-efficacy and perceived utility; and (3) enactment of behavior change through information seeking, problem solving, and resource utilization (Catania, Coates, & Kegeles, 1994; Family Health International, 2004). For example, a staged risk-reduction health-promotion approach could be used to reduce cardiovascular risk among rural adults by starting with a culturally situated hypertension awareness campaign, followed by the development of individual and family behavior change goals in consultation with community leadership, culminating in the engagement and activation of local health-promotion resources to effect change at the individual and community level.

Rural Health-Promotion Theory Highlight: Risk Reduction Behavioral Change Model

The risk reduction behavioral change model includes: (1) labeling the risk, (2) committing to change, and (3) enacting change (Catania, Coates, & Kegeles, 1994).

Rural communities and small towns are frequently home to intimately woven social networks. A pattern of close interaction among intergenerational extended families persists in much of rural America (Bushy, 2011; Lee & McDonagh, 2010). These interreliant extended family networks serve to provide social support, advice, caretaking, and resource sharing for family members and maintain significant influence over family and community function. Consistent with the persisting traditional gender roles in rural communities, women within the family and social network frequently assume much of the family caretaking and other supportive functions (Bushy, 2011; Leipert, 2010). As the primary caretakers, female identity within the more traditional rural community may be predominantly attached to family relationships, such as the roles of wife and mother (Bushy, 2011). Traditional male gender roles in the rural community may include much of the remunerated work outside of the home, and the male identity may be strongly attached to production and community leadership (Bushy, 2011). These potential patterns of family dynamics and gender role functioning in the rural community influence both the development and delivery of nursing health-promotion activities.

The social network in the rural community often operates much like an additional extended family. Residents of rural communities are known to "show up for one another," rallying around a local need and contributing to an identified cause with passion and commitment (Bales et al., 2010). Whereas "who you know" may be conceived as a competitive strategy in urban communities, in many rural cultures it is understood as a collaborative commitment (Klugman & Dalinis, 2008). Rural residents are accustomed to daily transactions involving social relationships and thus often prefer to seek support from acquaintances rather than strangers (Bushy, 2011). When given the option of utilizing services provided within the social network, by local organizations, or through government agencies, rural residents will often turn to the social network, and then local organizations, before relying on external resources (Bushy, 2011). Volunteered services rendered within the social network of the rural community are culturally understood to be reciprocal, and generally repaid in kind over time (Nelson, 2008).

The rural cultural commitment to "caring for your own" can be utilized in the development and implementation of family-centered health-promotion activities to further the well-being of the rural community. Engagement of extended family members and social networks into health-promotion planning is a potentially potent, and possibly essential, mechanism for improving the integration of health-promotion practices in the rural community. Ignoring the influence of family and social networks, instead treating individuals and families like singular or isolated nuclear units in a society with strongly embedded patterns of interrelationships, may result in the failure of health-promotion activities. Although rural residents have become progressively more connected and open to external resources, the introduction of new health-promotion activities can be difficult because new services may still be met with resistance and skepticism (Findholt, 2010; Lee & McDonagh, 2010). Rural residents frequently "don't take to" the perception of outsiders (city-folk, townies, flatlanders) dictating local community needs and solutions to rural residents (Lee & McDonagh, 2010). The aphorism "they won't care how much you know, until they know how much you care" may be even more acutely experienced in the small town environment. Thus, attempts at health-promotion interventions within the rural community should be carefully situated within the context of the local culture and social structure; community and religious leaders must be included in the assessment, planning, and implementation process for new health services; and referrals to external resources should demonstrate a clear connection back to the local community network.

Evidence suggests that the supportive social network of the rural community may provide health benefits for rural residents. Substantial research on social support and health has led to the general conclusion that individuals who perceive more social support experience better health outcomes (Berkman & Glass, 2000). It is important, however, to recognize that the benefits of social support within the rural community may be reserved for the well-integrated residents with sufficient social and financial capital, and the more marginalized populations may experience even further isolation as an outsider within a small community with few options and resources. Disruptions of established social expectations, including employment practices, family functioning, and gender roles, may be particularly stressful for residents of the traditional rural community. It is essential for the health of the entire rural community that the development of health-promotion activities does not simply facilitate the most engaged and empowered residents, but specifically address the needs of the more vulnerable, marginalized individuals.

Another potential liability of the small community environment in relation to the provision of health-promotion services is the lack of anonymity and resultant concerns for confidentiality. In a tightly knit small community, little resident activity proceeds unseen by friends and neighbors, and employees within the healthcare system are not uncommonly social acquaintances of their clients. This can create barriers to the provision of health-promotion services related to concerns for confidentiality (Bushy, 2011; Dunkin, 2000). This is particularly true for services that may push the boundaries of accepted social norms, such as confidential reproductive health services for minors and sexual minorities, or mental health and substance abuse programs. Although well connected to relationships within the community, it is not uncommon for rural residents to feel there is no one they can confide in concerning culturally sensitive subjects because a breach of confidentiality is perceived to have potentially devastating social consequences (Bushy, 2011). The advent of available electronic health information has improved the accessibility of anonymous support for sensitive concerns and should be employed in the rural community to improve the delivery of confidential health-promotion services (Lee & McDonagh, 2010).

From a Social Ecological perspective, the nurse planning health-promotion activities in the rural community must give careful consideration to the gamut of contextual factors and resources affecting the delivery of healthcare services (Stokols, 1996). Respect for the regionally specific rural culture, while avoiding overgeneralizations, simplifications, and the exclusion of marginalized subgroups, is essential for the successful development of rural health-promotion activities. It is important to identify the cultural assumptions and situated ways of being within the community and question how the subgroup populations interact and contribute to or inhibit the healthy practices of the individual and the community. Equally essential are considerations of epigenetic manifestations, including the developmental expression of genetic predispositions based on the regional population demographics as influenced by natural and constructed environmental factors. For example, assessment of the intergenerational risk for diabetes in a rural region with limited opportunities for recreational activities, limited accessibility of healthful food choices, and reduced access to health-promotion services is a necessity.

In planning for health-promotion services in the rural community, it is essential to evaluate the physical topography and infrastructure of the local community. Is the community remote, micropolitan, or directly connected to an urban center and resources? How does the physical terrain and climate create challenges and opportunities for health promotion? Evaluate the infrastructure, including the condition of the public and private facilities. How are the public spaces constructed and maintained? What are the patterns of transportation, and how are community resources connected by sidewalks, roads and public transportation? What opportunities does the small town infrastructure create for health promotion and what barriers exist?

Consider as well the local economic resources and employment opportunities. Identify fiscal resources and significant socioeconomic disparities within subpopulations in the same small community. How have the resources and opportunities changed with time and how has the community adapted to those changes? What are the predominant employment practices within the community? Rural communities often include employment with unique health risks, such as the agricultural industry, mining, logging, fishing, and recreational facilities. Consider the specific health risks these types of employment create and what opportunities for health-promotion activities exist within the regional workforce.

Rural Health Promotion Theory Highlight: Social Ecological Model

The Social Ecological Model considers the spectrum of individual, cultural, and environmental contexts influencing the health and health behavior of rural communities. (Stokols, 1996)

RURAL HEALTH PRIORITIES

The health of rural communities is a complex phenomenon involving tremendous regional variation and multiple causal factors including epigenetic influences, the environmental context, local culture, regional demographics, employment practices,

financial resources, and healthcare accessibility. Rural morbidity and mortality statistics in the United States vary considerably by race/ethnicity, socioeconomic status,
region, and degree of rurality (Wallace et al., 2004). However, in general when compared with urban populations, rural residents experience significant health disparities
including worse birth outcomes and higher rates of debilitating chronic disease (Gamm
et al., 2003). Overall, health disparities increase as the region of residence becomes
more remote. Available data also indicate that while risk behaviors among rural residents equal or surpass urban and suburban populations, engagement in prevention
practices and access to prevention services are comparatively limited (Bennett et al.,
2008; Gamm et al., 2003; IOM, 2005). Increased disease rates in rural communities
may be related to demographic, epigenetic, and cultural factors in conjunction with
barriers to healthcare services. Barriers to healthcare services in the rural community
may include a lack of financial resources, inadequate insurance coverage, an insufficient
healthcare workforce, substandard healthcare services, concerns about confidentiality, lower literacy rates, language barriers, geographic inaccessibility, and unreliable
public transportation (Wallace et al., 2004). Higher poverty rates among rural populations and increased dependence on lower-reimbursed publicly funded health insurance
programs reduce the viability and therefore availability of many healthcare services in
the rural community. Geographic inaccessibility of healthcare services, attributed to a
lower community density and a less-developed infrastructure, is further exacerbated by
the limited, inconvenient, and inconsistent availability of public transportation. Lower
literacy rates and language barriers are particularly problematic in the rural community
as the availability of bilingual providers and translation services is frequently limited.

Barriers to health care in the rural community include cost, inadequate insurance coverage, insufficient healthcare providers, concern for confidentiality,
lower literacy rates, language barriers, lack of culturally congruent healthcare services, geographic inaccessibility, and limited public transportation.

Identified health priorities of rural communities, corresponding with the Healthy
People 2020 objectives, in ranked order include: (1) heart disease and stroke; (2) diabetes;
(3) mental health; (4) oral health; (5) tobacco use; (6) substance use; (7) maternal, infant,
and child health; (8) nutrition and overweight; (9) cancer; and (10) immunization and
infectious disease (Gamm et al., 2003) (see **Box 8-1**).

In summary, significant health disparities exist in rural populations, calling for serious consideration of the resources and mechanisms necessary to improve the current
and future health of rural community. Much of the work to improve rural health is the

Box 8-1 Healthy People 2020 Rural Health Priorities (U.S. DHHS, 2011a)

1. Improve **cardiovascular health** and quality of life through prevention, detection, and treatment of risk factors for heart attack and stroke; early identification and treatment of heart attacks and strokes; and prevention of repeat cardiovascular events.
2. Reduce the disease and economic burden of **diabetes mellitus** and improve the quality of life for all persons who have, or are at risk for, diabetes.
3. Improve **mental health** through prevention and by ensuring access to appropriate, quality mental health services.
4. Prevent and control oral and craniofacial diseases, conditions, and injuries, and improve access to preventive services and **dental care**.
5. Reduce illness, disability, and death related to **tobacco use** and secondhand smoke exposure.
6. Reduce **substance abuse** to protect the health, safety, and quality of life for all, especially children.
7. Improve the health and well-being of **women, infants, children, and families**.
8. Promote health and reduce chronic disease risk through the consumption of healthful diets and **achievement and maintenance of healthy body weights**.
9. Reduce the number of new cancer cases, as well as the illness, disability, and death caused by **cancer**.
10. Increase **immunization rates** and reduce preventable infectious diseases.

purview of nursing practice within the community setting, schools, homes, and tertiary care centers. At some level, each of the identified rural health priorities can be addressed through culturally sensitive nursing health-promotion activities for rural residents that builds on the varied assets currently available within the rural community.

MATERNAL AND CHILD HEALTH PROMOTION

Prenatal Care

Improving birth outcomes and reducing maternal–child health disparities in the United States is a Healthy People 2020 goal and a leading health indicator (IOM, 2011; U.S. Department of Health and Human Services [U.S. DHHS], 2011a). Disparities in birth outcomes, including low birth weight, preterm birth, and infant death have been demonstrated to increase with the degree of residential rurality in the United States (Gamm et al., 2003; Lou & Wilkins, 2008). Ultimately, the population health effect of perinatal disparities is not just limited to the neonatal period. In accordance with the

---

Box 8-2 Disparities in Rural Health

- Rural residents more frequently report their health as only "Fair to Poor," and reporting of "Fair to Poor" health increases with the degree of rurality (Bennett et al., 2008).
- Rural adults report more chronic disease than urban residents, including heart disease, cancer, diabetes, COPD, asthma, arthritis, and poor dentition (Bennett et al., 2008; Gamm et al., 2003; Morton, 2004).
- Rural residents are more likely to be obese and not meet the CDC recommendations for moderate or vigorous physical activity than urban or suburban residents (Bennett et al., 2008).
- Tobacco use is more prevalent in rural areas (Gamm et al., 2003).
- Rates of substance use among rural youth are frequently higher and increasing more rapidly than in urban settings (Lorenz, Wickrama, & Yeh, 2004).
- Infant mortality is higher among rural populations and poor birth outcomes increase with the degree of rurality (Gamm et al., 2003; Lou & Wilkins, 2008).
- Rural residents are more likely to experience worse mental health outcomes, including higher rates of suicide, than urban or suburban residents (Hirsch, 2006).
- Residents in most rural counties are nearly twice as likely to die in a motor vehicle accident than are urban residents (Morton, 2004).
- Rural residents are less likely to participate in regular preventive care, including age-appropriate check-ups, mammograms, pap smears, colorectal screening, and dental care (Bennett et al., 2008; Gamm et al., 2003).
- Rural residents are exposed to unique occupational health risks including agricultural, logging, and mining accidents; particulate inhalation; and pesticide exposure (Schulman & Slesinger, 2004; Hodne, 2004).

Life Course Perspective of health, exposures and contexts in the perinatal period, and subsequently throughout the developmental lifespan, directly affect the trajectory of adult health and prevalence of chronic health issues (Osler, 2006). Therefore, optimum population health promotion in the rural community begins not only before birth, but even preconception.

Rural Health Promotion Theory Highlight: Life Course Perspective

From the Life Course Perspective of health, intervention at critical developmental periods is essential to affect the longitudinal trajectory of health and health behaviors.

Disparities in birth outcomes in rural regions may be attributed to the indirect effects of rural demographics, including higher poverty levels, lower levels of education, and more limited access to medical care, as well as cultural practices including risk behaviors, limited engagement in prevention services, and birthing practices (Gamm et al., 2003). In addition, there are more births in the rural community among women under age 20 and over age 40, subgroups who demonstrate an increased risk for poor birth outcomes regardless of residence (Gamm et al., 2003; RAC, 2011b).

Addressing disparities in birth outcomes in rural communities must begin first with the prevention of unintended pregnancy. Unintended pregnancies contribute to poor birth outcomes related to delayed prenatal care and prolonged risk behaviors, such as substance use and poor nutrition (Brown & Eisenberg, 1995). Rural women may be at increased risk for unintended pregnancy due to the disproportionate representation of socioeconomic disadvantage in the rural community, a demographic known to consistently correlate with higher rates of unintended pregnancy (Finer & Henshaw, 2006). Potential barriers to contraceptive services in rural communities may also contribute to unintended pregnancies, such as an inadequate supply of reproductive health providers, geographic inaccessibility of services, traditional gender roles and disparities in gender empowerment, and concerns for confidentiality related to sexual practices within a conservative social climate (RAC, 2011b).

Removing barriers to culturally sensitive reproductive health education and contraceptive services for rural residents of childbearing age is an essential step in effective maternal–child health promotion in the rural community. Federal Title X funding from the Public Health Service Act is available to provide funding for culturally congruent, confidential, reproductive health services for low-income women and men in underserved rural regions to address disparities in unintended pregnancies (Hart, Silva, Tein, Brown, & Stevens, 2009). Successful implementation of these services in rural and remote communities requires careful consideration of the regional culture, gender roles and relationships, specific reproductive health concerns and practices, and patterns of accessibility among subgroup populations. The provision of reproductive health services in the small community requires an artful balance of accessibility and confidentiality, commitment to cultural congruence and the protection of individual access to safe and effective care.

To improve birth outcomes in the rural community, the preparation of rural women of childbearing age for a successful pregnancy must occur simultaneously with the prevention of unintended pregnancy. Rural women may be more vulnerable to poor birth outcomes than urban and suburban populations in relation to modifiable pre-conception health behaviors including substance use, diet, and inadequate dental care (Gamm et al., 2003; D'Angelo et al., 2007). Rural populations include a disproportionate percentage of residents dependent on Medicaid, a population demonstrating the highest-risk pre-conception health behaviors (D'Angelo et al., 2007; Gamm et al., 2003).

Substance use in pregnancy, including tobacco, alcohol, and illicit drugs, contribute to spontaneous abortion, stillbirth, birth defects, developmental disorders, and sudden infant death syndrome (D'Angelo et al., 2007). Many of the effects of substance use occur early in gestation, before the woman may even be aware she is pregnant or before she is able to access prenatal health care (D'Angelo et al., 2007). Maternal obesity and related conditions, including diabetes and hypertension, can precipitate preeclampsia, hypertension, and thromboembolic disease in the mother (D'Angelo et al., 2007). It can also cause fetal death, stillbirth, and birth defects in the neonate (D'Angelo et al., 2007). Inadequate nutrition including anemia and folic acid deficiency may also contribute to poor birth outcomes in rural communities, particularly among lower income populations. Addressing the national concern for pre-conception nutrition, increasing the proportion of women of childbearing age with a daily who have a daily intake of 400 micrograms of folic acid and reducing the proportion of women with low red blood cell folate levels are Healthy People 2020 objectives (Centers for Disease Control and Prevention [CDC], 2010; U.S. DHHS, 2011). Hispanic women have demonstrated a significantly higher risk of delivering a child with a neural tube deficit, a condition related to folic acid deficiency (D'Angelo et al., 2007). Therefore, targeted folic acid supplement campaigns among Spanish-speaking women in the rural community are recommended. Dental care for low-income populations in the rural community is seriously lacking and periodontal disease has been linked to low birth weight and preterm births (D'Angelo et al., 2007; Gamm et al., 2003). Increasing the availability of regular pre-conception dental care for rural women is a warranted health-promotion activity that may contribute to both improved birth outcomes and reduced dental health disparities in rural communities (California Dental Association [CDA], 2010).

As evidence suggests that pre-conception interventions targeting maternal health behaviors can improve birth outcomes, the CDC has prepared several recommendations for pre-conception health, including the need to:

- Increase public awareness of pre-conception health behaviors within appropriate literacy and cultural/linguistic contexts.
- Perform pre-conception risk assessments and health counseling of childbearing-age females and provide appropriate pre-conception health behavior interventions with higher risk clients.
- Integrate pre-conception health into established public health programs (D'Angelo et al., 2007).

The importance of access to health-promotion services for both the prevention of unintended pregnancy and the preparation for a healthy pregnancy cannot be understated. Community-based reproductive health services in the rural community provide a potential venue for delivering pre-conception nursing health-promotion activities. Successful strategies for improving pre-conception health among low-income rural women have been demonstrated in the *Strong Healthy Women* clinical trial, an intervention study theoretically based in Social Cognitive Theory (Hillemeier, Downs, Feinberg, Weisman & Chuang, 2008). Participation in a group program targeting multiple health-related behaviors associated with pregnancy outcomes improved behavioral intentions and induced actual behavior change among the female participants (Hillemeier et al., 2008). Results of this investigation present a promising model for the improvement of pre-conception health to reduce birth disparities; however, it is important not to exclude the consideration of male partners in the development of perinatal health-promotion activities. Another study analyzing the health behaviors of rural low-income fathers whose pregnant partners were enrolled in Medicaid demonstrated significant health risks including tobacco use, hazardous drinking, very low physical activity, and poor dietary practices (Everett et al., 2006). Pre-conception, perinatal, and postpartal sustained behavior change to promote the long-term health of the family unit in the rural community may require a partnered approach to health-promotion activities for this high risk population.

Rural Health Promotion Theory Highlight: Social Cognitive Theory

Social Cognitive Theory assumes that behavior change is goal-directed, that people are capable of self-regulation, and that perceived self-efficacy is a primary mediator of change (Bandura, 1986).

Post-conception, rural women demonstrate a higher incidence of delayed or no prenatal care and may receive less adequate obstetric care when it is available (RAC, 2011b). This is particularly concerning given the higher prevalence of preventable risk factors that can potentially affect birth outcomes among rural populations that could be addressed with timely prenatal care. Limited financial resources in the rural community, an increased reliance on lower-reimbursed public health insurance, and the concurrent rising cost of obstetric malpractice insurance contribute to an inadequate supply of rural reproductive health practitioners and services (RAC, 2011). Data indicate that the absence of accessible obstetric services decreases the timely utilization of prenatal care and contributes to poor birth outcomes (RAC, 2011b). Lower literacy rates and impaired language fluency are additional barriers to prenatal services in the rural community, as they can delay the application process for publicly funded services, while obstetric providers may refuse to serve clients until a guaranteed method of reimbursement is secured. Rural women in female-headed single parent households may be at an increased risk for delayed prenatal care related to socioeconomic disadvantage and limited social support (IOM, 2005). Overcoming the obstacles to early prenatal care in the rural community and establishing accessible obstetric nursing health-promotion services are essential to addressing the Healthy People 2020 objective to reduce disparities in perinatal health and improve birth outcomes.

Perinatal maternal depression is a concern among rural populations that may have lasting effects on maternal–child and longitudinal population health (Price & Proctor, 2009). Low-income women, along with women with limited social support living in isolated settings, may be particularly susceptible to perinatal depression. Depression screening of all postpartal women, but particularly higher-risk populations, and appropriate referral to mental health services are essential to support positive birth outcomes. However, the relative inadequacy of available mental health services in the rural community may impede the delivery of necessary interventions to women experiencing perinatal depression and jeopardize the future well-being of both mother and child (Gamm et al., 2003; Price & Proctor, 2009).

Interdisciplinary teams of advanced practice nurses, public health nurses, school nurses, mental health providers, and obstetricians in the rural community are critical to successful health promotion of the childbearing family before, during, and after pregnancy. School nurses and public health nurses are essential to the dissemination of pre-conception health-promotion information, screening, and referral of high-risk women in the rural community. Advanced practice nurses can partner with obstetricians through the use of telehealth technologies to provide culturally congruent perinatal health promotion and prenatal care to low-income, remote, and otherwise underserved women (West, 2010). Certified nurse midwives should be supported by local healthcare organizations and the interdisciplinary healthcare team to facilitate the delivery of uncomplicated births in the rural community (West, 2010). In order to improve rural birth outcomes, nursing advocacy is required to counter the prohibitive medical liability costs that create barriers to the availability of obstetric services for low-income populations and underserved regions. The utilization of mental health advanced practice nurses can improve the accessibility of cost-effective mental health-promotion services for at-risk mothers, and public health nurses can provide the necessary surveillance, case management, and support for the rural family unit within the home and the community (Baldwin et al., 2002; Price & Proctor, 2009).

Immunizations and Infectious Disease

Infectious disease control through timely administration of routine immunizations is central to community health promotion and the reduction of acute and chronic disease in the rural community. Recommended immunization schedules begin in infancy and continue through adolescence to adulthood. In 1977, the American Academy of Pediatrics (AAP) delivered a policy statement advocating universal childhood immunizations in the United States. However, the goal of universal immunization is still unrealized and increasing immunization rates to reduce preventable disease persists as a Healthy People 2020 objective (U.S. DHHS, 2011a).

Identified barriers to timely immunizations in the rural community include the physical and social constraints of poverty; inadequate health insurance, which contributes to inconsistent routine comprehensive pediatric health exams; language and literacy barriers leading to insufficient health education and accentuated fear of unintended consequences of immunizations; less access to immunization services and large travel distances for health care, which increases the inconvenience of vaccine delivery; and inadequate mechanisms for the tracking of immunization records among less stable populations (AAP, 2003; Hutchinson & Peck, 2004). High-risk subpopulations of rural racial and ethnic minorities, immigrants, and residents of American border regions have demonstrated increased disparities in immunization rates (Hutchinson & Peck, 2004).

Nursing health-promotion strategies for improving immunization rates among rural pediatric populations include:

1. The development and delivery of culturally congruent and language-accessible vaccine awareness campaigns.
2. Collaboration with community organizations serving at-risk populations for the provision of on-site immunization services.
3. Utilization of nursing standard orders for the independent provision of immunizations across practice settings and within community-based organizations.
4. Utilization of alternative community-based immunization delivery methods such as mobile health vans and visiting health services.
5. Implementation of community-based electronic immunization records, including automatic patient and provider immunization reminders (AAP, 2003; Findley et al., 2006; Hutchinson & Peck, 2004).

Embedding pediatric immunization education and vaccine services within established community-based organizations has demonstrated effectiveness in increasing immunization rates among at-risk rural pediatric populations (Findley et al., 2006; Mayer, Housemann, & Piepenbrock, 1999). Integrating vaccine services into trusted community organizations not only addresses the barriers of access and inconvenience, it may also increase cultural acceptance of vaccine protocols (Wilson, 2000). Lack of accurate knowledge regarding immunizations and exaggerated fear of adverse events is a major deterrent to improving immunization rates. Contributing to this fear is the insidious availability of flawed or biased media sources inaccurately representing the statistical risks and benefits of routine immunizations for vaccine-preventable disease (AAP, 2003). Providing accurate vaccine information to parents through trusted community members, rather than relying solely on external professional agencies, has demonstrated success in increasing immunization rates among at-risk populations (Findley et al., 2006). This strategy may be particularly relevant in the rural community given the cultural inclination of rural residents to look to informal sources, including social relationships and community leaders, for guidance and support.

In accordance with the IOM *Future of Nursing* agenda to improve the provision of health care by reducing barriers to nursing practice, nurses should be empowered to actively direct the provision of immunization services in the rural community through the implementation of standing vaccine orders (IOM, 2010). These standing orders provide authority for nurses to screen residents and deliver immunizations using established standardized vaccine protocols (AAP, 2003; CDC, 1993; CDC, 2000). Community-based health centers, school campuses, home health visits, urgent care clinics, emergency departments, long-term care facilities, and mobile health clinics are all important venues for the direct provision of routine immunizations by nurses in the rural community. Nurses must assess the vaccine status of rural residents at every healthcare encounter and should be sanctioned with the authority and resources necessary to provide the indicated immunizations. Innovative nurse-managed immunization programs such as *Vaccinate Before You Graduate*, a school-based immunization program targeting graduating high school seniors, are potent mechanisms for improving population health in the rural community through the prevention of infectious disease (California School Nurse Organization [CSNO], 2011).

Cost should not be a barrier to the provision of pediatric immunization services, as the federal Vaccines for Children (VFC) Program provides reimbursement for vaccines for the uninsured, underinsured, and Medicaid eligible populations (CDC, 2011b). In addition, particularly relevant to rural communities, all American Indians and Alaskan Natives are eligible for VFC services under the Indian Health Care Improvement Act (CDC, 2011b). Although cost should not be a barrier to immunization services, it can definitely be an obstacle, as outreach programs in rural communities attempt to navigate convoluted reimbursement mechanisms with limited resources for administrative support. Nursing advocacy for healthcare policy reform, including universal coverage for vaccine services, is fundamental to minimizing financial and administrative barriers to the prevention of infectious disease in the rural community through the timely administration of vaccines.

The multiple healthcare access points of hard-to-follow, higher-risk clients in the rural community can result in a scattered immunization record, creating yet another obstacle to routine immunizations in the rural community (Deutchmann Brayden, Siegel, Beaty, & Crane, 2000). Rural public health nurses must facilitate the implementation of community-based health information technologies to establish electronic vaccine records providing not only accessible documentation of resident immunization status, but also to generate vaccine reminders for clients and providers (Gamm & Hutchinson, 2004).

FIGURE 8-2   2012 Recommended Immunizations for Children from Birth Through 6 Years Old

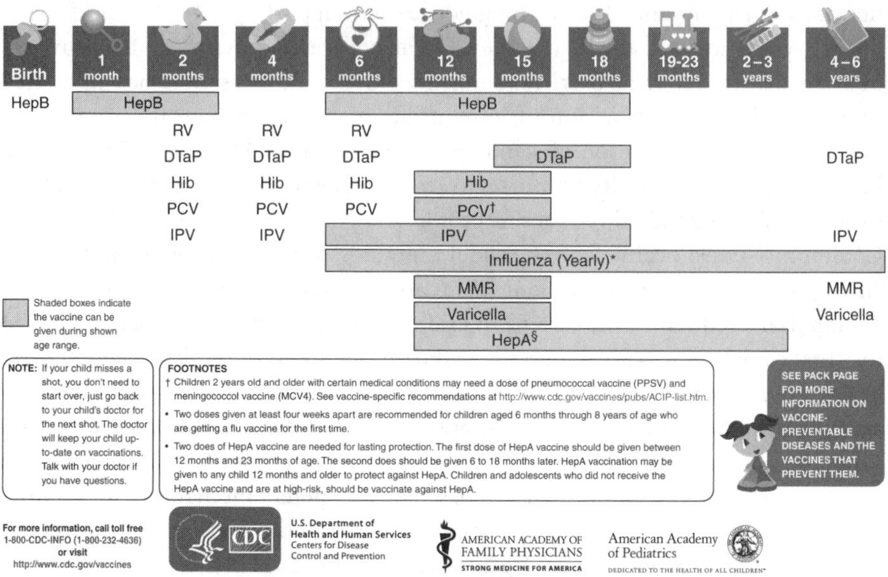

Source: Department of Health and Human Services, Centers for Disease Control and Prevention.

Childhood Obesity

Currently, one of the greatest risks to population health in the United States is the exponentially escalating obesity epidemic. In recognition of the diffuse biopsychosocial consequences of rampant obesity within the American population, Healthy People 2020 identifies the prevention of inappropriate weight gain among youth and adults, and the reduction of the proportion of children and adolescents who are obese, as two major national health objectives (U.S. DHHS, 2011a). Rural communities are inordinately afflicted by the obesity epidemic, demonstrating overall higher rates of obesity and obesity-related chronic disease than urban and suburban residents (Bennet et al., 2008; Gamm et al., 2003; Moore, Davis, Baxter, Lewis, & Zenong, 2008). This is a reversal from data obtained before 1980, when urban populations in the United States demonstrated a higher incidence of obesity than rural populations (Gamm et al., 2003). Available data suggest that the current obesity disparity in rural America is likely to continue, as the health patterns of youth are precursors to adult risk factors and obesity is more prevalent and rising more rapidly among children and adolescents in rural regions in the United States (Gamm et al., 2003; Liu et al., 2007; Wallace et al., 2004).

A progressive increase in body mass index is associated with a commensurate rise in the prevalence of chronic disease and a reduction in quality of life indicators (Sturm & Wells, 2001). In the long term, obesity directly correlates with the prevalence of adult chronic diseases including heart disease, hypertension, diabetes, cancer, and arthritis, all health issues of serious concern in the rural community (Bennet et al., 2008; Biro & Wein, 2010; Gamm et al., 2003; National Institutes of Health [NIH], 1998). In the short term, childhood obesity has demonstrated adverse effects throughout almost every organ system and can precipitate severe pediatric health consequences, including hypertension, dyslipidemia, insulin resistance, orthopedic problems, and psychological dysfunction (Han et al., 2010). Furthermore, the excess weight carried into adolescence tends to be perpetuated into adulthood, further potentiating the probability of adverse population health outcomes over time (Biro & Wen, 2010).

The causes of obesity are multifactorial, including potentially modifiable risk factors such as health behaviors and the constructed environmental context, as well as non-modifiable determinants including genetic predispositions and fixed contextual forces (Han, Lawlor, & Kim, 2010). It has been posited that the current obesity epidemic can be attributed to an anthropologic heritage of body composition and caloric utilization collapsing into to a sedentary, consumption-oriented, contemporary society (Han et al., 2010). Evidence to support this view includes data indicating that contemporary North American populations living traditional lifestyles, including dietary practices and imbedded physical activity, continue to experience lower rates of obesity (Basset, 2008). Internationally, rural populations in some countries still demonstrate a lower risk for obesity than urban populations, potentially related to a more persistent traditional lifestyle with culturally embedded physical activity and less access to cheap, calorie-dense food (Han et al., 2010).

The disproportionate prevalence of obesity in rural areas in the United States may be in part attributed to demographic trends and socioeconomic disparities in rural communities, including the genetic predispositions of racial and ethnic subpopulations residing in rural regions, an older and aging rural population, increased poverty, and less education, which are all epidemiologic determinants for an increased risk of obesity (Han et al., 2010; Lantz et al.,1998; Martikainen & Marmot, 1999). However, there is also evidence that rural culture and structure may present challenges to maintaining a healthy weight and preventing obesity (Gamm et al.. 2003). Cultural factors that may perpetuate rates of obesity in the rural community include an increased consumption of higher fat, higher calorie food (otherwise known as country cooking); specific subpopulation racial and ethnic cultural practices regarding dietary habits and food choices; declining physical activity in the daily of life of rural residents related to increasing use of technology and the mechanization of the agrarian lifestyle; and less pervasive collective social consciousness regarding weight maintenance (Gamm et al., 2003). Structural factors potentially affecting obesity rates in rural communities may include barriers to walking as a mode of transportation and recreation due to the lengthy distance between activities; lack of sidewalks, streetlights, and inadequate public transportation; lack of recreation facilities, particularly in more impoverished communities and regions that experience severe seasonal inclement weather; fewer opportunities and less support for organized physical activity; inadequate transportation for youth to engage in afterschool activities; limited choices for out-of-home dining and the increased availability of calorie-dense, cheap, fast food; and inadequate access to nutritionists and nutrition education (Gamm et al., 2003).

Consistent with the overall rural population, rural children in the United States are at greater risk for obesity than urban and suburban youth (Gamm et al., 2003; Liu et al., 2007). Current data from the United States indicate that rural youth living in micropolitan centers and regions adjacent to urban areas are at greater risk for obesity than youth living in more remote regions (Liu et al., 2007). Minority and poor rural youth have the highest incidence of obesity across regions, with rural Black youth demonstrating the highest rates of both overweight and obesity than other races/ethnicities (Liu et al., 2007). Rural children in the Southern United States have the highest rates of obesity (33.1%), followed by the Midwest (30.2%), the Northeast (29.5%), and the West (28.1%) (Liu et al., 2007).

Reduced physical activity and increased time spent in sedentary behavior, including use of electronic media, has been correlated with an increased risk for obesity among rural youth (Moore et al., 2008). Interestingly, an analysis of the 2003 National Survey of Children's Health (NSCH) indicates that, overall, rural children were more likely to meet the physical activity recommendations of at least 20 minutes of moderate to vigorous physical activity 3 or more days per week than urban children. This is an interesting finding given concurrent data indicating higher rates of obesity among rural youth (Liu et al., 2007). Perhaps, 20 minutes of activity 3 days per week is not enough activity to be protective against obesity, or is not an adequately sensitive predictor of obesity risk given the current dietary and overall behavioral patterns of rural youth. The Centers for Disease Control and Prevention and the American Academy of Pediatrics currently recommend that children engage in 60 minutes of primarily aerobic physical activity every day (AAP, 2011; CDC, 2011a). It is also important to note that although rural children report higher rates of "moderate to vigorous activity" than urban youth, the trend is not perpetuated into adulthood. After childhood, rural adults report less physical activity than urban adults (Bennet et al., 2008). Rural children in the West were the most active, with 23.5% of the youth population not meeting the recommended physical activity level. This was followed by children in the Northeast (23.7%) and then the South (26.0%), with children from the rural Midwest (26.1%) being the least likely to meet the physical activity recommendations (Liu et al., 2007). Data also indicate that older youth (ages 15–17), females, Hispanics, Blacks, and low-income youth were more likely to be inactive across geographic regions (Liu et al., 2007). Participation in organized sporting activities increases the opportunity for physical activity among rural youth and disparities exist in the athletic participation in the rural community. Rural Black and Hispanic children were found to be less likely to participate in afterschool athletics than rural or urban White children, decreasing their opportunity for physical activity and subsequently increasing the risk for obesity (Liu et al., 2007). Youth who report higher utilization of electronic media are more likely to be overweight or obese, and 48% of rural youth report at least 2 hours a day of electronic media use (Liu et al., 2007). Overuse of electronic media by rural youth may be precipitated by residential isolation, inclement weather, inadequate recreational facilities, and the lack of youth development opportunities in the rural community.

The best hope for combating the obesity epidemic to reduce the disproportionate impact of chronic disease and disability in the rural community is through health-promotion activities targeted at rural youth. However, to successfully impact the health and health behaviors of youth, primary prevention interventions must begin upstream at the level of the family and the constructed social environment (Han et al., 2010). Again, from a Life Course Perspective, prevention of childhood obesity begins pre-conception. Promoting a healthy pre-conception weight in rural women of childbearing age is important, as data suggest that maternal adiposity and diabetes may increase the risk of future obesity in subsequent offspring (Han et al., 2010). In addition, eliminating disparities in access to prenatal care in rural communities to reduce preterm and low birth weight deliveries is essential as these birth outcomes, found more frequently in rural regions, are also associated with later childhood obesity (Biro & Wen, 2010).

Addressing parental health behaviors is requisite to preventing childhood obesity, as the diet and exercise habits of children have been directly correlated with parental behaviors (Nicholson, 2000; Zive et al., 1998). Parents are the role models and gatekeepers of childhood nutrition and physical activity habits. Changing parental dietary practices, including limiting calorie-dense foods such as sweet drinks and fast foods, reducing food proportions, and incorporating healthy food choices into the daily menu, as well as facilitating increased adult physical activity and decreased media use, are potentially the most powerful points of intervention to prevent childhood obesity in the rural community. Health-promotion strategies to influence individual health habits may be based on a Theory of Planned Behavior perspective, emphasizing a cognitive evaluation of the significance of the behavioral change, a conscious determination of self-efficacy related to change, and intentionally constructed strategies for change such as goal setting and reward acquisition (Ajzen, 1985). Motivational interviewing techniques using open-ended questioning and reflective listening to clarify health goals and resolve ambivalence about change has been demonstrated to be a successful approach to increasing intrinsic motivation for behavior change and improving health-promotion outcomes (Irby, Kaplan, Garner-Edwards, Kolbash, & Skelton, 2010). The formation and implementation of dietary education, behavioral modification, weight surveillance, and weight management programs in the rural community is a health-promotion practice opportunity for nurses in a variety of settings, including community-based health centers, civic and religious organizations, occupational, and school sites. In addition, web-based intervention strategies for diet and exercise health-promotion activities might be particularly useful in rural and remote communities where distance and transportation may be a barrier to participation in organized, face-to-face, activities.

Rural Health Promotion Theory Highlight: The Theory of Planned Behavior Change

The Theory of Planned Behavior Change emphasizes cognitive recognition of the importance of behavior change, an appreciation for the potential of change, and intentional change strategies such as self-monitoring, goal setting, and reward acquisition (Ajzen, 1985).

Changing the course of childhood obesity in the rural community through behavior modification strategies involving the parents is an application of Social Cognitive Theory and the Theory of Learned Behavior (Bandura, 1989). From a Theory of Learned Behavior perspective, patterns of behavior are acquired through observation and reinforcement from role models within the social context—in other words, children are likely to repeat the health behaviors they observe and practice in the home. In addition, lack of parental support for physical activity has been identified as a barrier to increasing activity among rural youth (Hennessy et al., 2010). It is reasonable to surmise that increasing parental participation in behaviors to prevent obesity will result in both better role modeling and increased support for youth physical activity and healthy dietary practices.

Rural Health Promotion Theory Highlight: The Theory of Learned Behavior

From the perspective of the Theory of Learned Behavior, children are likely to repeat the health behaviors they observe in the home (Bandura, 1989).

The school setting is another potentially powerful level of intervention at which to address childhood obesity in the rural community (Zenzen & Kridli, 2009). The school setting may be the one place where youth living in more sparsely populated regions congregate on a regular basis and the most consistent point of professional contact among more marginalized, higher-risk, subgroup populations. The school setting presents opportunities to expose rural youth to alternative dietary and physical activity practices through health education curricula, organized school-based activities, and the introduction of adult and peer role models to reinforce behavior change. To facilitate success, the health-promotion activities developed for youth and adults in the rural community must take into consideration regional diversity and be developed in a culturally inclusive format. It is important to consider if the information, activities, and role models presented represent and engage the spectrum of diversity in the population or simply address the most dominant cultural voice. For example, a physical education curriculum involving American football with the exclusion of Latino futbol may discourage the participation of the Latino/Hispanic population. Likewise, nutrition education programs must be developed within the construct of established regional food preferences and dietary practices. Culturally incongruent health behavior interventions have little hope of transferability and sustainability among families back in the home setting.

From an ecological perspective, community-based structural interventions are essential to promote and sustain a reduction of obesity in the rural community. Structural school-based interventions could include improving the caloric balance of available food choices in the school setting, discouraging the sale of calorie-dense foods in locations adjacent to the schools, increasing the time allotted for physical activity during the school day, increasing the rigor and cultural inclusivity of physical education curriculum, improving school-based recreational facilities, and expanding the free use of school-based facilities to children and families outside of the established school schedule (Han et al., 2010; Nestle, 2010).

From a community perspective, previous studies have found that structural aspects of the rural community, such as inadequate sidewalks and street lights, the presence of high speed traffic, and inaccessible and poorly maintained recreational facilities are barriers to physical activity and correlate with an increased risk of population obesity (Casey et al., 2008; Dunton, Kaplan, Wolch, Jerret, & Reynolds, 2009; Hennessy et al., 2010). Therefore, nursing advocacy for structural improvements in rural schools and communities is an essential intervention for addressing the obesity and chronic disease disparities in the rural community.

Oral Health

Dental caries is the most prevalent preventable chronic disease, and unmet health need, among children in the United States (Hallas & Shelley, 2009; U.S. DHHS, 2000). The longitudinal impact of dental pathology is not solely limited to the oral cavity. Poor dental health can ultimately contribute to multisystem disorders including cardiovascular and respiratory disease, diabetes, poor maternal birth outcomes, and low self-esteem (Fos & Hutchison, 2004; U.S. DHHS, 2000). To combat dental health disparities, the Healthy People 2020 objectives call for an increase in preventive dental health care for children and adults and a reduction in untreated dental disease (U.S. DHHS, 2011).

Significant disparities exist in dental health between rural and urban populations. Rural residents receive less preventive dental care, experience more dental caries, and eventually experience more adult edentulism than urban residents (Fos & Hutchison, 2004). Independent of residence, low-income populations and racial and ethnic minorities receive less preventive dental care and experience more dental disease and untreated dental caries than nonminority and higher income populations (Bennett et al., 2008; Mertz & Mouradian, 2009; U.S. DHHS, 2003). Despite improvements in dental insurance coverage for youth, low-income children continue to experience barriers to dental care, resulting in an increase in dental caries among children aged 2–5 years (Dye et al., 2007; U.S. Government Accountability Office [U.S. GAO], 2008; Mertz & Mouradian, 2009; U.S. DHHS, 2000).

Multiple factors contribute to rural dental health disparities, including the systemic effects of poverty, cultural health practices, less water fluoridation, farther distances to travel for dental care and limited access to public transportation, an inadequate dental workforce in the rural community, and insufficient numbers of rural dental health providers willing to accept lower-reimbursed publicly funded insurance programs or provide lower cost dental services (Fos & Hutchison, 2004; Skillman, Doescher, Mouradian, & Brunson, 2010). Ultimately, the primary cause of dental health disparities in the rural community is attributed to the culminating effect of inadequate preventive dental care related to recalcitrant barriers to dental health services (Mertz & Mouradian, 2009; Skillman et al., 2010).

Recommended interventions to reduce chronic disease related to poor dental health in the rural community include increasing fluoridation of the available water supply and providing fluoride supplementation, increasing access to preventive services including fluoride varnishes and dental sealants, performing caries risk assessment and dental referrals as indicated among high-risk populations, the provision of oral health education and promoting behavioral changes such as the reduction of dietary sugar, improved dental hygiene practices, and tobacco cessation (CDA, 2010; Skillman et al., 2010). Prenatal dental care has become an essential component of preventive dental health, as research has demonstrated that the transmission of cariogenic bacteria from untreated maternal caries can increase the risk of dental caries among children (CDA, 2010). Maternal health providers should refer rural pregnant women for a dental examination and treatment. Routine childhood dental screening should begin by 12 months of age and then continue twice yearly throughout adulthood (American

Academy of Pediatric Dentistry [AAPD], 2011; CDA, 2010). Individual dental prevention and treatment plans are guided by a risk assessment tool such as "CAMBRA: Carries Management By Risk Assessment," which outlines intervention plans based on the classification of client risk for caries from low to extremely high (Featherstone, Domejean-Orliaguet, Jensen, Wolff, & Young, 2007; Ramos-Gomez, Crall, Gansky, Slayton, & Featherstone, 2007; Young, Featherstone, & Roth, 2007).

Rural dental health disparities are ultimately the result of the inadequate provision of preventive dental care in the community. Dental workforce shortages in rural regions are projected to increase in the future as older dentists retire and younger dental graduates choose more lucrative practice opportunities in urban and suburban settings, in part to pay off large dental school loans (Mertz & Mouradian, 2009). Solutions to improve access to dental care in rural communities include increasing the rural dental workforce through the recruitment and training of students within rural regions, providing loan repayment and scholarship options to reduce the burden of dental school expense for practitioners willing to work in underserved communities, the training and use of nondental medical providers to provide preventive dental health services, and offering preventive services through alternative modalities such as school-based clinics, community health centers, mobile health clinics, and telehealth technology (Skillman et al., 2010).

It has been noted that nondental child health practitioners generally have greater access to high-risk youth than dental providers (CDA, 2010). Therefore, it is recommended that nondental health practitioners be trained to provide early dental screening, apply some preventive treatments, and perform dental referrals for high-risk populations in underserved areas (CDA, 2010; Skillman et al., 2010). School nurses and community-based advanced practice nurses are perfectly situated to address the need for increased preventive dental services, and to improve the health of the rural community through the provision of routine dental screenings and prevention services to high-risk children and families. As noted previously, school settings may be the most consistent point of professional contact for high-risk youth in rural and remote communities. With appreciation for the potential the school setting has to improve access to dental health services, the Healthy People 2020 objectives call for an increase in the number of school-based preventive dental health programs in the United States (U.S. DHHS, 2011a). School-based, interdisciplinary collaboration between school nursing, advanced practice nursing at school-based health centers, pediatricians, and local dental providers could greatly increase the provision of cost-effective dental health preventive services in the rural community.

Likewise, Healthy People 2020 calls for the increased utilization of Federally Qualified Health Centers (FQHC) in the provision of dental health prevention services. FQHCs are organizations providing health care in medically underserved areas (MUA) or to medically underserved populations (MUP) using federal funding grants under section

330 of the Public Health Service Act (RAC, 2011c). Advanced practice nurses and other non-physician clinicians already provide much of the health care for MUA/MUP populations in FQHCs (Grumbach, Hart, Mertz, Coffman, & Palazzo, 2003). Additional training and utilization of advanced practice nurses in these settings to provide dental preventive services would be a logical and cost-effective mechanism to reduce barriers to dental care for high-risk populations. Nurse-managed mobile health vans and telehealth broadcasts are other viable options for providing dental health-promotion outreach to underserved residents of more remote rural communities.

Oral health curricula and practice competencies for nondental health professionals have been developed by academic dental health programs and the American Academy of Pediatrics. Although oral health curricula is currently integrated into the advanced practice nursing education, further interdisciplinary training and continuing education opportunities must be accessible to nursing providers to support proficiencies in the delivery of preventive dental care to high-risk populations (Hallas & Shelley, 2009). Interdisciplinary dental health-promotion training for nurses is currently available in some university settings in conjunction with the schools of dentistry (AAP, 2011; Hallas & Shelley, 2009; Mouradian et al., 2005). Public health organizations can also provide opportunities for interdisciplinary dental health education, such as "Into the Mouths of Babes," a program designed by the North Carolina Department of Health and Human Services (NCDHHS) to train medical providers in preventive oral health services (NCDHHS, 2011). Utilizing academic and public health mechanisms to train rural nurses to provide preventive dental care to high-risk populations in school and community-based settings holds tremendous potential to reduce dental health disparities and improve health promotion in underserved rural communities.

RURAL ADOLESCENT HEALTH PROMOTION

Adolescence is a critical developmental period from a Life Course Health Development perspective of nursing health promotion (Graber & Brooks-Gunn, 1996; Halfon & Hochstein, 2002; Savin-Williams, 1991). The timing and synchronization of experiences during the profound physiological metamorphosis and pivotal social transitions of adolescence distinctly inform the trajectory and ultimate outcome of healthy development (Halfon & Hochstein, 2002). The transformational expanse of adolescence is conceptually divided into substages: early adolescence (from 10–13 years), middle adolescence (from 14–17 years), and late adolescence or early adulthood (from 18–24 years) (Curtis, 2008). Each stage of this critical period presents unique, developmentally propelled, and contextually situated risks and opportunities for a healthy lifestyle.

The American Nurses Association (ANA) (1980) defines health as "a dynamic state of being in which the developmental and behavioral potential of an individual is realized to the fullest extent possible" (p. 5). Unfortunately, data indicate a potential for decline in health status during adolescence, which is primarily related to unhealthy lifestyle behaviors (Curtis, Waters, & Brindis, 2011; Harris et al., 2006; Mulye et al., 2009). The predominant causes of morbidity and mortality in adolescence are attributed to preventable risk factors including unhealthy dietary practices, inadequate exercise, emerging mental health concerns, substance use, unsafe sexual practices, violence, and physical risk-taking (CDC, 2010; Curtis et al., 2011; Harris et al., 2006; Mulye et al., 2009). These lifestyle behaviors and preventable risk factors generate both acute pathology among youth and perpetuate the risk for chronic disease in adulthood (Halfon & Hochstein, 2002). It is estimated that one-half of the deaths among

---

Box 8-3 Adolescent Health Snapshot

- Seventy percent of adolescent morbidity and mortality is attributable to preventable risk behaviors including risky driving behaviors, violence, unsafe sexual activity, substance use, poor nutritional habits, and inadequate physical activity (NRC, 1999).
- Unintentional injury, homicide, and suicide account for almost three-quarters of all deaths among adolescents (National Center for Injury Prevention and Control, 2007).
- The percentage of overweight adolescents has tripled since 1980, while routine physical activity among adolescents has decreased (MacKay and Duran, 2007; Park et al., 2006).
- There has been an increase in the prevalence of asthma and diabetes among American adolescents in recent decades (Akinbami, 2006; Duncan, 2006; Rudd & Moorman, 2007).
- The lifetime prevalence of mental health problems may be as high as 37% by age 16, and one-half of all cases of adult mental disorders start by age 14 (Costello et al., 2003; Kessler et al., 2005).
- National data indicate that approximately 40% of adolescents report recent alcohol consumption and 20% report recent marijuana use (CDC, 2010).
- Sexually transmitted infections are the most commonly reported infectious diseases in adolescents and the incidence of reported infections continues to increase (CDC, 2006; Halfon & Hochstein, 2002).
- Pregnancy rates among Hispanic and non-Hispanic Black adolescents continue to be twice as high as those among non-Hispanic White adolescents (Federal Interagency Forum on Child and Family Statistics, 2007; Halfon & Hochstein, 2002; Kost, Henshaw, & Carlin, 2010).

adults can be attributed to health-related behaviors that commonly originate during the critical developmental period of adolescence (National Research Council [NRC] & IOM, 2009; McGinnis & Foege,1993; Mokdad, Marks, Stroup, & Gerberding, 2004). To improve the trajectory of adolescent health, professional organizations, including the Society for Adolescent Health and Medicine, the American Academy of Pediatrics, and the U.S. Preventive Services Task Force, advocate routine health-promotion and disease prevention services for adolescents; however, data indicate that relatively few adolescents receive the recommended services (AAP, 2008; Halfon & Hochstein, 2002; Solberg, Nordin, Bryant, Kristensen, & Maloney, 2009).

Life Course Health Development theory reinforces the understanding that the critical developmental period of adolescence is inextricably affected by macrocontextual influences within the family, local community, and global society (Halfon & Hochstein, 2002). Adolescents are particularly susceptible to macrocontextual forces as they are progressively engaged in independent health practices and adult behaviors, yet lack social and financial capital, geographic mobility, and full autonomous capacity to access services for perceived health needs (Curtis, 2008). Rural youth may be more vulnerable to poor health outcomes in adolescence due to engagement in risk behaviors that equal or surpass urban and suburban populations while in environmental contexts with less availability of protective positive youth development opportunities and fewer adolescent-sensitive health services (Fahs et al., 1999; Levine & Coupey, 2003). Specific barriers to health promotion exist for adolescents in the rural community, including a lack of adolescent-sensitive health services and a general insufficiency of healthcare providers, limited autonomous consent capacity for minors, concerns for confidentiality regarding risk behaviors within the socially conservative small community, inaccessibility of care related to extensive distances between services and the unavailability of public transportation, and limited community and personal financial resources (Elliott & Larson, 2004). To address adolescent health concerns in the United States, the Healthy People 2020 Adolescent Health Topic area emphasizes not only increasing access to adolescent sensitive wellness and prevention services, but also outlines goals for improving the macrocontextual environments in which adolescents live in order to improve health outcomes for youth (U.S. DHHS, 2011a).

Rural Health Promotion Theory Highlight: Life Course Health Development

"Health development is shaped by the dynamic and continuous interaction between biology and experiences and is framed by the constantly changing developmental contexts over the lifetime." (Halfon & Hochstein, 2002, p. 457)

Injury

Motor Vehicle Accidents

Motor vehicle accidents (MVAs) are the leading cause of mortality among adolescents aged 10–24 years (Mulye et al., 2009). Contributing factors to MVAs and resultant injury among adolescents are age, experience, gender, risky driving behaviors such as unsafe speeds, in-vehicle distractions including cell phones and other passengers, alcohol, sleepiness, and unreliable seat belt use (Neyens & Boyle, 2008; NRC & IOM, 2009; NRC, IOM, & Transportation Research Board [TRB], 2007; Peek-Asa, Britton, Young, Pawlovich, & Falb, 2010; Rhodes & Pivik, 2010). It is estimated that MVA-related injury can be reduced by 50–60% through the proper use of seat belts, though adolescents have demonstrated the lowest use of seat belts of any age group (National Highway Traffic Safety Administration, 2001; Shope & Bingham, 2008). Adolescent males engage in more risky driving behaviors than females, are less likely to wear a seat belt, and are more likely to combine driving with alcohol use; therefore, adolescent males have predictably higher rates of MVA fatality (Mulye et al., 2009; NRC & IOM, 2009; Rhodes & Pivik, 2010). Data demonstrate that the incidence of MVAs diminishes progressively in adolescence with increasing age and cumulative experience behind the wheel (NRC, IOM, & TRB, 2007). The developmental changes in driving risks during the course of adolescence are explained by neurobehavioral science as the effects of cognitive maturation on impulse control and attentiveness (Dahl, 2008).

Alcohol use is a principal factor in the incidence of adolescent MVAs, contributing to 23% of fatal crashes for the 16–20 years age group, and 41% of fatal crashes among drivers 21–24 years (Mulye et al., 2009). Sleepiness can mimic the effects of alcohol on the teen driver, resulting in inattentiveness, lapses in judgment, and increased aggression (Dahl, 2008). It is estimated that after 17 hours of wakefulness (such as from 6:30 AM to 11:30 PM), the adolescent's driving performance is impaired comparable to a 0.05 blood alcohol level; after 24 hours awake, driving impairment reaches the 0.10 blood alcohol level (NRC, IOM, & TRB, 2007). Crashes attributed to sleepiness peak in adolescence because of a biological increased need for sleep and changes in sleep habits in response to physical, social, and academic demands (NRC & IOM, 2009; Pack, 1995).

Adolescent MVA fatalities declined considerably between 1990 (25.3/100,000) and 2005 (18.6/100,000). The reduction in adolescent MVA fatalities during that period may be in part attributed to improved adolescent driving behaviors, including the increased use of seat belts and decreased drinking and driving; a result of safety campaigns; and because of enhanced law enforcement (Mulye et al., 2009; NRC & IOM, 2009). The implementation of graduated driver licensing (GDL), typically including an extended supervised practice stage for newly licensed adolescents, followed by provisional licensure targeting adolescent-specific risk factors, has demonstrated marked reductions in adolescent crash rates in several states (NRC, IOM, & TRB, 2007; Shope & Bingham,

2008). However, MVA fatalities related to distracted driving, particularly cell phone use, have increased between 1999 and 2008 (Wilson & Stimpson, 2010). Although all adolescents are more likely to be severely injured by cell phone or passenger distractions than other markers of inattentiveness, female adolescent drivers sustain more severe injuries in distraction-related crashes than male drivers (Neyens & Boyle, 2008).

Motor vehicle accident injury and fatality rates are considerably higher among rural youth when compared to urban populations (Kmet & Macarther, 2006; Peek-Asa et al., 2010). Structural and environmental conditions of the rural community may contribute to increased adolescent MVA injury. More driving time on the road due to extended distances between destinations and inadequate public transportation, lower traffic density allowing for increased vehicular speeds, less traffic surveillance and law enforcement in remote communities, rural road safety features including narrow two lane roads with inadequate lighting and visibility, wildlife hazards, inclement weather, and delayed post-collision access to trauma care all may increase the risks of rural adolescent drivers (Kmet & Macarther, 2006; McDonald & Trowbridge, 2009). These structural factors, combined with adolescent risky driving behaviors including speeding, alcohol use, seat belt noncompliance, and a higher prevalence of underaged driving in the rural community, contribute to increased MVA morbidity and mortality (Kmet & Macarther, 2006; McDonald & Trowbridge, 2009). From a public health and economic perspective, adolescent MVAs impose an enormous cost to society (NRC, IOM, & TRB, 2007). In addition to the tragic loss of life, the CDC estimated that, in 2002, crashes involving drivers ages 15–20 years cost society $40.8 billion (NRC, IOM, & TRB, 2007).

Active engagement in the reduction of adolescent MVAs must be a rural nursing health-promotion priority. Comprehensive adolescent driving safety programs coordinated between interdisciplinary healthcare providers and community health programs are imperative to improve evidence-based safety interventions in the rural community (NRC, IOM, & TRB, 2007). Since driving legislation is enacted primarily at the state level, nursing advocacy for local community-specific contextual interventions targeting rural adolescent driving risk reduction is necessary. Nurses must consider if the local rural community could be better structured to reduce the driving risks for adolescents by altering the scheduling of adolescent events to reduce sleeplessness, increasing the availability of public transportation, improving drivers education training and adolescent licensing legislation to reflect rural-specific driving risks, increasing the presence of rural law enforcement during peak adolescent travel times, and improving the quality of local rural roads. Rural nurses must educate youth and counsel parents on the inherent adolescent driving risks in the rural community, initiate a family-based adolescent vehicular risk assessment, support families in making an accurate assessment of their individual child's developmental readiness to drive on rural roads, and facilitate the exploration of safer alternatives in adolescent transportation within the rural community.

Gun Related Mortality

Although youth in urban and rural regions demonstrate a relatively indistinguishable incidence of gun related mortality across the United States, the causative forces behind adolescent firearm deaths differ distinctly between communities (Nance, Carr, Kallan, Branas, & Wiebe, 2010). In urban counties, firearm deaths among youth are disproportionately attributed to homicide, whereas in rural counties firearm deaths are predominately related to unintentional injury and suicide (Nance et al., 2010). Firearms in the home and the recreational use of firearms by adolescents are more common in rural areas. Access to firearms within the home, along with inadequate firearm storage practices, have been linked to increased rates of unintentional firearm injury and suicide (Miller, Azrael, Hemenway, & Vriniotis, 2005; Nance et al., 2010; Sorenson & Vittes, 2004; Vittes & Sorenson, 2005).

The American Academy of Pediatrics affirms that the most effective measure to reduce firearm mortality among adolescents is to create gun-free environments in homes and communities (AAP, 2000a). That being said, gun ownership, for both recreational use and home and livestock protection, is a constitutionally protected cultural mainstay in rural and remote communities in the United States. Therefore, risk reduction measures for adolescent health promotion must be considered by rural nurses, including the assessment of gun accessibility among rural adolescents, active mental health evaluations of rural adolescents with specific discussions of suicidal ideation and use of appropriate mental health referral mechanisms as indicated, rural suicide awareness campaigns, education on the importance of gun safety and proper gun storage techniques within the family, and advocating for alternative, out-of-home, methods for storing guns used for recreational use, such as at community sport shooting centers.

Unintentional Injury

Unintentional injury is the leading cause of morbidity and mortality among adolescents in the United States (Sleet, Ballesteros, & Borse, 2010). The rates of fatal and nonfatal major injuries among youth attributable to mechanisms other than firearms are higher in rural communities than most urban communities (Cohen, Tiesman, Bossarte, & Furbee, 2009; Nance et al., 2010; Riley et al., 1996). Although the majority of severe unintentional injuries among adolescents in the rural community are caused by MVAs, a variety of other mechanisms of injury should be addressed with respect to the Healthy People 2020 objective of reducing fatal and nonfatal unintentional injuries (U.S. DHHS, 2011a).

An analysis of rural adolescent health found that one in five adolescents sustained an injury severe enough to be treated within the last year (Curtis, 2011). Sports injuries (44.9%) and falls (19.1%) were the most common causes of nonfatal adolescent injury among this rural sample. Bicycle accidents are another substantial source of youth morbidity across all regions of the United States. Young adolescents, 10–14 years of age, have the highest rates of bicycle-related fatalities, predominantly due to severe head injuries (Sleet, Ballesteros & Borse, 2010).

Other safety hazards of particular concern for rural youth include injuries sustained from large animals and agricultural work, drowning, and all-terrain vehicle (ATV) accidents (Curtis, 2011; Sleet et al., 2010). Adolescents living in rural regions are more likely to be exposed to hazards from agricultural, fishing, forestry, and mining work, including trauma from large animals, occupational falls and burns, drowning, machinery accidents, and pesticide exposure (Gamm et al., 2003; Sleet et al., 2010). Proper adult supervision, adequate safety training, and use of protective gear are essential interventions to reduce the incidence of agricultural injury among youth (Reed, Browning, Westneat, & Kidd; 2006). In addition, the Fair Labor Standards Act, designed to protect youth from hazardous work conditions, specifies minimum ages for particular types of agricultural work, prohibits work during hazardous times, and dictates an hourly maximum work day for adolescents (Sleet et al., 2010).

Drowning is the fifth leading cause of unintentional fatality in the United States and most drownings in adolescents over 15 years of age occur in natural water settings (Nasrullah & Muazzam, 2011; Sleet et al., 2010). Contributing factors to fatal drowning in rural and remote regions include cold water, traumatic injury preceding drowning, and delayed access to emergency treatment (Nasrullah & Muazzam, 2011). In addition to boating and swimming in natural waters, other risk factors for accidental drowning include swimming alone, swimming at night, aquatic risk taking, and swimming under the influence of alcohol, all male-dominated behaviors (Stiglets, 2001). The incidence of male drowning peaks in late adolescence, ultimately reaching a 10:1 male to female drowning ratio (Stiglets, 2001). Drowning prevention interventions specific to the rural adolescent population include water safety education emphasizing the dangers of combining alcohol with water activities, encouraging the use of personal flotation devices (PFDs), local public safety awareness campaigns identifying seasonally variable natural water hazards and providing education on cold water survival techniques, CPR training for adolescents, mandatory boating safety classes for adolescent boat operators, and increased law enforcement presence around bodies of natural water used for recreation (Weiss, 2010).

All-terrain vehicles (ATVs), four-wheeled off-road motorized vehicles, are common in rural communities for use in recreation and agricultural labor (Helmcamp, Aitken, & Lawrence, 2009; Jones & Bleeker, 2005). Data indicate a continued increase in human and societal costs related to ATV accidents, prompting serious public health concern, particularly in rural communities (Helmcamp et al., 2009; Jones & Bleeker, 2005). It has been advised that state and local governments with large rural populations carefully consider safety requirements for ATV use including age restrictions for operation, mandatory ATV hands-on training, and obligatory use of safety equipment

(Helmcamp et al., 2009). As youth are particularly at-risk for ATV injury, the AAP issued a policy statement recommending anticipatory guidance assessment and education regarding the safe use of ATVs, which should be reinforced by all rural nurses working with youth and families (AAP, 2000).

Mental Health

Although the overall data on rural–urban differences in the incidence of psychological distress and mental illness are equivocal and potentially related to factors other than the degree of residential rurality, disparities are identified in mental health outcomes and mental health service utilization in the United States based on geographic residence (Dhingra, Strine, Holt, Berry, & Mokdad, 2009; Elgar, Arlett, & Groves, 2003; Gamm et al., 2003; Hauenstein, 2008; Lorenz, Wickrama, & Yeh, 2004; Rohrer, Borders, & Blanton, 2005). Most strikingly, rural communities consistently demonstrate markedly higher rates of suicide in adolescent and adult populations when compared to urban regions, particularly among farmers and residents of the Western states (Biddle, Sekula, & Puskar, 2010; Hirsch, 2006; Lorenz et al., 2004; Nance et al., 2010). Evidence suggests a high prevalence of major depression in rural communities, especially among rural women, and it is frequently correlated with poverty, poor physical health, and a history of emotional, physical, and/or sexual abuse (Hauenstein & Peddada, 2007; Probst, Laditka, Moore, Harun, & Powell, 2008; Simmons, Braun, Charnigo, Havens, & Wright, 2008). Data also indicate a higher rate of comorbid externalizing disorders among rural populations, including substance use and intermittent explosive disorder associated with major depression, generalized anxiety, and lifetime antisocial disorder (Hauenstein, 2008). In addition, agricultural workers with a chronic exposure to organophosphate pesticides have demonstrated increased levels of tension, anger, anxiety, and depression (Hirsch, 2006). These proclivities, combined with economic stress, social isolation, the cultural stigmatization of psychological disorders, a lack of mental health services, substance use, and the presence of firearms in the home, proves to be a lethal combination for the rural community (Biddle et al., 2010; Hauenstein, 2008; Hirsch, 2006; Gustafson et al., 2009; Zigmond, 2010).

Adolescence is a critical period for lifecourse mental health development, as data indicate that one-half of all adult mental health disorders start by the age of 14 and it is estimated that the lifetime prevalence of mental health problems may be as high as 37% by age 16 (Costello et al., 2003; Kessler, 2005). The most common mental health problems in adolescence, in order of relative prevalence, are anxiety, depression, attention deficit hyperactivity disorder (ADHD), conduct disorder, and disordered eating (NCR & IOM, 2009). Unaddressed adolescent mental health concerns contribute to poor school performance, social isolation, substance use, and other risky behaviors, as well as suicide (Peden, Reed, & Rayens, 2005).

It has been suggested, and the disproportionately high suicide rates among rural adolescents support, that rural adolescents are more vulnerable to serious mental health outcomes than their urban peers, potentially related to the systemic effects of impoverished social environments and inadequate availability of support services (Nance et al., 2010; Peden et al., 2005). Research suggests that 40% of rural adolescents experience symptoms of depression weekly, with a high level of depressive symptoms indicated by approximately 30% of the rural adolescent population (Curtis et al., 2011; Peden et al., 2005). Data also indicate that depressive symptoms among rural adolescents peak among the 14–15-year-old age group, suggesting developmentally propelled mental health vulnerability during the early years of high school in rural communities (Curtis et al., 2011).

The World Health Organization (WHO) champions the stance that "there can be no health without mental health," and in recognition of the considerable social and economic burden mental illness levies across the globe, the WHO advocates intensive investment in community-based mental health-promotion and prevention strategies particularly targeting underserved and other vulnerable populations (WHO, 2005, p. 11). In addition, the WHO specifically advocates for the availability of mental health-promotion activities during vulnerable life stages, such as adolescence (WHO, 2005). Substantial evidence supports the use of mental health-promotion activities, community-based mental health screening, and early intervention strategies to reduce the inextricably enmeshed physical, psychological, and socioeconomic public health impacts of mental health disability (Parham, 2008; Wand, 2011; WHO, 2005). Current emphasis on intervening at the level of the social determinants of mental health, which include economic status, living environments, gender equity, and public policy, is especially pertinent to rural mental health and articulates directly with the contextually based Healthy People 2020 adolescent health framework (Yearwood & Siantz, 2010). Rural residents are disproportionately vulnerable to poor mental health outcomes related to the psychological effects of pervasive and persistent poverty, social isolation, a high prevalence of chronic disease, exposure to toxic environmental hazards such as organophosphate pesticides, culturally embedded inequities in gender empowerment contributing to interpersonal violence and depression, a lack of positive youth development resources and other recreational activities, and inadequate public health policies supporting the accessibility of evidenced-based mental health services in rural and remote communities (Hauenstein, 2008; Hirsch, 2006; Simmons et al., 2008; Zigmond, 2010). In conjunction with addressing the social and environmental risk factors for poor mental health, integration of strength-based interventions for mental health-promotion are advocated, including programs to facilitate the development of self-esteem, self-efficacy, communication, and coping skills for vulnerable populations in the rural community (Wand, 2011).

The World Federation for Mental Health admonishes that healthcare providers must develop more effective interdisciplinary models to address prevention, early detection, and intervention for mental health problems to circumvent disabling mental conditions within vulnerable populations (Wand, 2011). Currently, the mental health needs of rural populations in America are inadequately addressed due to insufficient funding, fragmentation of mental health services, and a lack of accessible mental health providers for underfunded, at-risk populations (Gustafson et al., 2009; Hauenstein, 2008). Nurses are the largest healthcare workforce integrated throughout multiple systems in the rural community, and are therefore ideally posed to address the populations' unmet mental health needs (Wand, 2011). It is incumbent upon the nursing profession to use its considerable visibility and credibility within the rural community to lead innovations in mental health promotion for vulnerable and underserved rural populations (Wand, 2011). Community-based nurses in schools, occupational settings, and religious and other civic organizations can provide mental health-promotion programs and perform mental health screening in underserved rural communities. Acute care nurses must screen all rural patients for undetected mental health comorbidities, including depression, substance use, and interpersonal violence. Public health nurses can provide case management services to address the fragmentation of mental health services in the rural community and promote continuity of care. Advanced practice registered nurses can work in interdisciplinary teams with counselors and psychiatrists to provide cost-effective management of the rural mental health client. Using evidenced-based mental health prevention, promotion, and policy models and employing innovative healthcare workforce and information technology solutions, nurses must lead the rural community in meeting the Healthy People 2020 goal of improving mental health through prevention by ensuring access to appropriate, quality mental health services (U.S. DHHS, 2011a; Yearwood & Siantz, 2010).

Substance Use

Substance abuse (including alcohol, illicit drug use, and nonmedical prescription drug use) is a common comorbidity of mental health disorders and an essential component of community-based mental health-promotion interventions in the rural community. Although significant differences in overall rates of substance abuse are not consistently demonstrated among rural, suburban, and urban populations, data indicate that alarming trends exist in substance use among specific rural populations and significant substance abuse-related health-promotion disparities exist in rural communities (Blanco et al., 2007; Gfroerer, Larson, & Colliver, 2007; Hutchinson & Blakely, 2003; Lambert, Gale, & Hartley, 2008; Van Gundy, 2006).

Tobacco and alcohol are the most commonly used substances among adults and adolescents, ultimately contributing to the first and third leading causes of actual death in the United States, respectively (Mokdad & Remington, 2010; Van Gundy, 2006). The use of cigarettes and smokeless tobacco has demonstrated steady declines in the

United States since the 1990s among both adolescents and adults. However, all tobacco products are used more frequently among rural residents, with the highest incidence of tobacco use documented among American Indian and Native Alaskan populations (Gfroerer et al., 2007; Nelson et al., 2006; NRC & IOM, 2009). Reports of alcohol use, abuse, and binge drinking are, for the most, part equally prevalent among adults in rural communities when compared to urban samples, with regional variations across the United States (Borders & Booth, 2007; Hutchinson & Blakely, 2003; Van Gundy, 2006). Alcohol abstinence is most common in the rural South, potentially related to religious affiliations and convictions, and excessive alcohol use is generally more problematic in both the rural and urban Midwest (Borders & Booth, 2007). Unemployed adults demonstrate increased vulnerability to excessive alcohol use across regions and rural communities include a disproportionate number of unemployed adult residents (Hutchinson & Blakely, 2003; Van Gundy, 2006). In addition, rural adults have documented higher rates of drinking and driving, increasing the safety risk associated with alcohol intake in the rural community (Hutchinson & Blakely, 2003). For illicit drug use in general, rural adults demonstrate less or equivalent prevalence rates. Even so, concerning trends in the data on rural adult substance use include evidence that nonmedical prescription drug abuse is dramatically increasing among adults in all regions, and methamphetamine use is more prevalent and continuing to escalate in rural communities (Blanco et al., 2007; Gfroerer et al., 2007; Hutchinson & Blakely, 2003; Lambert et al., 2008; Van Gundy, 2006).

Adolescence is a critical developmental period for the initiation of substance use, potentially inciting serious acute and chronic pathology including respiratory, cardiovascular, liver, and mental health disorders. Current trends in adolescent substance use in the rural community are disconcerting. Rural adolescents are more likely to use tobacco products than urban or suburban youth (Hanson et al., 2009; Heck, 2004; Nelson et al., 2006). The majority of adolescents who smoke continue the habit into young adulthood, with 82% of adult smokers starting the habit before age 18 (NRC & IOM, 2009). Underage drinking is more prevalent in rural communities and the disparity increases progressively with the degree of rurality (Gfroerer et al., 2007; Lambert et al., 2008; Swaim & Stanley, 2010; Van Gundy, 2006). At ages 12–13, rural youth are two times more likely than urban youth to report alcohol use (Van Gundy, 2006). A strong relationship exists between the age at onset of drinking and the risk of later alcohol-related problems. Thus, the disproportionately early age of alcohol consumption among rural youth increases the probability of alcohol-related health disparities in rural communities (Hingson & Kenkel, 2004; NRC & IOM, 2009). Rural youth are also more likely to report heavy drinking and binge drinking and more frequently engage in dangerous behaviors under the influence, including driving (Lambert et al., 2008). Data indicate that rural minority youth are at increased risk for drinking and getting drunk than non-minority adolescents, with American Indian, Alaskan Native, and Hispanic adolescents demonstrating a particularly high prevalence of problematic drinking behaviors (NRC & IOM, 2009; Swaim & Stanley, 2010).

Evidence now exists that rural youth are more likely to use illicit drugs, including marijuana, cocaine, methamphetamines, inhalants, and nonmedical prescription medications, than urban youth (Havens, Young, & Havens, 2011; Rhew, Hawkins, & Oesterle, 2011). In one analysis, eighth graders in rural America were 83% more likely to use crack cocaine, 50% more likely to use cocaine, and 34% more likely to use marijuana than urban youth (Center on Addiction and Substance Abuse [CASA], 2000). Another study of the nonmedical use of prescription medications demonstrated that rural adolescents, ages 12–17 years, were 26% more likely to have used prescription medications such as pain relievers, tranquilizers, sedatives, and stimulants for nonmedical use than urban youth (Havens et al., 2011). It is hypothesized that problems with drug use among rural youth may be attributed to the overall psychosocial effects of socioeconomic disadvantage, the social disorganization of underprivileged rural communities, an inadequacy of positive youth development opportunities, reduced access to drug education and treatment services, and the unavailability and cultural stigmatization of mental health services in the rural cultural environment (Rhew et al., 2011).

Clearly, there is a critical need for substance abuse prevention and treatment services for youth in the rural community specifically targeting tobacco, alcohol, methamphetamines, and nonmedical prescription drug use. As reflected in the Healthy People 2020 objectives, effective efforts to reduce the rates of substance abuse must address the social determinants of health in the rural community (U.S. DHHS, 2011). Opportunities for positive youth development activities including prosocial involvement in the community, school, family and peer domains have demonstrated positive effects in the reduction of adolescent substance use (Rhew et al., 2011). Likewise, protective factors for the prevention of substance use were found to be enrollment in school and living in a two-parent household (Havens et al., 2011; Van Gundy, 2006). Therefore, programs and policies supporting positive family engagement, the local school system, and other community-based prosocial activities for youth are integral to addressing the plague of rural substance abuse.

The IOM (2005) indicated an overall inadequacy of core medical services in the rural community contributing to persistent health disparities among rural residents. Accessible and culturally congruent substance abuse treatment programs are a medical service sorely needed and significantly lacking in rural America. Barriers to substance abuse treatment programs in rural regions include funding deficiencies, a lack of expert practitioners, extensive distances between services and residents, and insufficient development of evidence-based treatment programs specifically designed for rural communities (Van Gundy, 2006). Recommendations for the development of substance abuse services in the rural community include drawing on existing community strengths and resources such as the influence of community leaders, strong interpersonal relationships among community members, and faith-based community practices (Van Gundy, 2006). Telehealth methods should be incorporated into substance abuse prevention, health-promotion, and treatment programs in rural regions to increase the accessibility of services in remote communities and decrease barriers to care related to concerns for confidentiality in the small-town environment. Rural nurses must be proactively involved in substance abuse prevention programs throughout the community, including in schools, worksites, and religious and other civic organizations, to the promote the health and protect the vitality of the rural community.

Reproductive Health

The importance of accessible and culturally congruent reproductive health services in the rural community was discussed previously in this chapter in the section on maternal–child health. However, a few additional adolescent-specific reproductive health issues are worth reviewing. Rural adolescents may be at increased risk for early sexual debut and multiple sex partners, sexually transmitted infections, and early childbearing (Champion, Kelly, Shain, & Piper, 2004; RAC, 2011b). In addition, data indicate that minority rural adolescents engage in more sexual risk behaviors and experience more negative reproductive health outcomes than non-Hispanic White rural youth (Champion et al., 2004). Reproductive health disparities for rural adolescents may be related to poverty, lack of education, language barriers, inadequate access to prevention services, limited privacy and concerns for confidentiality, and sociopolitical barriers to adolescent reproductive health services related to the conservative nature of the rural community (Champion et al., 2004; Noone & Young, 2009). In order to address the Healthy People 2020 objectives of increasing sexual health education and access to reproductive health services, rural nurses must be prepared to advocate for sexual health-promotion services for rural youth in potentially unreceptive social and political climates. This can be a considerable challenge in isolated rural and remote communities, and rural nurses may need to turn to external support for adolescent health advocacy. Resources that may be helpful to the rural nurse in advocating for adolescent access to sexual health-promotion services include the Center for Adolescent Health and the Law: http://www.cahl.org/web/; the National Adolescent Health Information Center: http://nahic.ucsf.edu/; the American Civil Liberties Union (ACLU) Reproductive Freedom Project: http://www.aclu.org/reproductive-freedom; Advocates for Youth: http://www.advocatesforyouth.org/; and Planned Parenthood: http://www.plannedparenthood.org/.

Intimate Partner Violence

Intimate partner and adolescent dating violence are increasingly acknowledged as significant public health concerns across all regions of the United States (CDC, 2004).

Some studies have indicated a higher level of intimate partner violence (IPV) in rural areas, whereas other research demonstrates equal prevalence between rural and urban settings but identifies rural disparities related to a lack of mental health and domestic violence resources in the rural community (Adler, 1996; Brelding, Ziembroski, Black & 2009; Marquart, Nannini, Edwards, Stanley, & Wyman, 2007; McDonell, Ott, & Mitchell, 2010; Spencer & Bryant, 2000). Other factors that may increase the risk for IPV in the rural community include economic stress, substance use, more traditional gender roles, and social isolation (Adler, 1996; Brelding et al., 2009; Marquart et al., 2007; McDonell et al., 2010; Spencer & Bryant, 2000). Due to the prevalence of IPV across geographic regions in the United States, screening for IPV is a critical component of reproductive health-promotion practice. Since women in their 20s are most vulnerable to IPV, screening and education on IPV must begin at the very first reproductive health encounter and continue with each subsequent visit (CDC, 2004). Before implementing IPV screening in the rural community, it is essential that the nurse assess the available referral mechanisms and resources for victims of IPV, because improved IPV screening will certainly lead to increased violence detection and a plan for appropriate referral is crucial (CDC, 2004).

Adolescent Health-Promotion Services in the Rural Community

Adolescence is a critical developmental period for the reduction of health disparities in the rural community. Although the need for rural adolescent health-promotion services is great, barriers to developmentally sensitive adolescent health care in the rural community are considerable. Innovative solutions for the delivery of nursing health-promotion services for rural adolescents need to be developed and sustained, including interdisciplinary models utilizing primary care settings, school-based health centers, adolescent clinics within community health centers, and telehealth technologies (Burke, Bynum,Hall-Barrow, Ott & Albright, 2008; Clayton, Chin, Blackburn, & Echevarria, 2010; Pastore, Murray, & Juszczak, 2001). Data indicate that the most at-risk rural adolescents report the greatest reliance on community-based health services (Curtis, 2008). Therefore, the provision of community-based health-promotion programs targeting adolescent risks may have a significant impact on the reduction of health disparities in the rural community. Confidential health services for adolescents are a vital component of the effective delivery of adolescent health care as evidence demonstrates that confidential services increase the willingness of adolescents to seek care for critical issues such as reproductive health, mental health, and substance use (NCR & IOM, 2009). Community-based adolescent health services have historically provided a unique and developmentally sensitive platform for the provision of confidential adolescent services. Unfortunately, despite the considerable potential for improving population health, community-based services for adolescents are vulnerable to negative political and economic forces within the small community. Effective nursing advocacy for school and other community-based health services for adolescents must include a targeted community health assessment focused on the specific needs of youth and adolescent subgroups, public awareness campaigns presenting the potential benefits of community-based services for adolescents, the development of an integrated interdisciplinary adolescent healthcare team, creative and collaborative approaches to securing funding streams for adolescent health services, and data collection on adolescent health program outcomes to support the further development of best practices in the delivery of rural adolescent health care.

ISSUES OF ADULT AND OLDER ADULT RURAL HEALTH PROMOTION

Agricultural and Migrant Health Issues

The agricultural and extraction industries in the rural community present unique health risks to rural residents. These industries, including farming and livestock management, logging, mining, fishing, and hunting/trapping, consistently rank among the most hazardous industries for occupational morbidity and mortality (Schulman & Slesinger, 2004). The fishing, hunting, and trapping industries have the highest rates of fatality, followed by forestry, logging, and then mining (Schulman & Slesinger, 2004). Although farm workers have the lowest fatality rates of the other extractive industries, the fatality rate for the agricultural industry is still six times the national occupational average (Schulman & Slesinger, 2004). The majority of fatalities in the agricultural industry are caused by machine-related hazards including vehicle and equipment crashes and entanglements. Farmers and other extractive industry workers are also at increased risk for falls and entrapment; being struck by objects, animals, or electricity; noise-induced hearing loss; chronic pain syndromes related to overuse injuries; acute dehydration; and skin cancer from prolonged sun exposure (Connor, Layne, & Thomisee, 2010; Schulman & Slesinger, 2004). Older adult farmers and farm youth frequently contribute to the family-based agricultural industry and may be at increased risk for injury (Schulman & Slesinger, 2004). The unique mental health hazards of farming and extractive industry workers include stress related to a large number of uncontrollable environmental factors directly affecting productivity and revenue, periodic economic hardships, concerns for physical safety in more risky occupations, chronic exposure to organophosphate pesticides, social isolation, lack of available mental health services, and social stigma surrounding mental health issues in the rural community (Gustafson, Preston & Hudson, 2009; Hauenstein, 2008; Hirsch, 2006; Schulman & Slesinger, 2004). The varied occupational hazards of agricultural and extractive industries contribute to the disproportionate prevalence of chronic health conditions and disability in the rural community (Stamm et al., 2007).

Pesticides and other agricultural chemical exposures pose the potential for acute and chronic health problems among farm workers and rural community residents, particularly in the Midwest and California, where 80% of all the agricultural pesticides in the United States are applied (60% and 20%, respectively). Pathways of human exposure to agricultural chemicals in rural communities include occupational handling, ambient air inhalation, soil contamination, and ingestion through particulate accumulation in dietary and water sources, with acute symptoms related to agricultural chemical exposure being throat and eye irritation, fatigue, nausea, and diarrhea (Hodne, 2004). Chronic exposure to agricultural chemicals can cause lung and skin diseases, reproductive health issues, depression, neurobehavioral problems, and cancer (Hodne, 2004; Schulman & Slesinger, 2004; Ward & Atav, 2004). Inadequate sanitation and insufficient clean water sources, toileting, and hand-washing facilities present an additional environmental hazard to agricultural workers, potentially contributing to acute and chronic infections, parasites, dermatitis, and other illnesses (Schulman & Slesinger, 2004).

Seasonal and migrant workers comprise a significant sector of the agricultural workforce. Seasonal workers are employed on a temporary basis according to industry demand but maintain residence in one location, whereas migrant workers move from location to location following opportunities in agricultural employment (Ward & Atav, 2004). There are three major migrant worker streams in the United States. The Eastern migrant stream is based in Florida and moves up the coast into New England; the largest migrant stream originates in Texas, supplying the Midwest agricultural workforce; and the Western stream is based in California extending northward to Oregon, Idaho, and Washington (Ward & Atav, 2004). Much of the agricultural migrant workforce in the United States is foreign-born, predominantly emigrating from Mexico and other Latin American countries (Ward & Atav, 2004). Seasonal and migrant workers are vulnerable to the same health hazards as other agricultural and extractive workers, and share the disadvantages of much of the rural work force including underemployment, poverty, lack of insurance, low education levels, language barriers, inadequate transportation, and limited access to healthcare providers (Hoerster et al., 2011; Ward & Atav, 2004). Latinos in the United States in general experience a disproportionate burden of disease when compared to non-Hispanic White populations, including higher rates of infectious disease, diabetes, hypertension, liver disease, and HIV and poorer self-reported health status, in conjunction with less access to healthcare services (Liao, 2011; Torres, 2004). Migrant workers have demonstrated greater health problems than seasonal stationary agricultural laborers, and data indicate that 1 in 4 migrant farm workers are living with a chronic disease (Ward & Atav, 2004). Other specific health risks of migrant workers are poor dental health, occupational injury, musculoskeletal overuse conditions, dehydration and exposure syndromes, anxiety, depression, and substance use (Connor et al., 2010; Hiott, Grzywacz, Davis, Quandt, & Arcury, 2008; Hovey, 2001; Larson, 2001; Lombardi, 2001; Peoples et al., 2010; Torres, 2004). Disparities in health among migrant workers may be related to ecological determinants, including social and financial instability, fragmented health care and inadequate follow-up services, language barriers, crowded and substandard living conditions, limited freedom to leave work to seek needed care, decreased access to safe and reliable transportation, discrimination, and reticence to receive care due to a fear of contact with immigration authorities (Connor et al., 2010; Hoerster et al., 2011; Holden, 2001; Ward & Atav, 2004).

Cultural and philosophical beliefs among the migrant workforce also contribute to health and health behaviors. Data indicate that the Latino migrant population experience chronic disease as a holistic phenomenon involving biological, emotional, and psychological processes, and employ both biomedical and traditional folk remedies in self-care practices (Connor et al., 2010; Heuer & Lausch, 2006). Data support that traditional social behavior of immigrant Latino migrant farmworkers, including the supportive nature of the Hispanic culture, may be protective against some health risks, but the protective cultural traits appear to dissipate with progressive acculturation over time (Torres, 2004). Madeleine Leininger's Transcultural Care Theory is a viable theoretical framework for assessing cultural health practices and developing intervention strategies among immigrant populations (Alexander et al., 1986). Leininger promotes the understanding that cultural awareness, competence, and congruence is integral to the delivery of optimum healthcare services within diverse populations. Using the Transcultural Care framework, delivery of holistic care is dependent on an appreciation for biophysical, cultural, psychological, social, and environmental dimensions of health, incorporating a consideration of traditional practices into the development and implementation of nursing care (Alexander et al., 1986).

Rural Health Promotion Theory Highlight: The Transcultural Care Theory

The Transcultural Care Theory explores healthcare behaviors, healthcare goals, and nursing practice within the context of cultural beliefs and social structure (Alexander et al., 1986).

The Migrant Health Act of 1962, administered through the Bureau of Primary Health Care within the United States Department of Health and Human Services, established migrant health programs to provide medical and support services to farm workers and their families (Shi & Stevens, 2005). Primary and preventive migrant health services are frequently coordinated through local Federally Qualified Health Centers and Health Departments along the migrant worker streams. However, these limited resources only provide care to approximately 20% of the migrant population (Connor et al., 2010; Shi & Stevens, 2005). Additional healthcare resources are needed to adequately meet the needs of the migrant population, particularly during the peak agricultural seasons (Connor et al., 2010).

The nursing profession is well situated to provide culturally congruent health-promotion services to agricultural workers through the organization of interdisciplinary nurse-managed clinics providing health screenings, health education, psychosocial support counseling, preventive dental services, immunizations, physical therapy evaluations, primary care health management, and medical referral in collaboration with local health agencies and academic health institutions. During the peak agricultural season, these services must be delivered to the migrant population where and when the worker is available. Care should be brought to the farm fields, packing sheds, worker barracks, childcare centers, and schools sites, particularly after sunset and into the evening (Connor et al., 2010). In addition, to adequately promote and sustain optimum migrant worker health, nursing health promotion and advocacy must continue upstream with information sharing and education for agricultural employers, the consumer public, city administrators, and state and federal legislators in order to secure safe living and working conditions and adequate provision of healthcare services for this vulnerable population in rural America.

Health Promotion and Chronic Disease Management in the Rural Community

Chronic disease is the leading cause of morbidity and mortality in the United States, causing 7 out of 10 deaths each year (U.S. DHHS, 2011). The prevalence of chronic disease is a Healthy People population health indicator; however, despite targeted efforts, national goals for the prevention and reduction of chronic disease remain elusive (Chowdhury et al., 2010; U.S. DHHS, 2011). Rural adults experience more chronic disease than urban and suburban populations, including arthritis, asthma, heart disease, diabetes, hypertension, cancer, and mental disorders (Bailey, 2009; Bennett et al., 2008; Gamm et al., 2003; IOM, 2005). In addition, racial and ethnic disparities exist in the prevalence of chronic disease in the rural community. Rural Black, American Indian, and Hispanic populations are more at risk for many chronic disease conditions such as obesity, diabetes, and hypertension than rural White populations (Bennett et al., 2008; Liao, 2011; Peek & Zsembik, 2004; Rhoades & Cravatt, 2004; Torres, 2004). In rural Appalachia, the predominantly White population consistently demonstrates disproportionately high rates of cancer, in particular largely preventable lung and cervical cancers (Gatz, Graham, Rowles, & Tyas, 2004; Wingo et al.. 2008). The inception and progression of many of these chronic diseases afflicting rural America are preventable through the delivery of nursing health-promotion and early detection services. According to the American Nurses Association (2011), the role of nursing is "the protection, promotion, and optimization of health and abilities, prevention of illness and injury, alleviation of suffering through the diagnosis and treatment of human response, and advocacy in the care of individuals, families, communities, and populations" (para. 2). It is therefore the responsibility of the nursing workforce, the largest healthcare workforce in the rural community, to develop collaborative, interdisciplinary models of chronic disease prevention and management to alleviate the chronic disease burden in rural America (Hauenstein, 2008).

The Health Belief Model is a theoretical framework originally constructed in the 1950s to explore the utilization of preventive health services and subsequently applied to the development of prevention-related interventions for asymptomatic health concerns such as cancer, hypertension, and cardiovascular disease screening (Glanz & Bishop, 2010). As such, it is an applicable theoretical framework for the organization of nursing health-promotion services for the reduction of chronic disease in the rural community. The key constructs of the model are: (1) perceived susceptibility and perceived severity, (2) perceived benefits and perceived barriers, (3) cues to action, and (4) self-efficacy (Glanz & Bishop, 2010). The Health Belief Model theorizes that an individual's readiness to make a health behavior change is related to the perception of health risk in relation to the perceived benefit of making a behavior change (Glanz & Bishop, 2010).

Rural Health Promotion Theory Highlight: The Health Belief Model

The Health Belief Model theorizes that an individual's readiness to make a health behavior change is related to the perception of susceptibility to a health problem and the perceived benefit of making a behavior change (Glanz & Bishop, 2010)

Health Promotion for Older Adults in the Rural Community

Older adults are the fastest growing population, not only in the United States, but throughout much of the world (U.S. DHHS, 2011b; WHO 2002). By the year 2030, citizens aged 65 and over will constitute 20% of the American population, disproportionately represented in rural communities across the United States (IOM, 2005; Lang, Benson, & Anderson, 2005; Morton, 2004). The increased prevalence of chronic disease in rural communities is a function of this age gradient, as well as a complex interaction of other variables including racial and ethnic and socioeconomic demographics, environmental and occupational influences, culture, and healthcare resource allocation (Bennett et al., 2008; Gamm et al., 2003; IOM, 2005; Utz, 2008). Regardless of how it is construed, older adult health promotion through chronic disease management is the major health issue facing nursing in rural America in the upcoming decades.

The World Health Organization (2002) defines older adult health promotion as "the process of enabling people to take control over and to improve their health" and disease prevention as "the prevention and management of conditions that are particularly common as individuals age" (p. 21). The purpose of health promotion and disease prevention strategies are to both improve health status and maximize healthcare resource utilization across the age spectrum (WHO, 2002). Routine older adult immunization is an example of the cost-saving potential of health prevention strategies. In addition to reducing morbidity and mortality, the vaccination of older adults against influenza saves 30–60 healthcare dollars for every dollar spent (WHO, 2002). Yet despite the human and fiscal benefits, less than two-thirds of rural adults receive the recommended influenza (annual) and pneumonia (single dose for individuals over 65 years) vaccines (Bennett et al., 2008; WHO, 2002).

To address the articulated national goal of improving the "health, function, and quality of life of older adults," Healthy People 2020 has outlined the following health-promotion and disease prevention objectives: (1) increase the proportion of older adults who are up-to-date on clinical preventive services and (2) increase the proportion of older adults who report confidence in managing their chronic disease (U.S. DHHS, 2011b, OA-2–3). However, meeting these goals will necessitate a reorganization of the healthcare delivery system in rural communities from an acute and episodic care model to an interdisciplinary prevention and health-promotion model addressing the spectrum of well-being, functionality, and quality of life for older adults (WHO, 2002). Effective health-promotion methods for rural older adults within a redesigned healthcare delivery system will simultaneously promote the dignity and autonomy of older citizens while strengthening the knowledge and skills necessary for older adults to make informed health choices and engage in positive health behaviors (FallCreek, 2004). The U.S. Department of Health and Human Services Administration on Aging supports Health, Prevention, and Wellness programs to improve or maintain senior health and facilitate the management of chronic disease (U.S. DHHS, 2011c). The two core programs providing discretionary grants to state governments to implement community-based interventions for seniors are the Chronic Disease Self-Management Program and the Evidenced-Based Disease and Disability Prevention Program (U.S. DHHS, 2011c). Specific examples of evidence-based health-promotion programs for older adults and program design toolkits can be found on the Administration of Aging website at http ://www.aoa.gov/AoARoot/AoA_Programs/HPW/Index.aspx

Cardiovascular disease, diabetes, and related syndromes, including obesity and hypertension, are critical chronic health problems affecting older adults in the rural community. Cardiovascular disease is the leading cause of death and the most costly healthcare condition in the United States (Fahs & Kalman, 2008). Older adults comprise 44% of all cases of heart disease and 61% of all cases of stroke in America (Lang et al., 2005). Diabetes is a common comorbidity of heart disease and the sixth leading cause of death in the United States (Utz, 2008). Diabetes is also more prevalent in older adults, afflicting 20.9% of the over-65 population (Utz, 2008). The prevalence of both cardiovascular disease and diabetes is higher among residents in rural communities, and racial disparities have been documented, including increases in morbidity and mortality among American Indians, Blacks, and Hispanic Americans (Bennett et al., 2008; Fahs & Kalman, 2008; Utz, 2008; Zuniga, Anderson, & Alexander, 2003). As Americans age, the prevalence of cardiovascular disease will continue to increase as, ironically, improvements in cardiovascular care have incited an exponential increase in the prevalence of heart failure and arrhythmia patients in the rural community (Fahs & Kalman, 2008; Valderrama, Dunbar, & Mensah, 2005).

Healthy People 2020 identified goals to improve cardiovascular health through the prevention, detection, and treatment of risk factors for heart attack and stroke; early identification and treatment of heart attacks and strokes; and the prevention of repeat cardiovascular events (U.S. DHHS, 2011a). Likewise, Healthy People 2020 identified the reduction of diabetes as a national health priority (U.S. DHHS, 2011a). Research has indicated that much of the risk and associated morbidity and mortality of these chronic diseases can be attenuated through the adoption of healthy behaviors, early identification of symptoms, and adequate management of chronic disease symptoms (Lang et al., 2005). However, barriers exist to improving the cardiovascular and diabetes management outcomes among older adults in the rural community, including a paucity of specialty cardiovascular healthcare providers and services, particularly those willing to care for low-income populations; less access to diabetic health educators; a lower quality of health care in some rural settings; suboptimal interdisciplinary collaboration resulting in ineffectual communication between providers and poorly articulated follow-up services; physical isolation and inadequate public transportation systems equipped to accommodate senior residents; limited financial resources; and cultural factors affecting lifestyle behaviors (Fahs & Kalman, 2008; Goines, 2005; Utz, 2008; Zuniga et al., 2004).

To improve the health of older adults in the rural community, nursing innovations in primary and secondary prevention that address the risks of diabetes and cardiovascular disease are imperative. At the primary level of prevention, diet, physical activity, risk behavior (particularly obesity and smoking), and disease awareness education delivered within a culturally congruent format must be accessible to older adults through multiple media in the rural community (Carter, Gaskins & Shaw, 2005; Deskins et al., 2006; Fiandt, Pullen, & Walker, 1999; Ortiz, Arizmendi, & Cornelius, 2004; Skelly et al., 2007; Tessaro, Smith, & Rye, 2005). Data indicate that public information campaigns have been successful in increasing cardiovascular risk awareness, as in the case of heart disease among women, and the researchers conclude that future initiatives in disease prevention education should specifically target high-risk populations (Fahs & Kalman, 2008). Research has also demonstrated that nurse-managed cardiovascular disease prevention programs are effective in improving the cardiovascular risk profile of patients (Bove, 2011; Wood et al., 2008). Imperative to the success of primary prevention for the reduction of chronic disease among older adults in the rural community is vigorous political advocacy to secure the resources necessary for health-promotion program development and operation in the economically disadvantaged rural community (Eyler & Vest, 2002; Sanderson, Littleton, & Pulley, 2002).

Screening rural adults for diabetes and cardiovascular disease is an integral aspect of chronic disease secondary prevention (Carter, 2005; Deskins, 2006; Fiandt, 1999; Ortiz, 2004). Essential elements of community-based diabetes and cardiovascular disease screening include an assessment of risk behaviors, body mass index calculations and waist circumference measurements, testing blood glucose and serum cholesterol, and assessing blood pressure, as well as screening for other associated symptoms of disease. In the primary-care setting, advanced practice nurses should further the assessment with a more comprehensive cardiovascular history and physical exam, including a complete serum lipid analysis, HBA1C (glucose measurement over time) as indicated for the pre-diabetic, peripheral artery disease (PAD) screening using a Doppler to obtain an ankle brachial index (ABI), and a foot exam at every visit for all diabetic and PAD patients (Pearson, 2010). Concurrently, education on the early awareness of myocardial ischemia, stroke, heart failure, or cardiac arrhythmia symptomatology is necessary to reduce morbidity and mortality from an acute cardiovascular event (Alkadry, Wilson, & Nicholson, 2005; Eaves, 2000; Fahs & Kalman, 2008).

Time to treatment is a critical factor in the successful management of acute cardiovascular disease, and in rural and remote communities with extended distances to tertiary care centers, delays in early symptom identification and inappropriate patient response can precipitate poor patient outcomes. Particularly important to cardiovascular symptom awareness is the recognition of atypical symptomatology, such as the experience of unusual fatigue and anxiety as possible warning signs of acute myocardial infarction (McSweeny & Crane, 2000; Morgan, 2005). The nurse must counsel the older adult rural resident to seek timely medical evaluation for sub-acute symptomatology, as rural residents may experience an atypically high pain tolerance, attempt to manage symptoms from home, and proceed to seek treatment only when acute symptoms begin to interfere with daily function (McSweeny & Crane, 2000; Morgan, 2005; Waginold, Rowland, Dimmler, & Peters, 2004). One nurse-run, early identification stroke intervention program, FAST (an acronym for stroke symptoms "face," "arm," "speech," and the appropriate response "time to call 911") demonstrated success in improving stroke knowledge among rural dwellers (Fahs, 2006). More evidenced-based, nurse-developed community health-promotion programs to screen for and reduce cardiovascular risks and improve acute symptom awareness for older adult rural populations are indicated to reduce the impact of chronic disease in the rural community (Fahs & Kalman, 2008).

Secondary prevention activities are also indicated for rural adult populations previously diagnosed with a chronic disease or at increased risk for chronic disease. Nurse-run chronic disease management programs have demonstrated promise for reducing the impact of diabetes and cardiovascular disease, improving the quality of life for older adults in the rural community, and optimizing the expenditure of healthcare dollars (Bray et al., 2005a; Bray, Thompson, Wynn, Cummings, & Whetstone, 2005; Meng, Wamsley, Eggert, & Van Nostrand, 2007). Reduced cardiovascular risk factors in adults after an acute cardiac event and improvement in the achievement of diabetic treatment goals are two documented successes of nurse-run secondary prevention and case management interventions (Gabbay et al., 2006; Irmak & Fesci, 2010). Remote monitoring and nurse-led self-management programs for rural cardiology patients with pacemakers and intracardiac defibrillator devices are cost-effective methods for early detection of atrial and ventricular arrhythmias to prevent stroke and sudden cardiac death (Ricci, Morichelli, & Santini, 2008). Social support and self-care education have been noted to improve chronic disease self-management and should be implemented by nurses in both face-to-face and remote formats to accommodate the needs of older adults in more isolated rural areas (Anderson-Loftin et al., 2002; Bray et al., 2005b; McSweeney & Coon, 2004, Morris, 2007; Nagelkerk, Reick, & Meengs, 2006; Utz et al., 2006). Chronic disease nurse case managers, nurse-run chronic disease self-management programs, cardiac rehabilitation services, and remote telemetry and congestive heart failure monitoring are all nursing health-promotion programs with potential to make significant impact on the well-being of older adults in the rural community and reduce the stress on the under-resourced rural healthcare workforce (Evans & Kantrowitz, 2001; Suh, 2011; Waginold, Rowland, Dimmler, & Peters, 2004).

Less is available in the literature concerning the use of nurse-managed chronic disease programs for the treatment of asthma and chronic obstructive pulmonary disease (COPD), but the same principles and therapeutic potential apply (Jónsdóttir, 2008). The prevalence of asthma has been on the rise in the United States since 1980, currently affecting more than 23 million citizens and costing society approximately $20 billion a year in healthcare expenditures and loss of productivity (American Academy of Allergy, Asthma & Immunology [AAAI], 2011). Rural adults report higher rates of asthma than urban populations, with the highest rates documented among rural American Indians (Bennett et al., 2008). Asthma prevalence has also been noted to be 20.1% higher among Black Americans when compared to White populations, regardless of region of residence (AAAI, 2011).

COPD is the fourth-leading cause of death in the United States caused primarily by smoking, but it is also related to other environmental exposures such as occupational dust and chemicals (U.S. DHHS, 2011d). Rural older adults are more at-risk for

COPD and poor respiratory health outcomes as a result of higher rates of smoking, the increased prevalence of asthma in the rural community, increased exposure to occupational triggers through agricultural and extraction industries, and increased barriers to healthcare services (Bennett et al., 2008; Schulman & Slesinger, 2004; Stevens, Colwell & Hutchison, 2003).

The Healthy People goal of promoting respiratory health through "better prevention, detection, treatment, and education efforts" must be addressed through rural nursing health-promotion interventions specifically targeting these two chronic respiratory conditions, particularly among high-risk populations (U.S. DHHS, 2011d, para. 1). Primary prevention for respiratory diseases involves smoking cessation interventions and advocacy for safe occupational environments. Secondary prevention includes screening at-risk residents and early self-care chronic disease management to prevent disease exacerbations and improve quality of life, preserve lung function, and reduce hospitalizations (Jónsdóttir, 2008). Further consideration needs to be given to the use of nurse-managed chronic respiratory disease clinics in the underserved and aging rural populations to promote respiratory health and maximize healthcare resource utilization (Jónsdóttir, 2008).

Nurse-managed health centers are a promising mechanism for providing health-promotion, disease prevention, and chronic disease management in the rural community in order to meet the Healthy People 2020 objectives. These nurse-run delivery systems have been demonstrated to be effective in managing a broad range of health issues, are well received by local communities, and are a cost-effective method of addressing health disparities for underserved populations (Hansen-Turton, 2005; Ramsey, Edwards, Lenz, Odom, & Brown, 1993). Nurse-managed health centers are eligible for Federal Qualified Health Center funding and supported by the 2010 Patient Protection and Affordable Care Act, making them a fiscally viable option for the provision of collaborative, interdisciplinary disease prevention and health-promotion services in rural communities across the United States (English, 2010; Hansen-Turton, 2005). More nursing research is indicated on the disease management outcomes, patient satisfaction and cost-effectiveness of nurse-managed health centers in the delivery of health-promotion services in the rural community.

CONCLUSION

In 2005, the Institute of Medicine charged the United States healthcare system with the task of eliminating rural health disparities by curbing the increasing burden of chronic disease in rural communities. In 2010, the IOM challenged the nursing profession to optimize professional nursing practice and become leaders in healthcare redesign in order to meet the healthcare needs of America. An essential component of this healthcare redesign must involve utilizing the nursing workforce to transition the United States healthcare system to a health-promotion and disease-prevention service model. Arguably, there is no place more critically in need of the contributions of nursing health-promotion and disease-prevention services than in the underserved and often disadvantaged rural communities. The Patient Protection and Affordable Care Act of 2010 specifically recognized the importance of nursing services and community-based health centers in addressing the urgent health care needs of the American public (English, 2010). It is now up to the nursing profession to respond to the critical healthcare needs of rural America through nursing health-promotion practice, program development, nursing research and policy advocacy.

DISCUSSION QUESTIONS

1. How does the cultural climate and socioeconomic status of the rural community affect the provision of nursing health-promotion services?
2. Identify three theoretical frameworks, either from this chapter or another resource, that could be used in the development of rural nursing health-promotion services or a rural health research proposal. Explain how the theoretical frameworks might apply to a specific rural health issue and nursing health-promotion service or research problem.
3. Identify three Healthy People 2020 objectives that are particularly relevant to rural communities in America.
4. Identify three potential resources for improving the provision of nursing health-promotion services in relation to a specific rural health issue.

CHECK YOUR UNDERSTANDING

1. In general, how do the current and projected future demographics of the rural community differ from suburban and urban populations?
2. Identify five major health issues affecting rural populations.
3. Identify three potential influences that may increase health disparities among rural populations.
4. Identify three factors that may contribute to birth disparities among rural residents.
5. Identify three potential barriers to timely immunization in the rural community.
6. Explain why the significant disparities in rural dental health affect the overall health of the rural resident.

7. Identify three factors that may influence the obesity health disparity in the rural community.
8. Identify three adolescent health issues of particular concern to rural residents. What are some potential barriers to care experienced by rural adolescents?
9. Identify three social determinants of mental health pertinent to the rural community.
10. Identify three occupational health issues particularly pertinent to rural residents in America.
11. Identify three health issues particularly relevant to the migrant worker population and discuss potential barriers to care for these health concerns.
12. Describe primary, secondary, and tertiary nursing services to improve outcomes in the management of cardiovascular and respiratory chronic disease among older rural residents.
13. Design a nursing health-promotion proposal for a rural health issue within a specific population and an identified rural region. The proposal should include:

    A. a discussion of the health issue as it relates to the rural community and the Healthy People 2020 objectives,
    B. an ecological community assessment,
    C. a nursing health-promotion intervention plan based in an appropriate theoretical framework and reflective of applicable cultural concerns,
    D. a consideration of available resources and interdisciplinary collaboration opportunities to support the health-promotion interventions, and
    E. an outline of the desired outcomes of the health-promotion intervention and an outcomes evaluation plan.

WHAT DO YOU THINK?

1. How would you apply the principles of patient-centered care to the provision of nursing health-promotion services in the rural community? Describe a patient-centered care approach to the provision of nursing health-promotion services in relation to a particular rural health issue.
2. Consider current health policy trends in America in relation to the provision of nursing health-promotion services for a specific rural health issue. How would you pursue systems change in the delivery of healthcare services to reduce rural health disparities?
3. Identify a research problem or research question that could potentially add to the available literature to improve the provision of evidence-based nursing health-promotion services in the rural community. How might you design a research project to investigate the research problem?

REFERENCES

Abortion Access Project (2009). *Abortion Access and Opportunity in Rural Communities: A Survey of Clinicians.* Cambridge, MA: Abortion Access Project, Inc.

Adler, C. (1996). Unheard and unseen: Rural women and domestic violence. *Journal of Nurse Midwifery, 41*(6), 463–466.

Ajzen, I. (1985). From intention to actions: A theory of planned behavior. In J. Kuhl and J. Beckman (Eds.). *Action-control: From cognition to behavior* (pp. 11–39). Heidelberg, Germany: Springer.

Akinbami, L. J. (2006). The state of childhood asthma, United States, 1980–2005. *Vital Health Statistics, 381,* 1–24.

Alexander, J., Beagle, C. J., Butler, P., Dougherty, D. A., & Andrews-Robards, K. D. (1986). Madeleine Leninger: Transcultural Care Theory. In A. Marriner (Ed.). *Nursing theorists and their work* (pp. 144–160). St Louis, MO: The C.V. Mosby Company.

Alkadry, M. G., Wilson, C., & Nicholson, D. (2005). Stroke awareness among rural residents: The case of West Virginia. *Social Work in Health Care, 42*(2), 73–92.

American Academy of Allergy, Asthma & Immunology [AAAAI] (2011). *Asthma Statistics.* Retrieved from http://www.aaaai.org/media/statistics/asthma-statistics.asp

American Academy of Pediatric Dentistry [AAPD] (2011). *Regular Dental Visits.* Retrieved from http://www.aapd.org/publications/brochures/regdent.asp

American Academy of Pediatrics [AAP]. (2008). Achieving quality health services for adolescents. *Pediatrics, 121*(6), 1263–1270.

American Academy of Pediatrics [AAP]. (2011). *Oral Health Initiative.* Retrieved from http://www.aap.org/oralhealth/links-training.cfm

American Academy of Pediatrics [AAP]. (2011). *Promoting Physical Activity.* Retrieved from http://www.aap.org/family/physicalactivity/physicalactivity.htm

American Academy of Pediatrics [AAP], Committee on Community Health Services and Committee on Practice and Ambulatory Medicine. (2003). Increasing immunization coverage. *Pediatrics, 112,* 993–996. DOI: 10.1542/peds.112.4.993

American Academy of Pediatrics [AAP]. Committee on Injury and Poison Prevention. (2000). All-terrain vehicle injury prevention: Two-, three-, and four-,wheeled unlicensed motor vehicles. *Pediatrics, 105*(6), 1352–1354.

American Academy of Pediatrics [AAP]. Committee on Injury and Poison Prevention. (2000a). Firearm-related injuries affecting the pediatric population. *Pediatrics, 105*(4), 888–895.

American Academy of Pediatrics [AAP], Committee on Standards of Child Health Care. (1977). AAP National Immunization Policy. *AAP News and Comment, 28,* 7–8.

American Nurses Association [ANA]. (1980). *Nursing: A social policy statement.* Kansas City, MO: Author.

American Nurses Association [ANA]. (2011). *Definition of Nursing.* Retrieved from http://nursingworld.org/MainMenuCategories/ThePracticeofProfessionalNursing.aspx

Anderson-Loftin, W., Barnett, S., Sullivan, P., Bunn, P., & Tavakoli, A. (2002). Culturally competent dietary education for southern rural African Americans with diabetes. *The Diabetes Educator, 28*(2), 245–257.

Bailey, J. M. (2009). *The top 10 rural issues for health care reform: A series examining health care issues in rural America (No. 2).* Lyons, NE: Center for Rural Affairs.

Baldwin, L., Grossman, D. C., Casey, S., Hollow, W., Sugarman, J. R., Freeman, W. L., & Hart, L. G. (2002). Perinatal and infant health among rural and urban American Indians/Alaska Natives. *American Journal of Public Health, 92*(9), 1491–1497.

Bales, R. L. (2010). *Health perceptions, needs, and behaviors of remote rural women of childbearing and child-rearing age.* In C. A. Winters & H. J. Lee (Eds.), *Rural nursing: Concepts, theory and practice* (pp. 91–104). New York, NY: Springer.

Bales, R .L., Winters, C. A. & Lee, H. J. (2010). *Health needs and perceptions of rural persons.* In C. A. Winters & H. J. Lee (Eds.), *Rural nursing: Concepts, theory and practice* (pp. 57–71). New York, NY: Springer.

Bandura, A. (1989). Social cognitive theory. In R. Vasta (Ed.). *Annals of child development.* (Vol 6. Six theories of child development) (pp. 1–60). Greenwich, CT: JAI Press.

Bandura, A. (1986). *Social foundations of thought and action.* Englewood Cliffs, NJ: Prentice-Hall.

Basset, D. R. (2008). Physical activity of Canadian and American children: A focus on youth in Amish, Mennonite, and modern cultures. *Applied Physiology, Nutrition, and Metabolism, 33,* 831–835.

Bennett, K. J., Olatosi, B., & Probst, J. C. (2008). *Health Disparities: A Rural-Urban Chartbook.* Columbia, SC: Rural Health Research and Policy Centers.

Berkman, L .F. & Glass, T. (2000). Social integration, social networks, social support, and health. In L. F. Berkman & I. Kawachi (Eds.), *Social Epidemiology* (pp. 137–173). New York, NY: Oxford Press.

Biddle, V. S., Sekula, L. K. & Puskar, K. R. (2010). Identification of suicide risk among rural youth: Implications for the use of HEADSS. *Journal of Pediatric Health Care, 24*(3), 152– 167. doi:10.1016/j.pedhc.2009.03.003

Bigbee, J. L. (1991). The concept of hardiness as applied to rural nursing. *Rural Nursing, 1,* 39– 58.

Biro, F. M. & Wen, M. (2010). Childhood obesity and adult morbidities. *The American Journal of Clinical Nutrition, 91*(5), 1499S–1505S. Doi:10.3945/_ajcn.2010.28701B

Blanco, C., Alderson, D., Ogburn, E., Grant, B. F., Nunes, E. V., Hatzenbuehler, M. L., & Hasin, D. S. (2007). Changes in the prevalence of non-medical prescription drug use and drug use disorders in the United States: 1991–1992 and 2001–2002. *Drug and Alcohol Dependence, 90,* 252–260.

Borders, T. F. & Booth, B. M. (2007). Rural, suburban, and urban variations in alcohol consumption in the United States: Findings from the National Epidemiologic Survey on alcohol and related conditions. *The Journal of Rural Health, 23*(4), 314–321.

Bove, A., Santamore, W., Homko, C., Kashem, A., Cross, R., McConnell, T. R.,..Menapace, F. (2011). Reducing cardiovascular disease risk in medically underserved urban and rural communities. *American Heart Journal, 161*(2), 351.

Bray, P., Roupe, M., Young, S., Harrell, J., Cummings, D., & Whetstone, L. (2005a). Feasibility and effectiveness of system redesign for diabetes care management in rural areas: The Eastern North Carolina experience. *The Diabetes Educator, 31*(5), 712–718.

Bray, P., Roupe, M., Young, S., Harrell, J., Cummings, D., & Whetstone, L. (2005b). Self- monitoring of blood glucose in a multiethnic population or rural older adults with diabetes. *The Diabetes Educator, 31*(1), 84–90.

Bray, P., Thompson, D., Wynn, J., Cummings, D., & Whetstone, L. (2005). Confronting disparities in diabetes care: The clinical effectiveness of redesigning care management for minority patients in rural primary care practice. *The Journal of Rural Health, 21*(4), 317–321.

Brelding, M. J., Ziembroski, J. S., & Black, M. C. (2009). Prevalence of rural intimate partner violence in 16 US states, 2005. *The Journal of Rural Health, 25*(3), 240–246.

Brown, S. S., & Eisenberg, L. E. (1995). *The best intentions: unintended pregnancy and the well- being of children and families.* Washington, DC: National Academy Press.

Burke, B., Bynum, A, Hall-Barrow, J. Ott, R. & Albright, M. (2008). Rural school-based telehealth: How to make it happen. *Clinical Pediatrics, 47*(9), 926–929.

Bushy, A. (2009). A landscape view of life and health care in rural settings. In W. A. Nelson (Ed.), *Handbook for rural health care ethics* (pp. 17–40). Hanover, NH: Dartmouth College Press.

Bushy, A. (2011). *Rural nursing: Practices and issues.* Retrieved from http://www.nursingworld.org/mods /mod700/rural.pdf

California Dental Association [CDA]. (2010). *Oral health during pregnancy and early childhood: Evidenced- based guidelines for health professionals.* Retrieved from http://www.cdafoundation.org/library/docs /poh_guidelines.pdf

California School Nurse Organization [CSNO]. (2011). *Vaccinate before you graduate.* Retrieved from http://www.cdph.ca.gov/programs/immunize/Documents/IMM765(2-07).pdf

Carter, M., Gaskins, S., & Shaw, L. (2005). Employee Wellness Program in a small rural industry. Employee evaluation. *AAOHN Journal, 53*(6), 244–248.

Casey, A. A., Elliott, M., Glanz, K., Haire-Joshu, D., Lovegreen, S. L. & Sailens, B.E., . . . Brownson, R. C. (2008). Impact of the food environment and physical activity environment on behaviors and weight status in rural U.S. communities. *Preventive Medicine, 47,* 600–604.

Catania, J. A., Coates, T. J., & Kegles, S. (1994). A test of the AIDS Risk Reduction mode: Psychosocial correlates of condom use in the AMEN cohort survey. *Health Psychology, 13*(6), 548–555.

Center on Addiction and Substance Abuse [CASA]. (2000). *No place to hide: Substance abuse in mid-size cities and rural America.* Retrieved from http://www.casacolumbia.org/templates/publications_reports.aspx

Centers for Disease Control and Prevention [CDC]. (1993). Standards for pediatric immunization Practices. *Morbidity and Mortality Weekly Report, 42*(No. RR-5). Retrieved from http://www.cdc.gov/mmwr/preview/mmwrhtml/00020935.htm

Centers for Disease Control and Prevention [CDC]. (2000). Use of standing orders programs to increase adult vaccination rates. *Morbidity and Mortality Weekly Report, 49*(RR01), 15–26. Retrieved from http://www.cdc.gov/mmwr/preview/mmwrhtml/rr4901a2.htm

Centers for Disease Control and Prevention [CDC]. (2004). *Addressing violence against women: Results from a national survey of Title X family planning providers.* Atlanta, GA: Division of Reproductive Health.

Centers for Disease Control and Prevention [CDC] (2010). *CDC Grand Rounds: Additional Opportunities to Prevent Neural Tube Deficits with Folic Acid Fortification.* Retrieved from http://www.cdc.gov/mmwr/preview/mmwrhtml/mm5931a2.htm

Centers for Disease Control and Prevention [CDC]. (2010b). Youth Risk Behavior Surveillance United States, 2009. Surveillance Summaries, June 4, 2010. *Morbidity and Mortality Weekly Report, 59*(No. SS-5).

Centers for Disease Control and Prevention [CDC]. (2011a). *How much physical activity do children need?* Retrieved from http://www.cdc.gov/physicalactivity/everyone/guidelines/children.html

Centers for Disease Control and Prevention [CDC]. (2011b). *Vaccines for Children Program.* Retrieved from http://www.cdc.gov/vaccines/programs/vfc/default.htm

Champion, J. D., Kelly, P., Shain. N., R & Piper, J. M. (2004). Rural Mexican American adolescent sexual behavior. *The Journal of Rural Health, 20*(3), 279–285.

Chowdhury, P., Balluz, L., Town, M., Chowdhury, F. M., Bartoli, W., Garvin, W., . . . Giles, W. (2010). Surveillance of Certain Health Behaviors and Conditions Among States and Selected Local Areas—Behavioral Risk Factor Surveillance System, United States, 2007. *Morbidity and Mortality Weekly Report Surveillance Summaries,* 59(SS-1), 1–220.

Clayton, S., Chin, T., Blackburn, S. & Echevarria, C. (2010). Different setting, different care: Integrating prevention and clinical care in school-based health centers. *American Journal of Public Health, 100*(9), 1592–1596.

Cohen, J. H., Tiesman, H. M., Bossarte, R. M., & Furbee, P. M. (2009). Rural urban differences in injury hospitalizations in the U.S., 2004. *American Journal of Preventive Medicine, 36*(1), 49–55.

Connor, A., Layne, L. & Thomisee, K. (2010). Providing care for migrant farmworker families in their unique sociocultural context and environment. *Journal of Transcultural Nursing, 21*(2), 159–166, DOI: 10.1177/1043659609357631

Costello, E. J., Mustillo, S., Erkanli, A., Keeler, G., and Angold, A. (2003). Prevalence and development of psychiatric disorders in childhood and adolescence. *Archives of General Psychiatry, 60,* 837–844.

Curtis, A. C. (2008). Health and its Contextual Determinants in Rural California Adolescents (Doctoral Dissertation, University of California, San Francisco, 2008). *Dissertation Abstracts International, 68-11,* 7244.

Curtis, A. C., Waters, C. M., & Brindis, C. D. (2011). Rural adolescent health: The importance of prevention services in the rural community. *Journal of Rural Health, 27,* 60–71. doi:10.111/j.1748-0361.2010.00319.x

Dahl, R. E. (2008). Biological, developmental, and neurobehavioral factors relevant to adolescent driving risks. *American Journal of Preventive Medicine, 35*(3S), S278–S284.

D'Angelo, D., Williams, L., Morrow, B., Cox, S., Harris, N., & Harrison, L. (2007). *Preconception and Interconception Risk of Women Who Recently Gave Birth to a Live Born Infant: Pregnancy Risk Assessment Monitoring System (PRAMS), United States, 26 Reporting Areas, 2004.* Retrieved from http://www.cdc.gov /mmwR/preview/mmwrhtml/ss5610a1.htm

Deskins, S., Harris, C. V., Bradlyn, A. S., Cottrell, L., Coffman, J. W., Olexa, J., & Neal, W. (2006). Preventive care in Appalachia: Use of the theory of planned behavior to identify barriers to participation in cholesterol screenings among West Virginians. *Journal of Rural Health, 22*(4), 367–374.

Deutchman, M., Brayden, R., Siegel, C. D., Beaty, B. & Crane, L. (2000). Childhood immunization in rural family and general practices: current practices, perceived barriers, and strategies for improvement. *Ambulatory Child Health, 6*(3), 181–189.

Dhingra, S., Strine, T., Holt, J., Berry, J., & Mokdad, A. (2009). Rural-urban variations in psychological distress: Findings from the behavioral risk factor surveillance system, 2007. *International Journal of Public Health, 54*(Suppl 1), 16–22.

Duncan, G. E. (2006). Prevalence of diabetes and impaired fasting glucose levels among U.S. adolescents. National Health and Nutrition Examination Survey, 1999–2002. *Archives of Pediatric and Adolescent Medicine, 16,* 523–528.

Dunkin, J. W. (2000). Exemplar: A framework for rural nursing interventions. In A. Bushy (Ed.), *Orientation to nursing in the rural community* (pp. 61–70). Thousand Oaks, CA: Sage.

Dunton, G. F., Kaplan, J., Wolch J., Jerret, M., & Reynolds K. D. (2009). Physical environmental correlates of childhood obesity. *Obesity Reviews, 10,* 393–402. doi: 10.1111/j.1467-789X.2009.00572.x

Dye, B. A., Tan, S., Smith, V., Lewis, B. G., Barker, L. K., Thorton-Evan, G., . . . Li, C. H. (2007). Trends in oral health status: United States, 1988–1994 and 1994–2004. *Vital Health Statistics, 11*(248), 1–92.

Eaves, Y. D. (2000). "What happened to me": Rural African American elders' experiences of stroke. *Journal of Neuroscience Nursing, 32*(1), 37–48.

Elgar, F. J., Arlett, C. A. & Groves, R. (2003). Stress, coping, and behavioral problems among rural and urban adolescents. *Journal of Adolescence, 26,* 574–585.

Elliott, B. A., & Larson, J. T. (2004). Adolescents in mid-sized and rural communities: Foregone care, perceived barriers, and risk factors. *Journal of Adolescent Health, 35,* 303–309.

English, A. (2010). *The Patient Protection and Affordable Care Act of 2010: How Does it Help Adolescents and Young Adults.* Chapel Hill, NC: Center for Adolescent Health & the Law; and San Francisco, CA: National Adolescent Health Information and Innovation Center.

Evans, G. W., & Kantrowitz, E. (2001). Strategies for reducing morbidity and mortality from diabetes through health-care system interventions and diabetes self-management education in community settings. A report on the recommendations of the Task Force on Community Preventive Services. *Morbidity and Mortality Weekly Report Recommendations and Reports, 50,* 1–15.

Everett, K .D., Bullock, L., Gage, J. D., Longo, D. R., Geden, E. & Madsen, R. (2006). Health risk behavior of rural low-income fathers. *Public Health Nursing, 23*(4), 297–306.

Eyler, A. A. & Vest, J. R. (2002). Environmental and policy factors related to physical activity in rural White women. *Women & Health, 36*(2), 111–121.

Fahs, P. S. (2006). Raising stroke awareness in rural communities. *American Journal of Nursing, 106*(11), 42.

Fahs, P. S. & Kalman, M. (2008). Matters of the heart: Cardiovascular disease and rural nursing. In J. Fitzpatrick & E. Merwin (Eds.). *Annual review of nursing research (Vol. 26): Focus on rural health* (pp. 143–173). New York, NY: Springer.

Fahs, P. S., Smith, B., Atav, A. S., Britteen, M. X., Collins, M. S., Morgan, L. C., & Spencer, G. A. (1999). Integrative research review of risk behaviors among adolescents in rural, suburban, and urban areas. *Journal of Adolescent Health, 24,* 230–243.

FallCreek, S. J. (2004). Older adult health promotion in rural setting. *The Journal of Gerontological Social Work, 41*(3), 193–211, DOI: 10.1300/J083v41n03_01

Family Health International (2004). Behavior change: A summary of four major theories. Retrieved from http://www.fhi.org/nr/rdonlyres/ei26vbslpsidmahhxc332vwo3g233xsqw22er3vofqvrfjvubwyz clvqjcbdgexyzl3msu4mn6xv5j/bccsummaryfourmajortheories.pdf

Featherstone, J. D., Domejean-Orliaguet, S., Jensen, L., Wolff, M., & Young, D. A. (2007). Caries risk assessment in practice for age 6 through adult. *California Dental Association Journal, 35*(10), 703–713.

Federal Interagency Forum on Child and Family Statistics. (2007). *America's Children: Key National Indicators of Well-Being, 2007.* Washington, DC: U.S. Government Printing Office.

Fiandt, K., Pullen, C. H., & Walker, S. N. (1999). Actual and perceived risk for chronic illness in rural older women. *Clinical Excellence for Nurse Practitioners, 3*(2), 105–115.

Findholt, N. (2010). The culture of rural communities: An examination of rural nursing Concepts at the community level. In C. A. Winters & H. J. Lee (Eds.), *Rural nursing: Concepts, theory and practice* (pp. 373–383). New York, NY: Springer.

Findley, S. E., Irigoyen, M., Sanchez, M., Guzman, L., Mejia, M., Sajous, M., . . . Chimkin, F. (2006). Community-based strategies to reduce childhood immunization disparities. *Health Promotion Practice, 7,* 191S. DOI: 10.1177/1524839906288692

Finer, L. B. & Henshaw, S. K. (2006). Disparities in rates of unintended pregnancy in the United States, 1994 and 2001. *Perspectives on Sexual and Reproductive Health, 38,* 90–96.

Fos, P. & Hutchison, L. (2004). The state of rural oral health. In L. D. Gamm, L. L Hutchinson, B. J. Dabney & A. M. Dorsey (Eds.), *Rural Health People 2010: A Companion Document to Health People 2010. Volume 1* (pp: 199–203). College Station: The Texas A&M University System Health Science Center, School of Rural Public Health, Southwest Rural Research Center.

Gabbay, R., Lendel, I., Saleem, T., Shaeffer, G., Adelman, A. M., Mauger, D. T., . . . Polomano, R. C. (2006). Nurse case management improves blood pressure, emotional distress and diabetes complication screening. *Diabetes Research and Clinical Practice, 71*(1), 28.

Gamm, L. D., Hutchison, L. L., Dabney, B. J., & Dorsey, A. M. (Eds) (2003). *Rural Health People 2010: A Companion Document to Health People 2010. Volume 1.* College Station: The Texas A&M University System Health Science Center, School of Rural Public Health, Southwest Rural Research Center.

Gamm, L. D., & Hutchison, L. L. (Eds) (2004). *Rural Health People 2010: A Companion Document to Health People 2010. Volume 3.* College Station: The Texas A&M University System Health Science Center, School of Rural Public Health, Southwest Rural Research Center.

Gatz, J. L., Rowles, G. D. & Tyas, S. L. (2004). Health disparities in rural Appalachia. In N. Glasgow, L. W. Morton & N. E. Johnson (Eds.), *Critical Issues in Rural Health* (pp: 183–194). Ames, IA: Blackwell.

Gfroerer, J. C., Larson, S. L. & Colliver, J. D. (2007). Drug use patterns and trends in rural communities. *The Journal of Rural Health, 23*(Supp.), 10–15.

Glanz, K. & Bishop, D. B. (2010). The role of behavioral theory in development in implementation of public health interventions. *Annual Review of Public Health, 31,* 399–418. DOI:v10.1146/annurev.publhealth .012809.103604

Goines, R. T., Williams, K. A., Carter, M. W., Spencer, S. M., & Soloveiva, T. (2005). Perceived barriers to health care access among rural older adults: A qualitative study. *The Journal of Rural Health, 21*(3), 206–213.

Graber, J. A., & Brooks-Gunn, J. (1996). Transitions and turning points: Navigating the passage from childhood through adolescence. *Developmental Psychology, 32*(4), 768–776.

Grumbach, K., Hart, G., Mertz, E., Coffman, J,, & Palazzo (2003). Who is caring for the Underserved? A comparison of primary care physicians and nonphysician clinicians in California and Washington. *Annals of Family Medicine, 1*(2), 97–104.

Gustafson, D. T., Preston, K. & Hudson, J. (2009). *Mental health: Overlooked and disregarded in rural America.* Lyons, NE: Center for Rural Affairs.

Halfon, N. & Hochstein, M. (2002). Life course health development: An integrated framework for developing health, policy and research. *Milbank Quarterly: A Journal of Public Health and Health Care Policy, 80*(3), 433–79.

Hallas, D. & Shelley, D. (2009). Role of pediatric nurse practitioner in oral health care. *Academic Pediatrics, 9,* 462–466.

Han, J. C., Lawlor, D. A., & Kim, S. Y. (2010). Childhood obesity. *Lancet, 375*(9727), 1737– 1748.

Hansen-Turton, T. (2005). The nurse-managed health center safety net: A policy solution to reducing health disparities. *Nursing Clinics of North America, 40*(4), 729.

Hanson, C., Novilla, M., Barnes, M., Eggett, D., McKell, C., Reichman, P., & Havens, M. (2009). Using the rural-urban continuum to explore adolescent alcohol, tobacco, and other drug use in Montana. *Journal of Child & Adolescent Substance Abuse, 18*(1), 93–105.

Harris, K. M., Gordon-Larson, P., Chantala, K., & Udry, J. R. (2006). Longitudinal trends in race/ethnicity disparities in leading health indicators from adolescents to young adulthood. *Archives of Pediatrics & Adolescent Medicine, 160*(1), 74–81.

Hart, G. L., Larson, E. H., & Lishner, D. M. (2005). Rural definitions for health policy research *American Journal of Public Health, 95*(7), 1149–1155.

Hart, J, Silva, S., Tein, N., Brown, A., & Stevens, K. (2009). *Assessment of Strategies for Providing Culturally Competent Care in Title X Family Planning Clinics: Final Report.* Retrieved from http://www.hhs.gov/opa /pdf/304b-assessment-of-strategies.pdf

Hauenstein, E. J. (2008). Building the rural mental health system: From de facto system to quality care. In J. Fitzpatrick & E. Merwin (Eds.). *Annual review of nursing research (Vol. 26): Focus on rural health* (pp. 143–173). New York, NY: Springer.

Hauenstein, E. J. & Peddada, S. D. (2007). Prevalence of major depressive episodes in rural women using primary care. *Journal of Health Care for the Poor and Under-served, 18,* 185–202.

Havens, J. R., Young, A. M. & Havens, C. E. (2011). Nonmedical prescription drug use in a nationally representative sample of adolescents: Evidence of greater use among rural adolescents. *Archives of Pediatric and Adolescent Medicine, 165*(3), 250–255, DOI:10.1001/archpediatrics.2010.217

Helmcamp, J. C., Aitken, M. E. & Lawrence, B. A. (2009). ATV and bicycle deaths and And associated costs in the United States, 200–2005. *Public Health Reports, 124,* 409– 418.

Heck, K. E., Borba, J. A., Carlos, R., Churches, K., Donohue, S., & Fuller, A. H. (2004). *California's rural youth: A report for the 4H center for youth development.* Davis, CA: 4H Center for Youth Development.

Hennessy, E. Kraak, V. I., Hyatt, R. R., Bloom, J., Fenton, M., Wagoner, C., . . . Economos, C. D. (2010). Active living for rural children: Community perspectives using Photovoice. *American Journal of Preventive Medicine, 39*(6), 537–545.

Heuer, L., & Lausch, C. (2006). Living with diabetes: Perceptions of Hispanic migrant farmworkers. *Journal of Community Health Nursing, 23*(1), 49–64. doi:10.1207/s15327655jchn2301_5

Hillemeier, M. M., Downs, D. S., Feinberg, M. E., Weisman, C. S., Chuang, C. H., Parrott, R., . . . Chinchilli, V. M. (2008). Improving women's preconceptual health: Findings of a randomized Trial of the Strong Healthy Women intervention in the Central Pennsylvania Women's Health Study. *Women's Health Issues, 18*(6) Supplement 1, S87–S96.

Hingson, R. W., & Kenkel, D. (2004). Social health and economic consequences of underage drinking. In National Research Council, *Reducing Underage Drinking: A Collective Responsibility* (pp. 351–382). Washington, DC: The National Academies Press.

Hiott, A. E., Grzywacz, J. G., Davis, S. W., Quandt, S .A., & Arcury, T. A. (2008). Migrant farmworker stress: Mental health implications. *The Journal of Rural Health, 24*(1), 32– 39.

Hirsch, J. K. (2006). A review of the literature on rural suicide: Risk and protective factors, incidence, and prevention. *Crisis, 27*(4), 189–199. DOI 10.1027/0227-5910.27.4.189

Hodne, C. J. (2004). Rural environmental health and industrial agriculture: A case example of concentrated animal feeding operations. In N. Glasgow, L. W. Morton & N. E. Johnson (Eds.), *Critical Issues in Rural Health* (pp. 61–73). Ames, IA: Blackwell.

Hoerster, K. D., Mayer, J. A., Gabbard, S., Kronick, R. G, Roesch, S. C., Malcarne, V. L., & Zuniga, M. L. (2011). Impact of individual-, environmental-, and policy-level factors on health care utilization among US farmworkers. *American Journal of Public Health, 101,* 685–692. doi:10.2105/AJPH.2009.190892

Holden, C. (2001). Housing. In National Center for Farmworker Health, Inc., *Migrant Health Issues: Monograph Series (Monograph no. 8).* Bethesada, MD: Bureau of Primary Health Care: Migrant Health Branch.

Hovey, J. D. (2001). Mental health and substance abuse. In National Center for Farmworker Health, Inc., *Migrant Health Issues: Monograph Series (Monograph no. 4).* Bethesada, MD: Bureau of Primary Health Care: Migrant Health Branch.

Hutchinson, L & Peck, J. (2004). Immunizations and infectious diseases in rural areas: A literature review. In L. D. Gamm & L. L Hutchinson (Eds.), *Rural Health People 2010: A Companion Document to Health People 2010. Volume 3* (pp. 61–68). College Station: The Texas A&M University System Health Science Center, School of Rural Public Health, Southwest Rural Research Center.

Hutchinson, L & Blakely, C. (2003). Substance abuse: Trends in rural areas. In L. D. Gamm, L. L. Hutchinson, B. J. Dabney & A. M. Dorsey (Eds.), *Rural Health People 2010: A Companion Document to Health People 2010. Volume 1* (pp. 223–236). College Station: The Texas A&M University System Health Science Center, School of Rural Public Health, Southwest Rural Research Center.

Institute of Medicine [IOM] (2005). *Quality through collaboration: The future of rural health care.* Washington, DC: National Academies Press.

Institute of Medicine [IOM] (2010). *The future of nursing: Leading change, advancing health.* Washington, DC: National Academies Press.

Institute of Medicine [IOM] (2011). *Leading health indicators for Healthy People 2020: Letter report.* Washington, DC: National Academies Press.

International Parish Nurse Resource Center (2011). *Fundamentals of Parish Nursing.* Retrieved from http://parishnurses.org/Fundamentalsofpn.aspx

Irby, M., Kaplan, S., Garner-Edwards, D., Kolbash, S., & Skelton, J. A. (2010). Motivational interviewing in a family-based pediatric obesity program: A case study. *Families, Systems, and Health, 28*(3), 236–246.

Irmak, Z., & Fesci, H. (2010). Effects of nurse-managed secondary prevention program on lifestyle and risk factors of patients who had experienced myocardial infarction. *Applied Nursing Research, 23*(3), 147–152.

Jones, C. S. & Bleeker, J. (2005). A comparison of ATV related behaviors, exposures, and injuries between farm youth and non-farm youth. *The Journal of Rural Health, 21*(1), 70– 73.

Jónsdóttir, H. (2008). Nursing care in the chronic phase of COPD: A call for innovative disciplinary research. *Journal of Clinical Nursing, 17*(7B), 272–290.

Kessler, R. C., Berglund, P., Demler, O., Jin, R., Merikangas, K., and Walters, E. (2005). Lifetime prevalence and age-of-onset distributions of DSM-IV disorders in the National Comorbidity Survey Replication. *Archives of General Psychiatry, 62,* 593–602.

Klugman, C. M. & Dalinis, P. M. (2008). *Ethical issues in rural health care.* Baltimore, MD: Johns Hopkins University Press.

Kmet, L. & Macarthur, C. (2006). Urban-rural differences in motor vehicle crash fatality and Hospitalization rates among children and youth. *Accident Analysis and Prevention, 38,* 122–127.

Kost, K., Henshaw, S., & Carlin, L. (2010). *U.S. Teenage Pregnancies, Births and Abortions: National and State Trends and Trends by Race and Ethnicity.* Retrieved from: http://www.guttmacher.org/pubs/USTPtrends.pdf

Lambert, D., Gale, J .A., & Hartley, D. (2008). Substance abuse by youth and young adults in rural America. *The Journal of Rural Health, 24*(3), 221–228.

Lang, J. E., Benson, W. F. & Anderson, L. A. (2005). Aging and public health: Partnerships that can affect cardiovascular health programs. *American Journal of Preventive Medicine, 29*(5S1), 158–163.

Lantz, P., House, J., Lepkowski, J., Williams, D., Mero, R., & Chen, J. (1998). Socioeconomic factors, health behaviors, and mortality. *JAMA: Journal of the American Medical Association, 279*(21), 1703–1708.

Larson, A. (2001). Environmental/Occupational safety and health. In National Center for Farmworker Health, Inc., *Migrant Health Issues: Monograph Series (Monograph no. 2).* Bethesada, MD: Bureau of Primary Health Care: Migrant Health Branch.

Lee, H. L. & McDonagh, M. K. (2010). Updating the rural nursing theory base. In C. A. Winters & H. J. Lee (Eds.), *Rural nursing: Concepts, theory and practice* (pp. 19–39). New York, NY: Springer.

Leipert, B. (2010). Rural and remote women and resilience: Grounded theory and photovoice variations on a theme. In C. A. Winters & H. J. Lee (Eds.), *Rural nursing: Concepts, theory and practice* (pp. 105–129). New York, NY: Springer.

Levine, S. B., & Coupey, S.M. (2003). Adolescent substance use, sexual behavior, and metropolitan status: Is "urban" a risk factor? *Journal of Adolescent Health, 32,* 350–355.

Liao, Y., Bang, D., Cosgrove, S., Dulin, R., Harris, Z., Taylor, A., . . . Centers for Disease Control and Prevention [CDC]. (2011). Surveillance of health status in minority communities—Racial and ethnic approaches to community health across the U.S. (Reach U.S.) Risk Factor Survey, United States, 2009. *Morbidity and Mortality Weekly Report Surveillance Summaries, 60*(SS-6), 1–41.

Liu, J., Bennett, K. J., Harun, N., Zheng, X., Probst, J. C. & Pate, R. R. (2007). *Overweight and Physical Inactivity among Rural Children Aged 10–17: A National and State Portrait.* Retrieved from http://rhr.sph .sc.edu/report/SCRHRC_ObesityChartbook_Exec_Sum_10.15.07.pdf

Lombardi, G. R. (2001). Dental/Oral health services. In National Center for Farmworker Health, Inc., *Migrant Health Issues: Monograph Series (Monograph no. 1).* Bethesada, MD: Bureau of Primary Health Care: Migrant Health Branch.

Long K., & Weinert C. (1989). Rural nursing: Developing a theory base. *Scholarly Inquiry for Nursing Practice, 3,* 113–127.

Lorenz, F. O., Wickrama, K. A. S., & Yeh, H. (2004). Rural mental health: Comparing differences and modeling change. In N. Glasgow, L. W. Morton & N. E. Johnson (Eds.), *Critical Issues in Rural Health* (pp. 37–45). Ames, IA: Blackwell.

Lou, Z-C & Wilkins, R. (2008). Degree of rural isolation and birth outcomes. *Paediatric and Perinatal Epidemiology, 22,* 341–349.

MacKay, A. P., and Duran, C. (2007). *Adolescent Health in the United States, 2007.* Hyattsville, MD: National Center for Health Statistics.

Marquart, B. S., Nannini, D. K., Edwards, R. W., Stanley, L. R. & Wyman, J. C. (2007). Prevalence of dating violence and victimization: Regional and gender differences. *Adolescence, 42*(168), 645–657.

Martikainen, P. T & Marmot, M. G. (1999). Socioeconomic differences in weight gain and determinants and consequences of coronary risk factors. *American Journal of Clinical Nutrition, 69*(4), 719–726.

Mayer, J. P., Housemann, R., & Piepenbrok, B. (1999). Evaluation of a campaign to improve Immunization in a rural Headstart program. *Journal of Community Health, 4*(1), 13–27.

McDonald, N. & Trowbridge, M. (2009). Does the built environment affect when American teens become drivers? Evidence from the 2001 National Household Travel Survey. *Journal of Safety Research, 40,* 177–183.

McDonell, J., Ott, J., & Mitchell, M. (2010). Predicting dating violence victimization and perpetration among middle and high school students in a rural southern community. *Children and Youth Services Review, 32,* 1458–1463.

McGinnis, J. M., & Foege, W. H. (1993). Actual causes of death in the United States. *Journal of the American Medical Association, 270,* 2207–2212.

McSweeney, J. C. & Coon, S. (2004). Women's inhibitors and facilitators associated with making behavioral changes after myocardial infarction. *Medical-Surgical Nursing, 31*(1), 49–56.

McSweeney, J. C. & Crane, P. B. (2005). Challenging the rules: Woman's prodromal and acute symptoms of myocardial infarction. *Research in Nursing & Health, 23*(2), 135–146.

Meng, H. Wamsley, B. R. Eggert, G. M. & Van Nostrand, J. F. (2007). Impact of a health promotion nurse intervention on disability and health care costs among elderly adults with heart conditions. *Journal of Rural Health, 23*(4), 322–331.

Miller, M., Azrael, D. Hemenway, D. & Vriniotis, M. (2005). Firearm storage practices and the rates of unintentional firearm deaths in the United States. *Accident Analysis and Prevention, 37,* 661–667.

Mertz, E. & Mouradian, W. E (2009). Addressing children's oral health in the new millennium: trends in the dental workforce. *Academic Pediatrics, 9,* 433–439.

Mokdad, A. H., Marks, J. S., Stroup, D. F., & Gerberding, J. L. (2004). Actual causes of death in the United States, 2000. *Journal of the American Medical Association, 291,* 1238–1245.

Mokdad, A. H., & Remington, P. L. (2010). Measuring health behaviors in populations. *Preventing chronic disease: Public health research, practice, and policy, 7*(4). Retrieved from http://www.cdc.gov/pcd/issues/2010/jul/10_0010.htm

Moore, J. B., Davis, C. L., Baxter, S. D., Lewis, R. D. & Yin, Z. (2008). Physical activity, metabolic syndrome, and overweight in rural youth. *Journal of Rural Health, 24*(2), 136– 142.

Morgan, D. M. (2005). Effect of incongruence of acute myocardial infarction symptoms on the decision to seek treatment in a rural population. *Journal of Cardiovascular Nursing, 20*(5), 365–371.

Morris, D. (2007). A rural diabetes support group. *The Diabetes Educator, 24,* 493–497.

Morton, L. W. (2004). Spatial patterns of rural mortality. In N. Glasgow, L. W. Morton & N. E. Johnson (Eds.), *Critical issues in rural health* (pp. 37–45). Ames, IA: Blackwell.

Mouradian, W. E., Reeves, A., Kim, S. Lewis, C., Kerbs, A., Slayton, R. L., . . . Marshall, S. G. (2005). A new oral health elective for medical students at the University of Washington. *Teaching and Learning in Medicine, 18*(4), 336–342.

Mulye, T. P., Park, M. J., Nelson, C. D., Adams, S. H., Irwin, C. E., & Brindis, C. D. (2009). Trends in adolescent and young adult health in the United States. *Journal of Adolescent Health, 45*(1), 8–24.

Nagelkerk, J., Reick, K., & Meengs, L. (2006). Perceived barriers & effective strategies to diabetes self-management. *Journal of Advanced Nursing, 54*(2), 151–158.

Nance, M. L., Carr, B. G., Kallan, M. J., Branas, C. C., & Wiebe, D. J. (2010). Variation in Pediatric and adolescent firearm mortality rates in rural and urban U.S. Counties. *Pediatrics, 125,* 1112–1118.

Nasrullah, M. & Muazzam, S. (2011). Drowning mortality in the United States. *Journal of Community Health, 36,* 69–75.

National Center for Injury Prevention and Control. (2007). *Leading Causes of Death and Fatal Injury Reports* (2004 data). Retrieved from http://www.cdc.gov/ncipc/wisqars/ [July 30, 2007].

National Highway Traffic Safety Administration. (2001). *Motor Vehicle Traffic Crash Fatality and Injury Estimates for 2000.* Washington, DC: U.S. National Highway Transportation Safety Administration.

National Institute of Health [NIH], National Heart, Lung and Blood Institute [NHLBI]. (1998). *Clinical guidelines on the identification, evaluation, and treatment of overweight and obesity in adults: The evidence report.* Bethesda, MD: Author.

National Public Radio [NPR]. (2011). Census shows more Blacks, Hispanics moving to N.C. Retrieved from http://www.npr.org/2011/03/04/134253846/The-Census-And-The-South

National Research Council [NRC]. (1999). *Risks and Opportunities: Synthesis of Studies of Adolescence.* M. D. Kipke (Ed.). Washington, DC: National Academy Press.

National Research Council [NRC] & Institute of Medicine [IOM]. (2009). *Adolescent Health Services: Missing Opportunities.* Committee on Adolescent Health Care Services and Models of Care for Treatment, Prevention, and Healthy Development, R. S. Lawrence, J. Appleton Gootman, and L. J. Sim, (Eds.). Board on Children, Youth, and Families. Division of Behavioral and Social Sciences and Education. Washington, DC: The National Academies Press.

National Research Council [NRC], Institute of Medicine [IOM], and Transportation Research Board [TRB]. (2007). *Committee for a Workshop on Contributions from the Behavioral and Social Sciences in Reducing and Preventing Teen Motor Crashes. Preventing teen motor crashes: Contributions from the behavioral and social sciences, workshop report.* Washington, DC: National Academies Press; 2007. Retrieved from http://www.nap.edu/openbook.php?record_id=11814&page=1

Nelson, D. E., Mowery, P., Tomar, S. Marcus, S. Giovino, G. & Zhao, L. (2006). Trends in smokeless tobacco use among adults and adolescents in the United States. *American Journal of Public Health, 96*(5), 897–905.

Nelson, W. (2008). The challenges of rural health care. In C. M. Klugman & P. M. Dalinis (Eds.), *Ethical issues in rural health care* (pp. 34–59). Baltimore, MD: Johns Hopkins University Press.

Nestle, M. (2010). Strategies to prevent childhood obesity must extend beyond school environments. *American Journal of Preventive Medicine, 39*(3), 280–281.

Neyens, D. M. & Boyle, L. N. (2008). The influence of driver distraction on the severity of Injuries sustained by teenage drivers and their passengers. *Accident Analysis and Prevention, 40*, 254–259.

Nicholson, S. (2000). The effect of cardiovascular health promotion on health behaviors in elementary school children: An integrative review. *Journal of Pediatric Nursing, 15*(6), 343– 355.

Noone, J. & Young, H. M. (2009). Preparing daughters: The context of rurality on mothers' role in contraception. *The Journal of Rural Health, 25*(3), 282–289.

Nonnnemaker, J. M., McNeely, C. A., & Blum, R. W. (2003). Public and private domains of religiosity and adolescent health risk behaviors: Evidence from the National Longitudinal Study of Adolescent Health. *Social Science & Medicine, 57*(11), 2049–2054. DOI:10.1016/S0277-9536(03)00096-0

North Carolina Department of Health and Human Services [NCDHHS]. (2011). *Into the mouths of babes.* Retrieved from http://www.ncdhhs.gov/dph/oralhealth/partners/IMB.htm

Ortiz, L., Arizmendi, L., & Cornelius, L. J. (2004). Access to health care among Latinos of Mexican descent in colonias in two Texas counties. *Journal of Rural Health, 20*(3), 246– 252.

Osler, M. (2006). The lifecourse perspective: A challenge for public health research and prevention. *European Journal of Public Health, 16*(3), 320.

Pastore, D. R., Murray, P. J. & Juszczak, L. (2001). School-based health center: Position paper of the Society for Adolescent Medicine. *Journal of Adolescent Health, 29*(6), 448–450. DOI:10.1016/S1054-139X(01)00314-7.

Pack, A. I., Pack, A. M., Rodgman, E., Cucchiara, A., Dinges, D. F., & Schwab, C. W. (1995). Characteristics of crashes attributed to the driver having fallen asleep. *Accident Analysis and Prevention, 27*, 769–775.

Parham J. (2008) Keeping promotion and prevention on the agenda in mental health: issues and challenges. *Australian e-Journal for the Advancement of Mental Health, 7*, 1–5.

Park, M. J., Mulye, T. P., Adams, S. H., Brindis, C. D., & Irwin, C. E., Jr. (2006). The health status of young adults in the United States. *Journal of Adolescent Health, 39,* 305–317.

Pearson, T. (2010). Cardiovascular risk in minority and underserved women in Appalachian Tennessee: A descriptive study. *Journal of the American Academy Nurse Practitioners, 22*(4), 210–216.

Peden, A. R., Reed, D. B. & Rayens, M. K. (2005). Depressive symptoms in adolescents living rural America. *The Journal of Rural Health, 21*(4), 310–316.

Peek, C. W. & Zsembik, B. A. (2004). The health of African Americans living in nonmetropolitan areas. In N. Glasgow, L. W. Morton & N. E. Johnson (Eds.), *Critical issues in rural health* (pp. 141–154). Ames, IA: Blackwell.

Peek-Asa, C., Britton, C., Young, T., Pawlovich, M., & Falb, S. (2010). Teenage driver crash incidence and factors influencing crash injury by rurality. *Journal of Safety Research, 41*, 487–492.

Peoples, J. D., Bishop, J., Barrera, B., Lamas, O., Dunlap, J. L., Gonzalez, P. A., . . . Chamberlain, L. J. (2010). Health, occupational and environmental risks of emancipated migrant farmworker youth. *Journal of Health Care for the Poor and Underserved, 21*(4), 1215–1226.

Price, S. K. & Proctor, E. K. (2009). A rural perspective on perinatal depression: Prevalence, correlates, and implications for help-seeking among low-income women. *Journal of Rural Health, 25*(2), 158–166.

Probst, J. C., Laditka, S. Moore, C. G., Harun, N. & Powell, M. P. (2008). *Depression in rural populations: Prevalence, effects on life quality, and treatment-seeking behavior.* Columbia: SC: South Carolina Rural Health Research Center.

Probst, J. C., Samuels, M. E., Jespersen, K. P., Willert, K., Swann, R. S., & McDuffie, J. A. (2002). *Minorities in Rural America: An Overview of Population Characteristics.* Retrieved from http://rhr.sph.sc.edu/report /minoritiesInRuralAmerica.pdf

Ramos-Gomez, F. J., Crall, J., Gansky, S. A., Slayton, R. L., & Featherstone, J. D. (2007). Caries risk assessment appropriate for the age one visit (infants and toddlers). *California Dental Association Journal, 35*(10), 687–702.

Ramsey, P., Edwards, J., Lenz, C, Odom, J. E., & Brown, B. (1993). Types of health problems and satisfaction with services in a rural-nurse managed clinic. *Journal of Community Health Nursing, 10*(3), 161–170.

Reed, D. B., Browning, S. R., Westneat, S. C. & Kidd, P. S. (2006). Personal protective safety equipment use and safety behaviors among farm adolescents: Gender differences and predictors of work practices. *The Journal of Rural Health, 22*(4), 314–320.

Rhew, I. C., Hawkins, J. D. & Oesterle, S. (2011). Drug use and risk among youth in different rural contexts. *Health & Place, 17,* 775–783.

Rhoades, E. R. & Cravatt, K. (2004). American Indians and Alaska natives. In N. Glasgow, L. W. Morton & N. E. Johnson (Eds.), *Critical issues in rural health* (pp. 127–139). Ames, IA: Blackwell.

Rhodes, N. & Pivik, K. (2010). Age and gender differences in risky driving: The roles of positive affect and risk perception. *Accident Analysis and Prevention, 43*(3), 923–931.

Ricci, R. P., Morichelli, L., & Santini, M. (2008). Home monitoring remote control of pacemaker and implantable cardioverter defibrillator patients in clinical practice: impact on medical management and health care resource utilization. *Europace, 10,* 164–170, DOI:10.1093/europace/eum289

Riley, A. W., Harris, S. K., Ensminger, M. E., Ryan, S., Alexander, C., Green, B., & Starfield, B. (1996). Behavior and injury in rural and urban adolescents. *Injury Prevention, 2,* 266–273.

Rohrer, J. E., Borders, T. F. & Blanton, J. (2005). Rural residence is not a risk factor for frequent mental distress: A behavioral risk factor surveillance survey. *BMC Public Health, 5,* 46. DOI:10.1186/1471–2458-5-46

Rudd, R. A., and Moorman, J. E. (2007). Asthma incidence: Data from the National Health Interview Survey, 1980–1996. *Journal of Asthma, 44,* 65–70.

Rural Assistance Center [RAC] (2011a). *Frontier.* Retrieved from http://www.raconline.org/info_guides /frontier/

Rural Assistance Center [RAC] (2011b). *Women's Health.* Retrieved from http://www.raconline.org/info_ guides/public_health/womenshealth.php

Rural Assistance Center [RAC] (2011c). *Federally qualified health centers.* Retrieved from http://www.raconline .org/info_guides/clinics/fqhc.php

Rural Health Research Center [RAC] (2011d). *RUCA.* Retrieved from http://depts.washington.edu/uwruca /ruca-codes.php

Sanderson, B., Littleton, M., & Pulley, L. (2002). Environmental, policy, and cultural factors related to physical activity among rural, African American women. *Women & Health, 36*(2), 75–90.

Santelli, J. S., Nystrom, R. J., Brindis, C., Juszczak, L., Klein, J. D., Bearss, N., . . . Schlitt, J. (2003). Reproductive health in school-based health centers: Findings from the 1998-1999 census of school-based health centers. *Journal of Adolescent Health, 32*(6), 443–451.

Savin-Williams, R. C. (1991). Critical periods. In R. M. Lerner, A. Petersen & J. Brooks-Gunn (Eds.), *Encyclopedia of adolescence* (pp. 181–183). New York, NY: Garland Publishing.

Schulman, M. D. & Slesinger, D. P. (2004). Health hazards of rural extractive industries and occupations. In N. Glasgow, L. W. Morton & N. E. Johnson (Eds.), *Critical issues in rural health* (pp. 49–60). Ames, IA: Blackwell.

Shi, L. & Stevens, G. D. (2005). *Vulnerable populations in the United States.* San Francisco, CA: Jossey-Bass.

Shope, J. T. & Bingham, C. R. (2008). Teen driving: Motor-vehicle crashes and factors that contribute. *American Journal of Preventive Medicine, 35*(3S):S261–S271.

Simmons, L. A., Braun, B., Charnigo, R., Havens, J. R. & Wright, D. W. (2008). Depression and poverty among rural women: A relationship of social causation or social selection. *The Journal of Rural Health, 24*(3), 292–298.

Skelly, A., Dougherty, M., Gesler, W., Soward, A., Burns, D. & Arcury, T. (2007). African American beliefs about diabetes. *Western Journal of Nursing Research, 28*(9), 9–29.

Skillman, S. M., Doescher, M. P., Mouradian, W. E., & Brunson, D. K. (2010). The challenge to delivering oral health services in rural America. *Journal of Public Health Dentistry, 70*(Supp. 1), S49–57.

Sleet, D. A., Ballesteros, M. F., & Borse, N. N. (2010). A review of unintentional injury in adolescents. *Annual Review of Public Health, 31,*195–212.

Solberg, L. I., Nordin, J. D., Bryant, T. L., Kristensen, A. H., & Maloney, S. K. (2009). Clinical preventive services for adolescents. *American Journal of Preventive Medicine, 37*(5), 445– 454.

Sorenson, S. B. & Vittes, K. A. (2004). Adolescents and firearms: A California statewide survey. *American Journal of Public Health, 94*(5), 852–858.

Spencer, G. A. & Bryant, S. A. (2000). Dating violence: A comparison of rural, suburban, and urban teens. *Journal of Adolescent Health, 27*, 302–305.

Stamm, B. H, Lambert, D., Piland, N. F. & Speck, N. C. (2007). A rural perspective on health care for the whole person. *Professional Psychology: Research and Practice, 38*(3), 298–304.

Stevens, S., Colwell, B., & Hutchison, L. (2003). Tobacco use in rural areas. In L. D. Gamm, L. L. Hutchinson, B. J. Dabney & A. M. Dorsey (Eds.), *Rural Health People 2010: A Companion Document to Healthy People 2010. Volume 1* (pp. 237–240). College Station: The Texas A&M University System Health Science Center, School of Rural Public Health, Southwest Rural Research Center.

Stiglets, S. (2001). Unintentional injuries in the young adult male. *Journal of the American Academy of Nurse Practitioners, 13*(10), 450–454.

Stokols, D. (1996). Translating social ecological theory into guidelines for community health promotion. *American Journal of Health Promotion.* 10(4), 282–298.

Sturm, R. & Wells, K. B. (2001). Does obesity contribute as much to morbidity as poverty or smoking? *Public Health, 115*(3), 229–235.

Suh, M., Chen, C., Woodbridge, J., Tu, M., Kim, J., Nahapetian, A., . . . Sarrafzadeh, M. (2011). A remote patient monitoring system for congestive heart failure. *Journal of Medical Systems, 35*(5), 1165–1179.

Swaim, R. C. & Stanley, L. R. (2010). Rurality, region, ethnic community make-up and alcohol use among rural youth. *The Journal of Rural Health, 27*, 91–102.

Tessaro, I., Smith, S., & Rye, S. (2005). Knowledge and perceptions of diabetes in an Appalachia population. *Public Health Research, Practice, and Policy, 2*(2), 1–9.

Torres, C. C. (2004). Health of Rural Latinos. In N. Glasgow, L. W. Morton & N. E. Johnson (Eds.), *Critical issues in rural health* (pp. 155–167). Ames, IA: Blackwell.

U.S. Census Bureau. (2011a). *Census 2000: Urban and rural classification.* Retrieved from http://www.census.gov/geo/www/ua/ua_2k.html

U.S. Census Bureau (2011b). Geographic comparison table. Retrieved from http://factfinder.census.gov/servlet/GCTTable?_bm=y&-geo_id=01000US&-box_head_nbr=GCT-P1&-ds_name=DEC_2000_SF1_U&-format=US-1

U.S. Census Bureau. (2011c). *Metropolitan and micropolitan statistical areas.* Retrieved from http://www.census.gov/population/www/metroareas/metroarea.html

U.S. Census Bureau. (2011d). Urban and rural classifications. Retrieved from http://www.census.gov/geo/www/ua/urbanruralclass.html

U.S. Department of Health and Human Services [USDHHS] (2000). *Oral Health in America: A report of the Surgeon General.* Rockville, MD: U.S. DHHS], National Institute of Dental Craniofacial Research, National Institute of Health.

U.S. Department of Health and Human Services [U.S. DHHS]. (2011a). *Healthy People 2020.* Retrieved from http://www.healthypeople.gov/2020/default.aspx

U.S. Department of Health and Human Services [U.S. DHHS]. (2011b). *Healthy People 2020: Older Adults.* Retrieved from http://healthypeople.gov/2020/topicsobjectives2020/overview.aspx?topicid=31

US Department of Health and Human Services [U.S. DHHS]. (2011c). *Administration on Aging: Health, Prevention and Wellness Program.* Retrieved from http://www.aoa.gov/AoARoot/AoA_Programs/HPW/Index.aspx

U.S. Department of Health and Human Services [U.S. DHHS]. (2011d). *Respiratory Diseases.* Retrieved from http://www.healthypeople.gov/2020/topicsobjectives2020/overview.aspx?topicId=36

U.S. Department of Health and Human Services [U.S. DHHS], Public Health Service, Centers for Disease Control and Prevention [CDC]. (2003). A national call to action to promote oral health, Rockville, MD:

National Institutes of Health, National Institute of Dental and Craniofacial Research. (NIH Publication; no. 03-5303).

U. S. Government Accountability Office [U.S. GAO]. (2008). *Extent of Dental Disease in Children Has Not Decreased, and Millions Are Estimated to Have Untreated Tooth Decay.* Retrieved from http://www.gao .gov/products/GAO-08-1121

Utz, S. W. (2008). Diabetes care in rural America. In J. Fitzpatrick & E. Merwin (Eds.). *Annual review of nursing research (Vol. 26): Focus on rural health* (pp. 3–39). New York, NY: Springer.

Utz, S., Steeves, R., Wenzel, J., Hinton, I., Jones, R., Andrews, D., . . . Oliver, M. N. (2006). "Working hard with it": Self-management of type 2 diabetes by rural African Americans. *Family & Community Health, 29*(3), 195–205.

Valderrama, A., Dunbar, S., & Mensah, G. (2005). Atrial fibrillation: Public health implications. *American Journal of Preventive Medicine, 29,* 75–80.

Van Gundy, K. (2006). *Reports on Rural America: Substance abuse in rural and small town America.* Durham: University of New Hampshire, Carsey Institute.

Vittes, K. A. & Sorenson, S. B. (2005). Recreational gun use by California adolescents. *Health, Education & Behavior, 32,* 751–766.

Waginold, G., Rowland, J., Dimmler, L., & Peters, D. (2004). Differences between frontier and urban elders with chronic heart failure. *Progress in Cardiovascular Nursing, 19*(1), 12–18.

Wallace, R. B, Grindenau, L. A., & Cirillo, D. J. (2004). Rural/Urban contrasts in population morbidity status. In N. Glasgow, L. W. Morton & N. E. Johnson (Eds.), *Critical Issues in Rural Health* (pp. 37–45). Ames, IA: Blackwell.

Wand, T. (2011). Real mental health promotion requires a reorientation of nursing education, practice, and research. *Journal of Psychiatric and Mental Health Nursing, 18,* 131–138. DOI: 10.1111/j.1365-2850.2010.01634.x

Ward, L. S. & Atav, A. S. (2004). Migrant farmworkers. In N. Glasgow, L. W. Morton & N. E. Johnson (Eds.), *Critical issues in rural health* (pp. 169–181), Ames, IA: Blackwell.

Weinert, C. & Long, K. A. (1987). Understanding the health care needs of rural families. *Family Relations, 36,* 450–455.

Weiss, J., & the Committee on Injury, Violence, and Poison Prevention (2010). Technical Report: Prevention of drowning. *Pediatrics, 126*(1), 253–262.

West, K. S. (2010). Strategizing safety: Perinatal experiences of rural women. In C. A. Winters & H. J. Lee (Eds.), *Rural nursing: Concepts, theory and practice* (pp. 73–90). New York, NY: Springer.

Wilson, F. A. & Stimpson, J. P. (2010). Trends in Fatalities from Distracted Driving in the United States, 1999 to 2008. *American Journal of Public Health, 100,* 2213–2219.

Wilson, T. (2000). Factors influencing the immunization of children in the rural setting. *Journal of Pediatric Health Care, 14*(3), 117–121. DOI:10.1067/mph.2000.103835

Wingo, P., Tucker, T., Jamison, P., Martin, H., McLaughlin, C., Bayakly, R., . . . Richards, T. B. (2008). Cancer in Appalachia, 2001–2003, *Cancer, 112*(1), 181–192.

Winters C & Lee H. (2010), *Rural nursing: Concepts, theory and practice (3rd Ed.).* New York, NY: Springer.

Wong, Y. J., Rew, L., & Slaikeu, K. D. (2006). A systematic review of recent research on adolescent religiosity/spirituality and mental health, *Issues in Mental Health Nursing, 27*(2), 161–183, DOI:10.1080/01612840500436941

Wood, D., Kotseva, K., Connolly, S., Jennings, C., Mead, A., Jones, A., . . . EUROACTION Study Group. (2008). Nurse-coordinated multidisciplinary, family-based cardiovascular disease prevention programme (euroaction) for patients with coronary heart disease and asymptomatic individuals at high risk of cardiovascular disease: A paired, cluster-randomised controlled trial. *The Lancet, 371*(9629), 1999.

World Health Organization [WHO]. (2002). *Active Ageing: A policy framework.* Retrieved from http://whq libdoc.who.int/hq/2002/WHO_NMH_NPH_02.8.pdf

World Health Organization [WHO]. (2005). Mental health: facing the challenges, building solutions. *Report from the WHO European Ministerial Conference*. Copenhagen, Denmark: Author.

Yearwood, E. L. & Siantz, M. L. (2010). Global issues in mental health across the lifespan: Challenges and nursing opportunities. *Nursing Clinics of North America, 45,* 501–519. DOI:10.1016/j.cnur.2010.06.004

Young, D. A., Featherstone, J. B., & Roth, J. R. (2007). Curing the silent epidemic: Caries Management in the 21st century and beyond. *California Dental Association Journal, 35*(10), 681–685.

Zenzen, W. & Kridli, S. (2009). Integrative review of school-based childhood obesity prevention programs. *Journal of Pediatric Health Care, 23*(4), 242–258. DOI:10.1010/j.pedhc.2008.04.008.

Zigmond, J. (2010). Not such a pastoral setting. Rural-specific issues contribute to high suicide rates. *Modern Healthcare, 40*(30), 30–31.

Zive, M., Frank-Spohrer, G., Sallis, J., McKenzie, T., Elder, J., Berry, C., . . . Nader, P. R. (1998). Determinants of dietary intake in a sample of white and Mexican-American children. *Journal of the American Dietetic Association, 98*(11), 1282–1289.

Zuniga, M., Anderson, D., & Alexander, K. (2003). Heart disease and stroke in rural America. In L. D. Gamm, L. L. Hutchinson, B. J. Dabney & A. M. Dorsey (Eds.), *Rural Health People 2010: A Companion Document to Health People 2010. Volume 1* (pp. 133–136). College Station: The Texas A&M University System Health Science Center, School of Rural Public Health, Southwest Rural Research Center.

For a full suite of assignments and additional learning activities, see the access code at the front of your book.

CHAPTER 9

Nursing Informatics

Bonnie Raingruber and Amy Zausch

OBJECTIVES

At the conclusion of this chapter, the student will be able to:

- Define healthcare informatics.
- Explain the relevance of healthcare informatics for patients, health care, and the nursing profession.
- Articulate the advantages and disadvantages of telehealth.
- Discuss the advantages and disadvantages of using avatars and virtual reality environments for health promotion.
- Critique the use of simulation instruction.
- Discuss the advantages and disadvantages of Internet support groups and health promotion sites.
- Assess the impact of technological devices on health promotion and nursing practice.
- Analyze federal government initiatives pertinent to health informatics reform.
- Evaluate how technology has influenced the practice and definition of nursing.

INTRODUCTION

It would be difficult to find an area of the healthcare system today that does not use information systems. Broadly defined, health informatics refers to "the application of computer and information science . . . to facilitate the acquisition, processing, inter-pretation, optimal use, and communication of health-related data. The focus is the patient and process of care, and the goal is to enhance the quality and efficiency of care provided" (Hebda, Czar, & Mascara, 2005, p. 9). Health informatics is used to support population and public health, health protection and promotion, disease prevention, and health monitoring and surveillance (Hannah & Ball, 2006). Informatics is used in research, nursing education, patient education, social support interventions, and service delivery (Blake, 2008a).

The administrative costs of health care, health plan profits, billing, and insurance-related functions are estimated to account for about 25% of all healthcare spending in the United States. (Kahn, Kronick, Kreger, & Gans, 2005; Woolhandler, Campbell, & Himmelstein, 2003). Proposals to reduce administrative healthcare costs include a focus on improving efficiency in billing through the use of technology.

NURSING AND INFORMATICS

Nurses have always played an integral part in information systems and indeed comprise the largest group of healthcare workers utilizing informatics (Hannah & Ball, 2006). A typical work day for a nurse often includes managing patient care through the use of informatics, which assists the nurse in collecting, recording, and retrieving patient data (Hebda et al., 2005).

In 1994, the National League of Nursing (NLN) defined nursing informatics as "the specialty that integrates nursing science, computer science, and information science in identifying, collecting, processing, and managing data and information to support nursing practice, administration, education, research, and the expansion of nursing knowledge" (Dixon & Newlon, 2010, p. 86).

In 1992, the American Nurses Association (ANA) identified nursing informatics as a specialty area with standards of practice and performance (Graybeal, 2009). The ANA council on computers in nursing redefined nursing informatics (NI) based on the NLN definition as "a specialty that integrates nursing science, computer science, and information science to manage and communicate data, information, knowledge, and wisdom in nursing practice" (ANA, 2008, p. 65). Further, the ANA stated that the goal of NI was "to improve the health of populations, communities, families, and individuals by optimizing information management and communication" (p. 65). The utilization of information systems assists nurses in their decision-making and patient care activities (Hannah & Ball, 2006).

Nurses with degrees in healthcare informatics work in a variety of settings, including the hospital, home health and hospice agencies, nursing homes, public and community health agencies, universities, private companies, and ambulatory care centers (ANA, 2008). They assume various roles within the setting of industry, academia, and administration using information technologies to care for patients, to assist in healthcare administrative roles, and to educate existing and future nurses (Hannah & Ball, 2006).

Academic Preparation

Communication through computers is an essential skill for nursing students to possess (McGonigle & Mastrian, 2009). Nursing students are educated using a multitude of educational tools, including simulations, multimedia content, and virtual clinical scenarios (DeSantis, 2009). Thus, exposure to nursing informatics begins with academic preparation at the undergraduate nursing level. Beyond undergraduate exposure, nurses can obtain advanced degrees in NI. Nurses wishing to earn a degree in informatics should be acquainted with general NI principles and understand how they relate to health care and policy. Accredited graduate level nursing education in informatics exists online and in universities. The first graduate program for nursing informatics was established in 1988 at the University of Maryland (Hannah & Ball, 2006). In 1995, the American Nurses Credentialing Center (ANCC) began offering the nursing informatics certification exam.

Professional Organizations and Initiatives Related to Nursing Informatics

The Alliance for Nursing Informatics (ANI) represents 5,000 nurses who specialize in informatics. ANI advocates for meaningful use of health information technology and evidence-based care for all Americans and encourages nurses to provide input into designing systems that capture data, support decision making, fit with workflow needs, and ensure privacy. Examples are electronic health records (EHRs), which are able to pull significant information from a past medical record and integrate it with current admission data to ensure patient safety and quality of care (Sensmeier, 2010).

The Technology Informatics Guiding Education Reform (TIGER) initiative is a national collaborative of nursing organizations, universities, and industry partners working together to promote informatics workforce development. Another goal is to engage nurses in contributing to development of technology that supports safer, more efficient, and accessible care. The TIGER initiative stresses the need for basic computer competency, information literacy, and information management skills for all nurses (Sensmeier, 2010). It encourages nursing participation in the "development, selection, implementation, adoption, and use of informatics in health care" (Dixon & Newlon, 2010, p. 82). Issues regarding how to develop faculty competencies, whether information technology competencies are mandated, where resources to support health information technology will come from, and what content could be deleted from existing nursing curricula to make room for information competence are still being debated. ANA and TIGER are working collaboratively to identify core informatics competencies (Dixon & Newlon, 2010).

ELECTRONIC HEALTH RECORDS

Many healthcare stakeholders believe that technology holds promise for improving quality and efficiency. The Health Information Technology for Economic and Clinical Health (HITECH) Act of 2009 encouraged the use of EHRs in part because their use was believed to be more efficient than the use of paper medical records (Hebda et al., 2005). The EHR is defined as "a secure, real-time, point-of-care, patient-centric information resource for clinicians" (Hebda et al., p. 252). The Institute of Medicine (IOM) formulated five criteria to guide the process of identifying core functionalities of the EHR, which include a commitment to improve patient safety, to support the delivery of effective patient care, to facilitate management of chronic conditions, to improve efficiency, and to support implementation of key functionalities within EHR systems (IOM, 2003).

Benefits of Electronic Health Records

There are a host of benefits associated with the use of EHRs. Patient benefits center on increased safety, improved quality of care, and electronic accessibility to medical information when moving from one city or one medical practice to another. Patient portals, which allow individuals to view laboratory and test results in a timely fashion, email their provider with a question, renew a prescription, or make an appointment, are popular options (Thede, 2008).

The benefits to nurses include fewer medical errors, less time spent on charting, less repetition in charting, electronic decision-making prompts, automation to facilitate more complete care, and the ability to electronically monitor compliance with prevention and disease management guidelines (Taylor et al., 2005). E-prescribing for physicians and nurse practitioners eliminates errors related to difficult-to-decipher handwriting. E-prescribing also allows real-time access to formulary options, drug–drug interactions, allergies, and the patient's past medication history (Balfour et al., 2009).

Electronic health records allow for monitoring patient-level and population-level data and simplifying data collection for quality improvement initiatives. Comparative effectiveness research, which establishes the best intervention for a given condition, requires efficient collection of data from EHRs. Eventually, genetic databases, electronic medical record data, and large population-based registries will allow researchers to examine which interventions work best for people with a given background (Scheuermann & Milgrom, 2010).

When population-level databases are created and linked with EHRs, they have the potential to increase coordination of care between systems. Patient-level data can be shared between hospitals, private physicians, home health agencies, physical therapy practices, pharmacies, long-term care facilities, and other healthcare agencies. However, this feature has not yet been realized. Not all systems have transitioned to EHRs and many existing systems are incompatible with one another because they have been purchased from competing private companies (Balfour et al., 2009). If open source EHR software were adopted, multiple providers would be able to share data. An example of an open source EHR is the one used by the Department of Veteran's Affairs (Yellowlees, Marks, Hogarth, & Turner, 2008).

Challenges and Unintended Consequences Associated with EHR Implementation

Initial startup costs; lack of standardization among platforms, which interferes with data sharing; lack of technical support; loss of productivity during implementation; and increased documentation time of up to 17.5% (for physicians) have been identified as some of the challenges associated with EHR implementation (Balfour et al., 2009).

To ensure that EHR data can be shared, the same information must be collected from multiple health agencies, including accurate information on race and ethnicity. However, different institutions often use varied race and ethnicity designations. Because common data elements must be collected, drop-down menus with standardized options rather than free text entries are favored (Scheuermann & Milgrom, 2010). Lack of financial incentives for and the extra time required to share patient data has been emphasized as another challenge interfering with coordination of care between systems (Middleton, 2005).

Once they are established, EHRs lack flexibility, making it difficult to add a screening tool, an outcome measure, or a clinical parameter without costly revision of the system and involvement of computer programmers. System downtime, server problems, and viruses/cyberthreats necessitate having a backup option that allows for the use of a paper medical record during crisis situations (Bloomrosen et al., 2011).

Authors have commented that automatic alerts programmed into EHRs can both prevent errors and interrupt nurses' and physicians' workflows. An overabundance of alerts can result in practitioners ignoring the automated notifications. More importantly, an overreliance on automated safety checks can lead to not taking the time to think through clinical decisions and documentation (Bloomrosen et al., 2011).

Large paper records that are converted to electronic formats can make it difficult to find relevant patient data. It can be time consuming to read through multilevel, drop-down lists. It is also the case that automated drop-down menus (even lengthy ones) are limited. Some clinicians select the closest option from the drop-down menu even if it is less precise than what they would have used for narrative charting. This can result in confusion about and misrepresentation of a patient's condition. In addition, for certain sections of charting more than one provider can access and edit the same EHR, which can result in duplicative or contradictory entries (Bloomrosen et al., 2011).

Significantly, research has shown the highly structured electronic format of EHRs has changed the clinical assessment and reasoning patterns of physicians. This guiding and narrowing of the clinical options that are considered can be a positive or an unanticipated negative consequence of using a highly structured charting format (Bloomrosen et al., 2011). It will be interesting to see if nursing research shows the same pattern of changes in critical thinking and a movement away from reliance on clinical expertise (Benner, Tanner, & Chesla, 1996) as has been seen in medicine.

Some clinicians have expressed a worry that the amount of time directed to health information technology will have a negative impact on professional autonomy and patient–provider relationships. Others have suggested a main driving force for EHRs is a move toward pay-for-performance reimbursement and care that is driven exclusively by evidence-based guidelines rather than provider expertise and individualized care (Lee & Lau, 2009). Inadequate policies about billing for e-visits are another challenge that needs to be addressed (Taylor et al., 2005).

Financial Factors Associated with Electronic Health Record Use

It is worth noting that medical errors have a tremendous impact on the costs of care. There were at least 1.5 million measurable medical injuries caused by errors in 2008; the average cost per error was $13,000, for a total annual cost of $19.5 billion (Shreve et al, 2010). "Medication errors alone are responsible for an estimated 1.5 million injuries and $3.5 billion in excess costs" (Balfour et al., 2009, p. S13). Estimates suggest that $156 million could be saved by avoiding adverse drug events and $410 million would be saved by standardized e-prescription of generic medications (Balfour et al., 2009).

Efforts to reduce medical errors are not only a moral imperative, but are a critical part of the larger effort to control healthcare spending. EHRs offer a very promising answer to the reduction of medical errors. A systematic review (Chaudhry et al., 2006) found that health information technology decreased ordering of laboratory tests and radiographic studies, some of which may have been duplicative. However, quality of care and safety were not considered (Balfour et al., 2009; Lee & Lau, 2009).

It is interesting to note that not-for-profit hospitals have "50% higher relative adoption rates for electronic medical records than do for-profits" (Taylor et al., 2005, p. 1236). Practices affiliated with a hospital or university are more likely to use EHRs, while small and rural hospitals and ambulatory practices are slower at adopting EHRs (Taylor et al., 2005). Reimbursements for EHR depend on payer type. "Of the estimated $77 billion that could be saved at a level of 90% EHR adoption, $23 billion would be allocated to Medicare and $31 billion to private payers" (Balfour et al., 2009, p. S15).

HEALTH INSURANCE PORTABILITY AND ACCOUNTABILITY ACT

One of the concerns that patients and healthcare professionals express in regards to EHRs is confidentiality of medical information. Patient privacy is of utmost importance to health professionals and it is their duty to ensure privacy rights are not breached. The Health Insurance Portability and Accountability Act (HIPAA) was passed in 1996 to ensure vital patient record protection (Hebda et al., 2005). HIPAA requires that patient information remains secure, including demographic data and specifics related to a patient's physical or mental health condition.

The Health Information Technology for Economic and Clinical Health Act (HITECH) adopted as part of the American Recovery and Reinvestment Act (ARRA) in 2009 broadened the reach of HIPAA and strengthened privacy and security standards. Beginning in 2009, covered entities were required to notify individuals whose health information had been disclosed as a result of a security breach that was determined to be above the little or no risk of harm levels. Sharing of a data set stripped of patient identifiers does not require notification, however (Goldstein & Thorpe, 2010).

Electronic Health Records and the Future

Many healthcare systems are embracing implementation of EHRs. Unfortunately, it is up to individual hospitals and outpatient practices to choose from the many forms of EHRs that currently exist. Without uniformity it is difficult for hospitals and clinics to share vital patient information or establish best-practice interventions based on patient outcomes. Government intervention to ensure uniformity EHR systems used in hospitals is generally accepted among many healthcare providers, but large scale implementation of consistent types of electronic medical records would require a substantially increased investment in time and money in an already costly system (Yellowlees et al., 2008).

The Role of the Government

The United States has been slow to implement EHRs; however, that transition has been accelerated by governmental involvement. President George Bush established a goal that by 2014 the majority of Americans would have an electronic medical record. "On July 15, 2008, Congress overrode a presidential veto and enacted the Medicare Improvements for Patients and Providers Act (MIPPA)" (Balfour et al., 2009, p. S13). That act included incentives for hospitals and physicians who adopt e-prescribing as well as penalties for those who do not. Exceptions for rural practitioners and agencies with limited Internet access exist, while additional bonuses are available to physicians in health professional–shortage areas (Goldstein & Thorpe, 2010).

In February 2009, President Obama signed the American Recovery and Reinvestment Act (ARRA), which included $23 billion for implementation of health information technology over a 5-year timeframe. Funds were to be used to enhance clinical decision making by including electronic prompts, expanding collection of patient demographic information, incorporating physician order entry, providing for quality control monitoring, and mandating electronic exchange of health records (Lee & Lau, 2009). A federal office, the National Coordinator for Health Information Technology, was established to be in charge of information technology including preventing medical errors, increasing efficiency, and reducing unnecessary costs (Bloomrosen et al., 2011).

The HITECH act included in ARRA stated that meaningful use of EHR technology for Medicare Part D will provide bonuses of up to 2% of annual charges for physicians beginning in 2011. The incentives continue for 5 years, with bonuses decreasing over time. Physicians who do not use e-prescribing by 2015 will lose at least 1% of Medicare revenues. Hospitals will also have bonuses beginning in 2011, which will decrease by 25% per year over a 4-year period. Beginning in 2015, hospitals will receive less than the current Medicare reimbursement rate and face penalties for not adopting meaningful use of EHR technology. Meaningful use requires e-prescribing, exchange of health information to improve quality, and reporting clinical quality outcome measures (Goldstein & Thorpe, 2010).

Likewise, the HITECH Act included in ARRA encouraged use of EHRs for Medicaid providers; however, implementation is optional depending on state choice. To qualify for Medicaid bonuses a provider must be a rural health clinic, a federally qualified health center, or have 30% of their patients receive Medicaid, State Children's Health Insurance, or uncompensated care. Providers may receive up to $25,000 beginning in 2011 and $10,000 each year for 5 years. An initial payment for equipment of $21,250 and $8,500 per year for 5 years can be received. Acute care hospitals with 10% Medicaid patients and all children's hospitals can receive incentives if EHRs are adopted before 2016 (Goldstein & Thorpe, 2010).

The Center for Medicaid Services (CMS) established stages of compliance: stage 1 requires electronic capture of information; stage 2 (implemented at the end of 2011) requires quality improvement measures and exchange of information; and stage 3 requires promoting health at a population level, clinical decision support for priority conditions, and patient access to self-management tools (implemented in 2013). Hospitals qualifying for stage 1 meaningful use must document that they are improving quality, becoming more efficient, reducing health disparities, engaging patients in their care, coordinating care, improving public health, and adhering to privacy standards. To encourage exchange of information across electronic systems, CMS will specify formats for documenting clinical summaries, prescriptions, clinical problem descriptions, procedures, laboratory tests, and medication orders (Goldstein & Thorpe, 2010). Because it is likely that pay-for-performance incentives will become more common, a national structure for reporting quality measures and comparative performance data will be needed (Balfour et al., 2009).

Through ARRA, the government has provided substantial funding and stimulated adoption of EHRs. It has also created statutory requirements that will require that private, state, and federal agencies devote time and resources to implementing and adhering to those standards (Goldstein & Thorpe, 2010).

The Drug Enforcement Agency (DEA) is working on e-prescribing regulations for controlled substances that would allow pharmacies to receive, dispense, and archive electronic prescriptions (Balfour et al., 2009). Taylor and colleagues (2005) suggested that Medicare and Medicaid have the most to gain from movement towards the use of health information technology. Because their payment guidelines tend to drive reimbursement from other sources, it is likely in time that private insurance reimbursement will also be patterned after Medicare and Medicaid guidelines.

Healthy People 2010 offers guidance regarding the quality of websites, health literacy levels for online content, and standards for research and evaluation of e-health (U.S. Department of Health and Human Services, 2000). A governmental agency, the Agency for Health Care Research and Quality, endorses and supports barcode medication administration (O'Malley, 2008).

Given the levels of governmental involvement in health care in recent years, it is vital that nurses enhance their knowledge of informatics. Nurses of the future must become active in lobbying Congress and varied professional organizations if they are going to have a voice in shaping how information technology influences health care, nursing practice, and health promotion activities.

TELEHEALTH AND MEDICAL HOMES

A vast number of ideas for containing healthcare expenditures have been proposed and will continue to be debated in the foreseeable future (Max, 2007). These proposals include those seeking to reduce medical costs and those seeking to shift demand away from expensive hospital-based medical care to primary and preventive health. Telehealth and the creation of medical homes both offer opportunities to improve the current healthcare system.

Telemedicine and Telehealth

Telemedicine or telehealth is one form of healthcare technology that is believed to have potential to improve quality of patient care in addition to reducing costs. Telemedicine is defined by the American Telemedicine Association (2012) as "the use of medical information exchanged from one site to another via electronic communications to improve patients' health status" (American Telemedicine Association, 2012, Telemedicine Defined, para. 1).

Although still in its early stages, telemedicine and telehealth have been associated with providing care to individuals in rural communities, homebound persons, areas where access to specialized care is limited, and locations that lack adequate numbers of healthcare providers. An advantage of telehealth is that it increases access to care among underserved communities while reducing appointment scheduling delays and minimizing patient travel costs (Reed, 2005).

Two types of technology are used in telemedicine. First, an audio or video file can be sent from one location to another through a telephone line for review at a later time. Second, synchronous telecommunication use allows both the patient and healthcare provider to see one another in real time. A computer with a built in camera and a stethoscope/blood pressure monitor can be placed in the patient's home or a clinic office. Peripheral monitors for heart rate, body weight, pulmonary function, blood sugar, temperature, and electrocardiogram evaluation are also available so that the provider can conduct a comprehensive patient assessment from a distant location (West & Milio, 2004).

In homecare settings, telehealth has been used by nurses to conduct insulin dosage checks during the initial phase of patient education. In addition, wound care management at home has been enhanced by nurses using telehealth. Each new wound care picture can be compared with previous pictures to yield an exact measurement of progress or the lack of healing (Simpson, 2002).

In Texas, telehealth has been used to provide medical management and nursing triage of prisoners, thereby reducing costs, avoiding unnecessary emergency room visits, and decreasing mortality. Nurse practitioners have been trained to do colorectal screenings in community clinics via telehealth, thus increasing gastrointestinal cancer detection rates—cost associated with the colorectal screening by nurse practitioners is less while

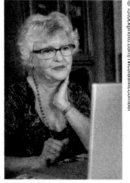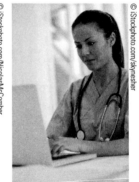

quality is comparable to care provided by gastroenterologists. A Telehealth asthma management provided by nurses has used technology to monitor patient's medication compliance and peak flow values resulting in an 83% reduction in hospitalizations. Advanced practice nurses (APNs) have transmitted digital images of retinas to ophthalmologists to screen for diabetic retinopathy in remote Native American tribal lands, which eliminates costly travel and increases the number of patients who actually engage in preventative care (Reed, 2005).

Telemedicine has been used to augment care provided in intensive care units (ICU) by providing consultation to less-experienced ICU staff. Evidence-based care protocols and decision trees are built into the technology to help identify needed interventions. A remotely based critical care team consisting of a critical care physician and a nurse work with the bedside ICU team. The mean staffing ratio for the remote team is approximately 1 telemedicine intensivist to 30 to 40 patients and 1 e-RN and 1 clerical assistant per 50 to 125 patients. High resolution zoom cameras and microphones allow for assessment of patient's skin color and breathing as well as monitoring labels on infusing medications. The cameras do not record images or conversations—they only allow for real-time monitoring. For example, tele-ICU staff can view bedside alarms but cannot reset them (Goran, 2010).

Software programs monitor bedside vital signs, laboratory results, medications, and charted data as well as flag situations that require immediate intervention. Data are encrypted and transmission is secured between sites to provide for confidentiality of patient-level data. Tele-ICUs have resulted in a 29% reduction in patient mortality and shorter lengths of stay in the 200 hospitals where they have been implemented. Cost-to-benefit calculations are still pending (Goran, 2010).

TeleKidcare, a telehealth program implemented in schools, allows nurses from different schools to consult with one another. A digital otoscope and electronic stethoscope are used along with interactive television screens. TeleKidcare brings services to rural schools and enables nurses to bring parents, teachers, and physicians together simultaneously to evaluate the need for the child to be seen by a physician. (Mackert, & Whitten, 2007).

Some limitations with telehealth that have been reported include the need for multiple phone lines and more reliable telecommunications infrastructure in rural areas. Some authors have questioned whether the provision of telehealth medicalizes a person's home and changes the character of what had been a healing environment. Whether the nature of the nurse–patient relationship is changed by distance rather than in-person communication has also been discussed (McGarry & Nairn, 2005). Finally, challenges associated with billing for services across state lines makes the use of telehealth interventions more complex (West & Milio, 2004).

Reimbursement for Telehealth Services

Billing for telehealth services is governed by the nurse practice act in each state. What a registered nurse (RN) or APN can do and bill for is not consistent in all states. The National Council of State Boards of Nursing has developed a mutual recognition model of licensure that allows a nurse to be licensed in his or her state of residence and maintain the requirements of that state board but practice across state lines. However, the challenge is that the scope of practice in the nurse's state of residence may not be the same as in the state where he or she is providing a telehealth intervention (Simpson, 2002).

Different payors have unique rules about reimbursement for telehealth. The 1997 Balanced Budget Act mandated that Medicare Part B pay for telehealth consultation and allowed nurse practitioners to both request and provide consultations. The payment to the distance practitioner is equal to the current fee schedule for the given service in the state in which the patient resides. In addition, the site where the patient is being treated receives a facility fee (Reed, 2005).

Nurses' Roles in Telehealth

Telehealth nurses are able to conduct telephone triage and provide follow-up calls to patients, which is especially important for patients in rural and underserved areas that lack convenient access to health care. Nurses can monitor chronic health conditions via telehealth and ease the transition from hospital to home. Both APNs and RNs can serve as telehealth consultants if they are acting within their scope of practice (Hannah & Ball, 2006).

Telehealth and the Nursing Shortage

The critical shortage of nurses remains an obstacle to providing quality health care. Efforts to supply more professional nurses have included importation of foreign-trained registered nurses, incentives to increase nursing schools' capacities, encouraging healthcare aides and licensed vocational nurses to become RNs, and enticing inactive nurses to return to work. Surprisingly, raising wages alone does not result in an increase in the number of hours nurses choose to work. One study found a backward-bending supply curve in which nurses who are being paid above a certain threshold actually choose to work less (Tellez, Spetz, Seago, Harrington, & Kitchener, 2008). While a shortage of nurses compromises the ability of the healthcare system to meet the demand for services, telehealth offers a time-savings realization for both the healthcare system and nurses. With the use of telehealth, nurses can efficiently see additional patients while eliminating the need for costly travel (Tellez et al.).

Medical Homes

Myriad health policy recommendations have been embraced by the primary care movement that would shift the bulk of U.S. health care from hospitals to outpatient "medical homes." The underlying rationale is that increased utilization of relatively inexpensive primary health care (PHC) will improve population health and decrease the need for costly, technology-intensive hospital care (Gruber, 2007).

Several barriers exist that prevent greater utilization of PHC in the United States, including a shortage of providers (attributed in part to low reimbursement rates), lack of insurance, and underinsurance (Gruber, 2007; Majette, 2009). The Patient Protection and Affordable Care Act (PPACA) includes many aspects intended to improve accessibility of PHC. Among these are incentives to increase the primary healthcare workforce, increased Medicaid reimbursement rates for PHC, and eliminate cost-sharing for Medicare beneficiaries receiving preventive services (Congressional Research Service, 2010).

VIRTUAL REALITY AND AVATARS

Avatars are created personalities that can talk, convey emotion, walk, and interact with other avatars in virtual environments. These humanlike visual representations of the user's identity vary from being three-dimensional in complexity with a persona (avatar) to a two-dimensional, animated talking head that has speech, gestures, and facial expressions (embodied conversational agent or ECA). Both can be used to provide health education and health promotion. The user is often given an option of selecting a humanlike avatar, a cartoon character, or some other self-representation. The user inhabits or adopts the point of view of the avatar (Moore, Cheng, McGrath, & Powell, 2005). The inclusion of emotional content and the active nature of participation required in a virtual reality environment engages the user's full attention (Park et al., 2009). Virtual reality programs can be visited multiple times and a range of scenarios for practice can be provided. This makes it possible for the user to feel anonymous and safe while learning from mistakes (Moore et al., 2005).

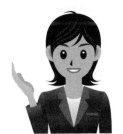

Some ECAs do not interact with a user, but instead only present health promotion-related content. Other ECAs provide health education by interacting and responding to patient questions and comments. A major programming challenge dealt with conveying when the avatar or ECA had stopped speaking by use of voice pitch, gaze, facial expressions, gestures, and mouth movements. Technology developed for online/telephone lip-reading support for hard-of-hearing individuals was used to address this challenge and allow the animated character to synchronize conversation with other avatars or the user. The avatar or ECA can be programmed to look straight ahead with raised eyebrows, signaling a willingness to listen (Edlund & Beskow, 2009).

Avatars are being used in a variety of areas. Researchers have examined self-presentation by having abused and nonabused girls create avatars to examine risk factors for online sexual victimization (Noll, Shenk, Barnes, & Putnam, 2009). As another example, researchers have used virtual reality programs to treat individuals with social phobia (Gregg & Tarrier, 2007).

Other researchers have conducted exploratory research (n = 34) to examine whether autistic children can make inferences from facial expressions and understand basic emotions conveyed by an avatar (Moore et al., 2005). This study found that 90% of autistic children could accurately recognize and understand an avatar's facial expressions (happy, sad, angry, and frightened). Because autistic individuals often have difficulty understanding subtle social rules, simplified communication via avatars was less overwhelming and allowed the autistic person to feel in control of their interactions where they would normally feel out of control (Moore et al., 2005). What are other possible advantages and disadvantages of using avatars with autistic children?

Healthcare professionals are being trained to prepare for a mass casualty event by using virtual reality programs. In another application, a student nurse's avatar can investigate a three-dimensional electrocardiogram tracing and name the rhythm (Hansen, 2008). Avatars are also being used to promote empathy among nursing students and nurses for individuals with conditions such as schizophrenia, autism, and aphasia by allowing the student or nurse to step into the world and perspective of someone with a disease process they themselves have not experienced.

Virtual reality platforms, in contrast to simulation, are relatively inexpensive. They are also available 24/7 and provide opportunities for online users to explore, create, collaborate, interact, and learn in a safe and engaging environment. A limitation is that the vivid nature of the experience may overshadow and diminish the impact of educational objectives. Unresolved issues regarding authorship are also a concern for faculty members and other individuals who use this technology (Hansen, 2008).

SIMULATION AND VIRTUAL PATIENTS

Increasingly, simulation is being used in nursing education and in training new nurses within hospital settings. Federal agencies such as the Health Resources and Services Administration are making funds available to purchase simulators and integrate simulation into the curriculum of nursing schools and into hospital-based continuing education programs. Simulation makes use of high-, mid-, and low-fidelity simulators, or human-sized mannequins that have been programmed to talk and have a blood pressure, heart rate, pupil reaction, lung sounds, and oxygen saturation monitoring capability.

Simulation allows students and new nurses to practice skills and evaluate the outcomes of critical thinking without risking making an error on a human patient. Simulator responses depend on student interventions and choices, so they provide a way for the learner to gain immediate feedback about the effectiveness of a clinical decision. Simulation has

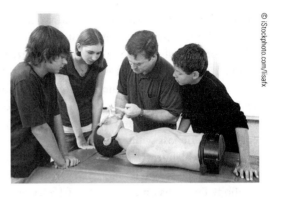

been described as an active learning strategy that requires thinking on your feet in real time. An advantage is that a variety of simulations can be developed by faculty members to meet the learning needs of any group of students or nurses. Typically, simulation has not been used to teach health promotion concepts, but instead is used to teach decision making in critical situations. When students have adequate knowledge and the ability to make sound clinical decisions, they are better prepared to help patients with their health promotion goals at some future point in their career.

Even though many nursing schools and hospital systems are adopting simulation in their curricula, some disadvantages have been identified. A variety of authors have reported lack of transfer of skills learned in simulation to clinical practice (Parr & Sweeney, 2006; Schoening, Sittner, & Todd, 2006; Reilly & Spratt, 2007). A false sense of learner self-efficacy can be created in a simulation even when it is not warranted (Pike & O'Donnell, 2010). Students have commented that real clinical situations and actual patient interactions differ substantially from simulation, given that voice tones, facial expressions, gestures, body posture, skin tone changes, and a number of other clinical indicators are missing in simulation (Bantz, Dancer, Hodson-Carlton, & Van Hove, 2007; Baxter, Akhtar-Danesh, Valaitis, Stanyon, & Sproul, 2009; Pike & O'Donnell, 2010). Since the quality of patient simulators has improved radically in recent years, it will be interesting to see what advances occur in the next decade with this technology. It will also be interesting to see if over time the federal government continues to provide the same amount of funding for simulation equipment for nursing schools.

INTERACTIVE GAMES AND HEALTH PROMOTION

Interactive Internet and computer-based health games help users evaluate health risks and their consequences, obtain needed health education, and engage in an enjoyable activity. One example, Dr. Health'nstein's Body Fun software, is used by school districts in several states (California, Georgia, Massachusetts, and Alabama) to teach health promotion. Body Fun begins with a 10-year-old character that grows into adolescence, adulthood, and who then becomes a senior citizen. Topics such as nutrition, fitness, and substance abuse are covered as the character makes health-related decisions. Users begin with 50 points and lose or gain additional points based on lifestyle decisions they make. Included are arcade-style games such as "Fat and Fiber Shootout," which requires the player to recognize low and high fiber foods; "Calorie Match Up," which tests knowledge of calorie loss with a spectrum of physical activities; and "The Purple Anatomy Machine," which teaches what happens to the body after exposure to cigarette smoke and alcohol. Body Fun is tailored to varied health literacy levels (Geiger et al., 2002).

Body Fun runs on a CD-ROM. Challenges associated with Body Fun include the fact that some schools don't allow teachers to load software onto networked computers without completing a lengthy permission process, and competition to use scarce computers is substantial in certain school districts (Geiger et al., 2002).

A video game that teaches cancer care has been used with adolescents and young adults (aged 13 to 29 years) diagnosed with leukemia, lymphoma, and soft-tissue sarcomas. In the game, players control a nanobot that operates in "a three-dimensional environment destroying cancer cells, managing common treatment-related adverse effects such as bacterial infections, nausea, and constipation by using chemotherapy, antibiotics, antiemetics, and a stool softener as ammunition" (Kato, Cole, Bradlyn, & Pollock, 2008, p. 306).

To win, players ensure the nanobot selects positive self-care behaviors including taking medications, engaging in good mouth care, reducing stress, and selecting a healthy diet. None of the nanobots die in the game; rather, the computer powers down and can be rebooted if too many poor health choices are made. This randomized, controlled study of 375 patients demonstrated that enhanced adherence to prescribed medications, increased self-efficacy, and improved cancer-related knowledge were associated with using the game at least 1 hour per week for a 3-month period (Kato et al., 2008). What are possible reasons participants experienced an increased self-efficacy after playing this video game?

The Smoking Zine website includes self-assessment tools, action planning for resisting and cutting down on smoking, interactive games, and an online bulletin board. One interactive game allows youth to select the packs-per-day someone might smoke; the program then calculates the cost per year of smoking at that level and takes the youth to a virtual shopping mall

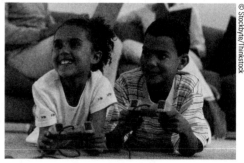

© Stockbyte/Thinkstock

where they can select to purchase other items costing up to that amount. Through this exercise, the Smoking Zine teaches the economic consequences of smoking. Another value clarification exercise allows youth to identify factors that might prompt them to begin smoking, reasons to quit, and reasons not to start smoking. Youth can design a personalized plan for quitting, or if they say they are not ready to quit, they are linked to quizzes that explore physical and social consequences of continuing to smoke (Skinner, Maley, & Norman, 2006). Which type of youth do you think would be most likely to respond favorably to the Smoking Zine and which might be less likely to enjoy the game?

Although use of some video games has been linked to childhood obesity, researchers have studied whether active video games increase energy expenditure. Researchers have reported active video games use a level of energy expenditure that is similar to mild to moderate intensity physical activity (Biddiss & Irwin, 2010; Foley & Maddison, 2010). Two specific games, Dance, Dance Revolution (DDR) and Nintendo's Wii bowling and boxing (played using a handheld controller) were compared to watching television or walking in terms of energy expenditure, heart rate, and step rate for a small sample of 14 boys and 9 girls (Graf, Pratt, Hester, & Short, 2009).

The DDR game requires children to move their feet to match step patterns displayed on a television screen. Points are allocated for matching the timing and accuracy of footsteps using a pressure-sensitive floor mat. Use of the Wii bowling and the beginner level DDR resulted in a two-fold increase in energy expenditure compared to watching television. The Wii boxing and the DDR level 2 games resulted in a two- to three-fold increase in energy expenditure compared to watching television. The authors concluded active video game play is comparable to moderate intensity walking (Graf et al, 2009).

A similar game has been developed for senior citizens to use at home. By manipulating a motion-sensitive controller, the senior citizen completes exercises that mimic the routine of a traditional physical therapy exercise program (Hansen, 2008).

E-HEALTH AND HEALTH PROMOTION

Electronic health, or e-health, includes the use of cell phones, portable computers, email, Internet postings, and Internet support groups to motivate patients to engage in preventative or restorative measures, to track early warning symptoms, to monitor health, to manage disease, and to collect data for health-related research studies. E-health messages sent by cell phone or text messaging can be used to monitor test results, prompt self-care behaviors, encourage self-monitoring of disease progress, remind patients to take necessary medications, and track patients with dementia who are likely to wander off by the use of a global positioning system (GPS). Messages can be personalized to match the needs of the target group or the individual (Blake, 2008b).

Cell Phones, Mobile Computers, and Text Messaging

Cell phones, palm pilot computers, and text messaging provide a way for a nurse to maintain contact with patients who have been discharged from the hospital and have returned home. An advantage of cell phones, palm pilot computers, and text messages is that individuals are receiving the intervention in real time in the midst of their everyday life. Therefore, behavior change is more likely to be incorporated into the patient's daily routine (Heron & Smyth, 2010).

Messages can be sent at predetermined times selected by the participant as convenient or at an at-risk moment. Messages can be tailored to individualized factors such as readiness to change, locus of control, self-efficacy, self-identified barriers to change, and previous health history. Messages can also be tailored to a population subgroup, such as African Americans at risk of high blood pressure. Tailored information increases the likelihood that people will consider the message to be meaningful and initiate behavioral change as a result (Heron & Smyth, 2010).

Cell phones and palm pilot computers can also be used to capture real-time research data, avoiding the bias associated with retrospective recall. Health promotion messages and research questionnaires sent via palm pilot computer or text messaging have the potential to reach large numbers of individuals at a minimal cost (Heron & Smyth, 2010). For example, collecting data on exercise levels, eating patterns, and insulin use, then creating colorful histograms from that data and returning it to patients, has been shown to improve glycemic control among diabetic patients. The resulting histograms also allow providers to identify individuals who are not testing their blood sugar or who have values outside preestablished norms. Communication between parents and diabetic children has also been improved using cell phones that transfer readings from the child's blood glucose monitor directly to the parent's mobile phone (Blake, 2008b).

Text message appointment reminders have been shown to decrease canceled appointments. Both cell phones and text messaging have been effectively used for diet and weight management, increasing physical activity levels, minimizing drug and alcohol use, and smoking cessation (Blake, 2008b). Interventions include tips for dealing with cravings that are sent at predetermined times identified as critical by the participant (Heron & Smyth, 2010).

One example of a cell phone intervention called Wellnavi allowed participants to photograph all food consumed and forward the electronic picture to a registered dietitian, who then calculated caloric and nutrient intake. Participants felt this method was the easiest way of recording food intake. This application can be used not only to monitor individual food intake and improve weight loss, but also to gain dietary information from a large population (Blake, 2008a; Wang, Kogashiwa, & Kris, 2006).

One randomized clinical trial compared a mobile phone-based smoking cessation program to physician advice, written patient education materials, and nicotine replacement therapy. Participants in the cellular telephone intervention were 3.6 times more likely than those in other arms of the study to quit smoking. A strength of the study was that results were biochemically verified (Blake, 2008a; Vidrine, Arduino, Lazev, & Gritz, 2006).

A mobile phone-based fitness journal was devised to track and share progress with increasing step counts. Participants were asked to share their success with 13 friends on a daily basis. Participants rated the intervention as effective and practical given their multiple daily commitments (Blake, 2008a; Consolvo, Everitt, Smith, & Landay, 2006).

King and colleagues (2008) studied the use of palm pilot computers to deliver messages designed to increase activity level in adults. Participants were signaled to complete a questionnaire at 2 PM and 9 PM daily. Caloric expenditure, number of active minutes, and pedometer steps increased in the group that received electronic educational materials and completed the palm pilot computer questionnaires.

Both palm pilot computers and desktop computers have been used to provide lifestyle, health, and risk assessments. Access can be provided in waiting areas of primary care offices, schools, or any location where screening would be convenient. Research is clear that individuals prefer revealing either highly personal or potentially embarrassing information to a computer rather than to a healthcare provider. Computerized assessments for alcohol consumption, smoking, diet, and physical activity exist and are often an effective way to encourage patient disclosure about lifestyle habits. In addition, computerized education that is cost effective can be provided immediately based on the health or risk assessment information that the patient provides (Carlfjord et al., 2009).

Limitations Related to Cell Phone and Text Messaging Interventions

Studies have shown older individuals are more likely to use cell phones than the Internet when communicating about their health (Blake, 2008b). However, a limitation of using cell phones is that information sent via mobile devices can be accessed by other individuals (Blake, 2008a). Security needs to be considered before implementing a cell phone intervention for sensitive issues such as HIV/AIDS and substance abuse. For what other health conditions would use of cell phones and text messaging not be appropriate?

ELECTRONIC SELF-CARE EDUCATION MATERIALS

The Internet has greatly increased access to medical and health promotion content. About 50% of Americans use the Internet to access health-related information. Income and age (< 65 years) are the strongest predictors of Internet activity. In a healthcare system that is increasingly complex and fragmented, seeking additional online education is a practical option (Perez, 2009). Use of the Internet to access health information is its third most popular use, following e-mailing and researching a product online before buying it (Bull, Gaglio, McKay, & Glasgow, 2005).

However, cases abound of biased, incomplete, and inaccurate information being posted online for a variety of health conditions. There has not been adequate research to evaluate how the content that is posted on websites is actually used or incorporated into the health behaviors of users. In evaluating websites, it is important to consider the credentials of the individual(s) creating the website, whether conflict-of-interest issues exist (such as products or services being sold on the website), the visual presentation of the site, the ease of access and navigation, the reputation of the site sponsor (government, university, private business, not-for-profit organization, professional organization, health plan), how often information is updated, and whether content is provided at an appropriate literacy level (Godin, Truschel, & Singh, 2005). Nurses need to empower patients to become active partners in maintaining their own health by providing lists of reputable Internet sites and recommending sites that individualize content based on patient needs (Perez, 2009).

Research indicates that Internet discussion boards and support groups are used more often than websites that only provide education and are not participatory or interactive. This may be because websites that provide both education and support groups help build relationships between people (Wang, Walther, Pingree, & Hawkins, 2008). As one user commented, "Physicians and websites can provide the facts, but other patients can tell you what it really feels like and what to expect next" (Preece, 1999, p. 63). Although credibility is important, it is not "what differentiates influential from uninfluential advice" (Wang et al., 2008, p. 365). Empathetic communication and feeling understood are highly valued by patients. Often, the opinions of "similar others are evaluated as more powerful than expert advice" (Wang et al., 2008, p. 366). In addition to providing a feeling of being understood, support groups contribute to a sense of social identity, in that one belongs to a group of similar individuals who are managing to cope with a given health condition (Wang et al., 2008).

Internet Discussion Boards and Support Groups

Interactivity of Internet discussion boards and support groups is a key feature. Other valuable tools that are commonly seen online are: (1) assessments about health and when to contact a doctor; (2) tailored interventions based on health history, health knowledge, patient need, risk assessments, or literacy level; (3) action plans and goal-setting assistance, along with feedback to maintain behavioral change; (4) peer support; (5) personal data tracking using graphic displays: (6) monitoring by professionals or the ability to "Ask an expert" or email a healthcare professional; (7) privacy and security statements; (8) site maps, search options, glossaries, and help sections to promote ease of site navigation; and (9) a "What's new" section for updated content (Bull et al., 2005).

Various sites, including the comprehensive health enhancement support system (CHESS), provide education and support to people living with HIV/AIDS, Alzheimer's, breast cancer, heart disease, and alcoholism. An advantage that has been reported from Internet support groups is that patients are more effective at managing disease at home, schedule fewer ambulatory clinic visits, and are better prepared to talk with physicians and nurses during healthcare visits after participating in a support group (Flatley-Brennan et al., 2001).

Nevertheless, authors continue to debate the advantages and disadvantages of Internet discussion boards and support groups. Some have highlighted the poor quality of information and suggested that not all content is as accurate as education that would be obtained from a healthcare provider. Meta-analyses have shown that there is no evidence to suggest Internet discussion boards and support groups cause harm and likewise there is no substantial evidence that they provide clear benefits. One obvious advantage of Internet discussion boards is in "recalibrating power relations between patients and health professionals" and empowering patients to become active participants in their own health care (Armstrong & Powell, 2009, p. 314).

Some patients have pointed out that when inaccurate information is posted, it is quickly corrected by other patients who use the discussion board. Health professionals have expressed the opposite opinion: that inaccurate content found in Internet discussion boards and support groups can remain online for days before it is corrected (Armstrong & Powell, 2009). Patients have responded that they selectively evaluate information posted on Internet discussion boards based on their own circumstances and experience, disregarding some content and making use of other information. Online content is viewed as providing a starting point for learning that requires active and reflective engagement as well as careful consideration. Patients view online content as a way to complement formal health care rather than as an alternative to seeking professional care.

Advantages discussed by patients of online support groups include reducing the feeling of being different, creating a space for vicarious learning, and providing role modeling from peers. Internet discussion boards allow patients to feel that others can empathize with them when family and friends cannot. By hearing other people's stories, patients feel that hope exists since those individuals have been able to manage life with the same condition. Patients also point out that Internet discussion boards are a way to receive practical advice from people who have lived with the given condition for a substantial period of time (Armstrong & Powell, 2009).

Wang and colleagues (2008) suggested that the lack of physical cues in discussion boards and support groups encourages greater self-disclosure than exists in face-to-face interaction, resulting in a feeling of greater intimacy and support even though the participants are strangers. Advantages of discussion boards and support groups include access to diverse sources of information, reduction of a sense of obligation one might expect in a friendship, anonymity and stigma control, ease of access, and the ability of shy members to learn by reading postings without actively participating in the dialogue (Wang et al., 2008).

Examples of Internet Support Groups Described in the Literature

HeartCare, an Internet-based education and support service for patients recovering from coronary artery bypass graft surgery, was developed by Patricia Brennan, a leader in nursing informatics at the University of Wisconsin-Madison. It is tailored to the graduated information needs of patients based on their recovery trajectory. An individual risk profile is completed by each patient, which includes key words that link to relevant web pages to provide individualized health education (Flatley-Brennan et al., 2001).

Weeks 1 and 2 focus on recovery tasks such as wound management, identifying adverse symptoms, and personal care issues. Weeks 3 through 6 focus on activities of daily living, while weeks 7 through 12 target returning to work or school. Weeks 13 to 26 focus on lifestyle changes, including reducing risk for heart disease. Email access and an online support group are also available. Patients can post and respond to messages from other patients. Patients can also communicate via email with a cardiac recovery nurse. Why is it a good idea to provide information that is tailored to weekly patient needs?

WebTV is used to connect to the Internet, avoiding access fees. Preprogrammed access keys make navigation easy. The authors summarized that "although some may criticize computerized nursing interventions for diminishing the holistic, interpersonal nature of nursing . . . such options allow nurses to reach patients previously not reached by traditional educational approaches" (Flatley-Brennan et al., 2001, p. 706).

An Internet listserv was used to create a worldwide support group for women diagnosed with lupus. Postings were broad in scope, including those that had to do with the disease process and treatment as well as social postings about significant life events. Participants posted requests for opinions about when to seek medical care, how to manage symptoms, which research studies to believe, and how to navigate the healthcare system. Since women from around the world participated, individuals described differences among healthcare systems in multiple countries. Women discussed how lupus had affected their daily life, how they managed stresses, and how they coped with negative comments from others. Since few individuals without lupus understand the level of fatigue that can occur, women took comfort from sharing with others who had also experienced extreme fatigue and knew how that can affect daily life. Women also posted friendly banter, descriptions of major life events, recipes, and discussions of movies they had seen. New participants were welcomed by a moderator and other women then introduced themselves. An introduction was provided about avoiding computer viruses and etiquette about not reposting or sharing content from the listserv. Advantages included the fact that women had access to a variety of opinions and experiences, could access content in a timely manner, and could check the posting at a convenient time (Mendelson, 2003).

Cautions associated with using a listserv identified by Mendelson (2003) included the fact that certain search engines can link postings back to email addresses, undermining the privacy of individuals. Because membership is fluid, it is often not possible for researchers to obtain consent from participants. Extreme care must be taken when conducting studies to avoid publishing quotations that could be tracked back to an original post (Mendelson).

USE OF TECHNOLOGICAL DEVICES TO PROMOTE HEALTH

A number of technological devices have been developed that are being used to promote health and reduce medical errors in a variety of populations and settings. Mobile electronic devices (microsensors) that are woven into clothing or attached as an accessory (computerized watches, belts, glasses, key chains) are now being researched and will likely become more widely used to monitor the health of senior citizens. The advantage of these devices is that they are unobtrusive, do not interfere with physical activity, require minimal to no cognitive effort to operate, and are hands-free. A spoken command can activate or turn off the devices. Devices are being developed to monitor food consumption; falls; blood pressure; pulse rate; physical activity levels; possible emergency situations, such as not turning off the stove; hours of sleep; and wandering (Lukowicz, Kirstein, & Troster, 2004).

Data can be collected over time and healthcare providers can use the information to monitor individual patients or research how disorders develop over time in a given population. Critical data can also be transmitted to a caregiver, a family member, a neighbor, or a home-health nurse, who then checks on the elderly person (Lukowicz et al., 2004).

Pacemakers have been in use for many decades, but mobile treatment systems such as the Functional Electrical Stimulator, which uses transcutaneous electrodes made out of conductive textiles embedded in pieces of clothing, are being developed. The electrodes contract paralyzed muscles of patients with stroke and spinal cord injuries to generate or improve lost motor function (Lukowicz et al., 2004). With healthy adults, big-screen televisions and an armband can be used to track calories and activity levels during workouts. Feedback is provided about whether a target heart rate has been achieved (Snider, 2011).

The AMON wrist worn monitor is currently being researched in Europe with high-risk cardiac patients. Multiple vital signs are collected, evaluated, and transmitted to a nearby medical center when emergency conditions are recorded. The device can also assess contextual factors; for example, an increase in pulse accompanied by physical activity is evaluated as normal, while an increase in pulse during sleep triggers an alarm and emergency notification (Lukowicz et al., 2004).

In Hong Kong, a wireless motion-monitoring system placed in the home of an elderly person compares current activity to their typical activity patterns. If, for example, motion is detected in the living room at 3 AM, a monitoring center or a family member is contacted. A motion-monitoring device worn over the ear is able to detect falls and notify preidentified caregivers (Lai, Chung, Leung, Wong, & Mak, 2010). In the United States, Lifeline, My Guardian Angel Service, and a number of other monitoring devices are readily available. An emergency notification alarm, concealed in either a necklace or watch, can be pushed if the elderly person falls or needs help. Typically, the monitoring station contacts family members first, followed by neighbors and friends who have volunteered to be available to check on the person.

Microprocessors are also being placed in the caps of pill bottles (medication event monitor systems) to assess whether individuals are taking their medication as prescribed. Each time the bottle is opened, the assumption is that the person has taken their medication. Data can be downloaded monthly or at a given interval by connecting the pill bottle to a computer (Olivieri, Matsui, Hermann, & Koren, 1991). In addition, plastic, waterproof wristbands can be programmed at whatever frequency desired to signal a person to take one's medications. Such devices help control overdosing and underdosing so that medication side-effects can be avoided and compliance increased (Cramer, Mattson,Prevey, Scheyer, & Quellette, 1989).

Vocera, a wireless communication device, is being used to enable nurses to contact other healthcare professionals, communicate with individuals outside of the hospital, and receive voice mail messages. A communication badge the size of a small, lightweight cell phone can be clipped to the nurse's clothing or worn on a lanyard around one's neck. A nurse who wishes to make a call has to press a button but otherwise communication is hands-free. One does not need to know a phone number to use Vocera, as a command like "Call the pharmacy" will connect you to a given department. A name or title will also connect the nurse with the person they wish to reach. Time spent playing "phone tag" is reduced because Vocera allows for nearly immediate communication between nurses and other healthcare professionals (Breslin, Greskovich, & Turisco, 2004; Vandenkerkhof, Hall, Wilson, Gay, & Duhn, 2009).

Because communication errors have been identified as "the leading cause of in-hospital mortality, far exceeding mortality due to inadequate clinical skill," the Vocera is a welcome addition to nursing practice that results in more efficient workflow (Vandenkerkhof et al., 2009, p. 254). Studies have shown a time reduction of up to 25% for communication-related activities, a 57% decrease in time spent walking to the telephone, a 45% decrease in time spent locating other staff, a 54% decrease in time spent looking for assistance, and a 32% decrease in time spent searching for medication keys (Breslin et al., 2004; Vandenkerkhof et al.).

Barcoding has been used in grocery stores since 1930 and now has been introduced into nursing. The amount of time necessary to develop the National Drug Code, which lists the name, dose, production company, and type of packaging for each drug, explains why it took time to integrate this technology into nursing units (O'Malley, 2008).

Barcode medication administration makes use of electronic handheld devices for scanning patient identification bands to increase the safety of medication administration. The nurse reviews the medication administration record online, checks the traditional five patient rights, and scans the patient identification band and the barcode on the unit-dose medication package. The medication is then automatically recorded in the electronic medication administration record and a scan is performed to ensure accuracy of the medication. Only then is the patient given the medication (O'Malley, 2008).

Limitations associated with this method of medication administration include the small size of many patient rooms, which make it difficult to move the computer on wheels to the bedside. The paper on the patient identification band must be fluid- and stain-resistant. Sometimes multiple scans are necessary because of the curved nature of the identification band circling the wrist (McRoberts, 2005). Barcode administration of medications can decrease errors, but it can also take longer to complete all the necessary steps. Things can go wrong, such as the wrong barcode being attached to a medication or the server going down. Nevertheless, a 97% decrease in adverse drug events has been reported when every dose is scanned using this method (O'Malley, 2008).

On a population level, the Genes and Environment Initiative's Exposure Biology Program, funded by the National Institute of Environmental Health, is supporting development of a number of unobtrusive health sensors. One device that is worn by children measures gases such as ozone while recording activity data. Spatial information is simultaneously collected by a global positioning system. Another study involves measuring residential particle counts, ozone levels, and tobacco smoke, as well as endotoxin levels and metabolic activity levels, for children with asthma while also graphing the children's geographic location. An air sampling device is being developed that fits inside the nostril of a field technician who is vacuuming dust from the beds of 4- to 5-year-old children at risk of allergies or asthma. Allergens and bacterial and fungal pathogen levels are transmitted using wireless technology (http://www.gei.nih.gov /exposurebiology).

ADVANTAGES AND DISADVANTAGES OF USING TECHNOLOGY FOR HEALTH PROMOTION

A variety of advantages have been identified associated with using interactive e-health technologies to promote health. These advantages include:

1. more opportunities to tailor information to the specific needs of individuals or groups,
2. improved capability to tailor the intervention to the learning styles of the users, user interest, and particular health risks,
3. increased possibility for users to remain anonymous while seeking information and support from peers or experts about a sensitive health issue,
4. increased access to information and support on demand, and
5. enhanced ability for users to update and maintain current scientific knowledge (Atkinson & Gold, 2002, p. 495; Robinson, Patrick, Eng, & Gustafson, 1998).

In simulation, Internet gaming, and virtual reality, participants can vicariously experience the positive and negative consequences of behavioral choices without having to engage in risky behavior. Simulation, Internet gaming, and virtual reality scenarios require active involvement and can be revisited to reinforce learning. Online support groups, telehealth, and text messaging allow for asynchronous communication that fits the schedules of busy individuals. "Technology has enabled people unable to hear to watch television (captioning technology), people unable to see to read (screen readers), and people unable to speak to communicate their ideas (Stephen Hawking)" (Atkinson & Gold, 2002, p. 499). Virtual reality experiences, cell phone communication, text messaging, and online support groups have the potential to reach large numbers of people at relatively low cost while encouraging active engagement in health promotion activities.

It is also the case that many technological interventions are costly to develop, update, and maintain. Several are reliant on the user being able to afford fast Internet access. Being able to select and use proper search terms, along with having the skill to distinguish actionable from questionable content, is a necessity. Some patients can become overwhelmed with the amount of information that is online. Acceptability of Internet use varies depending on the age, literacy level, and learning style of the user (Atkinson & Gold, 2002). It is likely that issues of unequal access will diminish over time, but at present there are still socioeconomic, geographic, gender, age and ethnic/racial inequities that exist. Unless access issues are addressed, technology could exacerbate health disparities rather than narrow them (Skinner, Maley, & Norman, 2010).

Some authors have suggested that while technological approaches "are useful in provoking an initial reaction, they are inferior to other forms of health-promotion instruction, without the appropriate follow-up and support services" (Clarke, 1999; Whitehead, 2000, p. 809). Others have questioned when reminders and tips sent by cell phone and text messaging move from being motivational to being intrusive or to advice giving (Thede, 2008). Overreliance on technology can result in transferring excessive responsibility for maintaining health to patients while undermining funding for care that is provided by healthcare professionals. Finally, delays in seeking medical and nursing care can result because a person has tried a product or service advertised on the Internet based on misleading or false claims. Furthermore, users have "little knowledge or control over what happens to personal information" entered on Internet health assessment sites, which may place them at risk (Robinson et al., 1998, p. 1265).

CONCLUSION

A major driving force in the use of informatics is increased demand for services, limited numbers of healthcare providers, inconsistent access to care, and a need to manage escalating healthcare costs and improve the quality of care that is to be provided. With 17% of the U.S. gross domestic product being spent on health care, it is important now more than ever for nursing professionals to take an active role in improving the quality of patient care and influencing meaningful healthcare reform through the use of informatics.

Some authors believe technology is a neutral tool that can be used in whatever way the creator desires. Still others suggest that technology has a life of its own that ends up changing the character of nursing practice (Johnson, 2000). Individuals have also suggested that technology is just a natural extension of nursing that can be easily integrated into daily practice. Others argue that technology is irreconcilable with the culture and values of nursing, which emphasize the connection between nurse and patient (Sandelowski, 1997). However, everyone agrees that technology will change the ways that nursing and health promotion are practiced. As C. Everett Koop, a former U.S. Surgeon General, commented, "Cutting edge technology, especially in communication and information transfer, will enable the greatest advances yet in public health" (Geiger et al., 2002, p. 401).

The relationship between nursing and technology is so complicated that Dr. Margarette Sandelowski, a leader in the area, has devoted two books and a multitude of articles to the subject. Schulz (1980) reflected that nursing and technology are symbiotically and "inexorably linked" (p. 211). Nurses "serve as the primary users and machine-body tenders in health care" (Sandelowski, 1999, p. 198). This close connection is viewed at varied times as one of two opposing paradigms that see nursing as either synonymous with technology or as being in conflict with technology.

Connected with the first view are historical precedents in which nurses were seen as performing manual labor, as mindlessly carrying out physician orders, as being part of the instrumentation of hospitals, and "acting as monitors of the unit or ward atmosphere" (Barnard & Sandelowski, 2001, p. 372). These perspectives began to change after World War II, when nurses began to embrace technology to make their work more visible, to increase their social and scientific standing, and to increase their power and prestige. Technology came to be seen as the embodiment of both scientific progress and professional development. Best practices were adopted; conformity was valued; sameness of product, process, policy, and thought were highlighted; and efficiency became the goal (Barnard & Sandelowski, 2001).

According to the second paradigm, technology was presented as a culprit and dehumanizing force as well as a driving force behind impersonal nursing care. Technology was credited with separating nurses from their moral mandate of providing humane care, as turning the focus to care of the machines rather than the patient, as shaping the way nursing is done, as blurring the boundaries between animate and inanimate, and creating a schism between self and body (Barnard & Sandelowski, 2001; Sandelowski, 1999). In this perspective, technology was viewed as having agency, biography, "language, idiosyncratic quirks, and inclinations" (Barnard & Sandelowski, 2001, p. 369). Machines in this perspective took on the work of the nurse, de-skilled the profession, and diminished the expertise within nursing practice. Intuition and expertise were marginalized by technology. Nurses were moved farther and farther from the bedside. Patients were objectified. Nurses treated the re-representation of the patient "in the form of a rhythm strip" or an X-ray, not the patient (Barnard & Sandelowski, 2001, p. 369).

These two perspectives and the debates that surround them are central to the identity of nursing. But it is also important to remember that the role ascribed to technology depends on historical, social, cultural, and perhaps gender-based perspectives. The "potential and power of a technological device to shape an interaction is not pregiven but is realized in practice" (Timmermans, 1998, p. 148). It is "not technology per se but rather how individual technologies operate in specific user contexts, the meanings attributed to them, and how any group defines what is human as well as the organizational, human, political and economic technological systems (technique)" that matter (Barnard & Sandelowski, 2001, p. 367).

It is technique, not technology, that is of primary importance. Technique emphasizes the rational, the efficient, the standardized, and the specialized over individual uniqueness, cultural differences, and human dignity. Technique is a stance that results in treating patients as extensions of or proxies for machinery. Nurses do not need to allow technique to dominate their practice irrespective of the level of technology that is used (Barnard & Sandelowski, 2001).

Many nursing leaders have stressed that nurses can choose to navigate the space between technology and caring. They have claimed that nurses can maintain "humane care in technological environments" (Barnard & Sandelowski, 2001, p. 372). Do you agree it is possible to navigate this balance? In order to navigate the space between technology and caring, it is clear that nurses must create for themselves the space to reflect on their practice. They must make time to sit on committees and hold positions that influence how technology will shape their everyday life and the culture of their workplaces. Nurses must become active at the national level, lobbying for change that promotes the health of the nation, opens access for all people, and shapes how technology will impact practice.

DISCUSSION QUESTIONS

1. Which informatics intervention described in this chapter would be the most costly to provide? Which is likely to be the least expensive?
2. Which technology or intervention would be the most likely and least likely to be accepted by older adults?
3. What are the main considerations nurses should weigh when designing a health promotion program using informatics?
4. What are the advantages and disadvantages of active governmental involvement in the development and implementation of healthcare technology?
5. How does technology shape the very definition and nature of nursing practice?
6. How might the increasing focus on technology have a negative impact on professional autonomy, patient–provider relationships, and individualized care?

7. Are pay-for-performance incentives in nursing and medicine a good idea or not? Explain your answer.

8. Why do Medicare and Medicaid guidelines influence private insurance reimbursement practices?

9. How does telehealth address the problem of a lack of healthcare providers?

10. How might telehealth influence nurse–patient ratios in the future?

11. Given that the scope of nursing practice varies by state, how should telehealth interventions be monitored if provided across state lines?

12. Why would people be more likely to share embarrassing or sensitive health information with a computer rather than a provider?

13. How does the availability of health information online affect the power balance between patients and providers?

14. Which nursing organizations and initiatives advocate for greater use of informatics?

15. How have EHRs influenced malpractice litigation as it relates to nursing charting?

16. How have EHRs facilitated collection of population-level data and evidence-based medicine?

17. Why are EHRs often incompatible between healthcare systems?

18. Are automated safety checks as part of an EHR a good thing or not? Explain your answer.

19. Do dropdown menus in EHR charting systems save time and increase precision or not? Explain your answer.

20. Can the structured format of an EHR charting system change the critical thinking of nurses or physicians? How might that happen?

CHECK YOUR UNDERSTANDING: EXERCISE ONE

What disadvantages might there be in the adoption of a national scope of practice for RNs and APNs? Which duties would be eliminated from the scope of practice of RNs and APNs in your state if national licensure were enacted based on the most conservative scope of practice within any state in the United States? Which lobbying groups might become involved in decisions to change nursing practice acts in the states?

CHECK YOUR UNDERSTANDING: EXERCISE TWO

Match the following laws and agencies with their primary purpose.

Laws/Agencies
1. Medicare Improvements for Patients and Providers Act of 2008
2. Healthy People 2010
3. The Nurse Practice Act
4. American Recovery and Reinvestment Act of 2009
5. The National Coordinator For Health Information Technology
6. HITECH Act
7. Stage 3 of the Center for Medicaid Services

Purposes
A. Increasing efficiency and reducing cost
B. Requiring patient access to self management tools
C. Providing incentives and penalties for hospitals and physicians who adopt or do not adopt e-prescribing
D. Providing guidance regarding the quality of health-related websites
E. Governing the billing of telehealth services for nurses
F. Providing Medicare bonuses to physicians who use e-prescribing and report quality outcome measures
G. Providing funding for clinical decision-making prompts and electronic exchange of healthcare records

CHECK YOUR UNDERSTANDING: EXERCISE THREE

Match the informatics innovations that follow with the most appropriate description of the innovation.

Informatics Innovation

1. Avatars
2. Simulators
3. Interactive health games
4. Embodied conversational agents
5. Wellnavi
6. The AMON monitor
7. Medication event monitor systems
8. VOCERA

Description of the Innovation

A. Activities to evaluate health risks and consequences
B. Three-dimensional personalities used to teach health education
C. A wireless communication device for providers
D. Microprocessors to access whether individuals open a pill bottle
E. An animated talking head with facial expressions
F. Human-sized mannequins that have vital signs and a voice
G. A cell phone for photographing food consumption
H. A wristwatch that collects and transmits vital signs

CHECK YOUR UNDERSTANDING: EXERCISE FOUR

Interview a nurse who did paper charting and then converted to electronic charting. Ask the nurse whether he or she felt it takes more or less time to chart after implementation of EHRs. Inquire about whether the nurse has ever been questioned about an EHR entry.

WHAT DO YOU THINK?

1. How would you use informatics to promote health if you had the funds to design any intervention you wanted to implement? What population would you target?

2. Think about how you locate health-related information when you want to manage a health issue. What sources do you use to seek health-related information? Which of those sources rely on or make use of technology?

3. Do you think the most critical preparation for a career in informatics would be a degree in nursing or a degree in computer science? Provide rationale for your answer.

4. How will future development and expansion of healthcare technology impact your nursing practice?

5. Do you think telehealth monitors within a person's home "medicalizes" his/her home? Explain your answer.

6. If you had a simulation lab in your nursing program, comment on what you liked and did not like about simulation.

7. Which EHR functions have your used in obtaining your own health care?

8. Have you worked in a hospital during a period when the EHR was "down" or "unavailable?" What backup systems were used for charting?

9. Have you or any of your family or friends ever been notified that your health information had been inadvertently disclosed? How would you feel if that happened?

10. Have you ever seen inaccurate or incomplete health education online? Describe what you found.

11. Have you ever taken a health risk assessment online? What was that like?

12. Do you agree that nursing and technology are symbiotically linked? Why or why not?

REFERENCES

American Nurses Association. (2008). *Nursing informatics: Scope and standards of practice*. Silver Spring, MD: Author.

American Telemedicine Association. (2012). *Telemedicine defined*. Retrieved from http://www.american telemed.org/i4a/pages/index.cfm?pageid=3333

Armstrong, N., & Powell, J. (2010). Patient perspectives on health advice posted on Internet discussion boards: A qualitative study. *Health Expectations, 12*, 313–320.

Atkinson, N. L., & Gold, R. S. (2002). The promise and challenge of e-Health interventions. *American Journal of Health Behavior, 26*(6), 494–503.

Balfour, D. C., Evans, S., Januska, J., Lee, H. Y., Lewis, S. J., Nolan, S. R., . . . Thapar, K. (2009). Health information technology: Results from a roundtable discussion. *Journal of Managed Care Pharmacy, 15*(1 Suppl A), S10–S17.

Bantz, D., Dancer, M. M., Hodson-Carlton, K., & Van Hove, S. (2007). A daylong clinical laboratory: From gaming to high-fidelity simulators. *Nurse Educator, 32*(6), 274–277.

Barnard, A., & Sandelowski, M. (2001). Technology and humane nursing care: (Ir)reconcilable or invented difference? *Journal of Advanced Nursing, 34*(3), 367–375.

Baxter, P., Akhtar-Danesh, N., Valaitis, R., Stanyon, W., & Sproul, S. (2009). Simulated experiences: Nursing students share their perspectives. *Nurse Educator Today, 29*(8), 859–866.

Benner, P., Tanner, C., & Chesla, C. (1996). *Expertise in nursing practice: Caring, clinical judgment and ethics*. New York, NY: Springer.

Biddiss, E. & Irwin, J. (2010). Active video games to promote physical activity in children and youth: A systematic review. *Archives of Pediatric and Adolescent Medicine, 164*(7), 664–672.

Blake, H. (2008a). Innovation in practice: Mobile phone technology in patient care. *British Journal of Community Nursing, 13*(4), 160–165.

Blake, H. (2008b). Mobile phone technology in chronic disease management. *Nursing Standard, 23*(12), 43–46.

Bloomrosen, M., Starren, J., Lorenzi, N. M., Ash, J. S., Patel, V. L., & Shortliffe, E. H. (2011). Anticipating and addressing the unintended consequences of health IT and policy: A report from the AIMA 2009 Health Policy Meeting. *Journal of the American Medical Informatics Association, 18*, 82–90.

Breslin, S., Greskovich, W., & Turisco, F. (2004). Wireless technology improves nursing workflow and communications. *Computers, Informatics, Nursing, 22*(5), 275–281.

Bull, S. S., Gaglio, B., McKay, H. G., & Glasgow, R. E. (2005). Harnessing the potential of the Internet to promote chronic illness self-management: Diabetes as an example of how well we are doing. *Chronic Illness, 1*, 143–155.

Carlfjord, S., Nilsen, P., Leijon, M., Andersson, A., Johansson, K., & Bendtsen, P. (2009). Computerized lifestyle intervention in routine primary health care: Evaluation of usage on provider and responder needs. *Patient Education and Counseling, 75*(2), 238–243.

Chaudhry, B., Wang, J., Wu, S., Maglione, M., Mojica, W., Roth, E., . . . Shekelle, P. G. (2006). Systematic review: Impact of health information technology on quality, efficiency, and costs of medical care. *Annuals of Internal Medicine, 144*(10), 742–752.

Clarke, A. (1999). Changing attitudes through persuasive communication. *Nursing Standard, 13*(30), 45–47.

Congressional Research Service (2010). Bill summary & status: H.R.3590. Retrieved from http://thomas.loc .gov/cgi-bin/bdquery/z?d111:HR03590:@@@D&summ2=m&

Consolvo, S., Everitt, K., Smith, I., & Landay, J. (2006, April). *Design requirements for technologies that encourage physical activity*. Paper presented at the CHI: Designing for Tangible Interactions, Montreal, Quebec, Canada.

Cramer, J. A., Mattson, R. H., Prevey, M. L., Scheyer, R. D., & Quellette, V. L. (1989). How often is medication taken as prescribed? A novel assessment technique. *JAMA, 261*(22), 3273–3277.

DeSantis, S. (2009). Nursing informatics and nursing education. In D. McGonigle & K. Mastrian (Eds.), *Nursing informatics and the foundation of knowledge.* (pp. 339–340). Sudbury, MA: Jones and Bartlett.

Dixon, B. E., & Newlon, C. M. (2010). How do future nursing educators perceive informatics: Advancing the nursing informatics agenda through dialogue? *Journal of Professional Nursing, 26*(2), 82–89.

Edlund, J., & Beskow, J. (2009). Mushy Peek: A framework for online investigation of audiovisual dialogue phenomena. *Language and Speech, 52*(2/3), 351–367.

Flatley-Brennan, P., Moore, S. M., Bjornsdottir, G., Jones, J., Visovsky, C., & Rogers, M. (2001). HeartCare: An Internet-based information and support system for patient home recovery after coronary artery bypass graft surgery. *Journal of Advanced Nursing, 35*(5), 699–708.

Foley, L. & Maddison, R. (2010). Use of active video games to increase physical activity in children: A virtual reality? *Pediatric Exercise Science, 22*(1), 7–20.

Geiger, B. F., Petri, C. J., Myers, O., Lan, J., Binkley, D., Aldrige, C. R., & Berdebes, J. (2002). Using technology to teach health: A collaborative pilot project in Alabama. *Journal of School Health, 72*(10), 401–407.

Godin, S., Truschel, J., & Singh, V. (2005). Assessing quality assurance of self-help sites on the Internet. *Journal of Prevention And Intervention In The Community, 29*(1/2), 67–84.

Goldstein, N. M. & Thorpe, J. H. (2010). The first anniversary of the health information technology for economic and clinical health (HITECH) act: The regulatory outlook for implementation. *Perspectives in Health Information Management, 7*(pii.), 1c. PMCID: PMC2921301.

Goran, S. F. (2010). A second set of eyes: An introduction to tele-ICU. *Critical Care Nurse, 30*(4), 46–56.

Graf, D. L., Pratt, L. V., Hester, C. N., & Short, K. R. (2009). Playing active video games increases energy expenditure in children. *Pediatrics, 124*, 534–540.

Graybeal, K. B. (2009). A winning course with nursing informatics. *Nursing Management,* 19–22.

Gregg, L., & Tarrier, N. (2007). Virtual reality in mental health. *Social Psychiatry and Psychiatric Epidemiology, 42*, 343–534.

Gruber, J. (2007). *Public Finance and Public Policy* (2nd ed.). New York, NY: Worth.

Hannah, K., & Ball, M. (2006). *Introduction to nursing informatics.* New York, NY: Springer-Verlag.

Hansen, M. M. (2008). Versatile, immersive, creative, and dynamic virtual 3-D health care learning environments: A review of the literature. *Journal of Medical Internet Research, 10*(3), e26. doi: 10.e196/jmir.1051

Health Information Technology for Economic and Clinical Health (HITECH) Act, Title XIII of Division A and Title IV of Division B of the American Recovery and Reinvestment Act of 2009 (ARRA), Pub. L. No. 111-5, 123 Stat. 226 (Feb. 17, 2009), *codified at* 42 U.S.C. §§300jj *et seq.*; §§17901 *et seq.*

Hebda, T, Czar, P, & Mascara, C. (2005). *Handbook of informatics for nurses and healthcare professionals.* Upper Saddle River, NJ: Pearson Prentice Hall.

Heron, K. E., & Smyth, J. M. (2010). Ecological momentary interventions: Incorporating mobile technology into psychosocial and health behavior treatments. *British Journal of Health Psychology, 15*, 1–39.

Institute of Medicine [IOM]. (2003). *Key capabilities of an electronic health record system.* Retrieved from http://www.iom.edu/Reports/2003/Key-Capabilities-of-an-Electronic-Health-Record-System.aspx

Johnson, P. G. (2000). Considering technology: Living and working in a technocratic society. *Journal of Midwifery and Women's Health, 45*(1), 79–80.

Kahn, J., Kronick, R., Kreger, M. & Gans, D. (2005). The cost of health insurance administration in California: Estimates for insurers, physicians, and hospitals. *Health Affairs, 24*(6), 1629–1639.

Kato, P. M., Cole, S. W., Bradlyn, A. S., & Pollock, B. H. (2008). A video game improves behavioral outcomes in adolescents and young adults with cancer: A randomized trial. *Pediatrics, 122*, 305–317.

King, A. C., Ahn, D. K., Oliveria, B. M., Atienza, A. A., Castro, C. M., & Gardner, C. (2008). Promoting physical activity through hand-held computer technology. *American Journal of Preventive Medicine, 34*, 138–142.

Lai, C., Chung, J., Leung, N., Wong, J., & Mak, D. (2010). A survey of older Hong Kong peoples' perceptions of telecommunication technologies and telecare devices. *Journal of Telemedicine and Telecare, 16,* 441–446.

Lee, J. C. & Lau, D. T. (2009). Health information technology and the American Recovery and Reinvestment Act: Some challenges ahead. [Editorial]. *Clinical Therapeutics, 31*(6), 1276–1278.

Lukowicz, P., Kirstein, T., & Troster, G. (2004). Wearable systems for healthcare applications. *Methods of Information in Medicine, 43,* 232–238.

Mackert, M., & Whitten, P. (2007). Successful adoption of a school-based telemedicine system. *Journal of School Health, 77*(6), 327–330.

Majette, G. (2009). From concierge medicine to patient-centered medical homes: International lessons & the search for a better way to deliver primary health care in the U.S. *American Journal of Law & Medicine, 35*(4), 585–619.

Max, W. (2007). Economic analysis in health care. In C. Harrington & C. Estes (Eds.), *Health policy: Crisis and reform in the U.S. health care delivery system* (5th ed., pp. 260–270). Sudbury, MA: Jones and Bartlett.

McGarry, J., & Nairn, S. (2005). Is telemedicine effective? *Primary Health Care, 15*(2), 21–23.

McGonigle, D., & Mastrian, K. (2009). *Nursing informatics and the foundation of knowledge.* Sudbury, MA: Jones and Bartlett.

McRoberts, S. (2005). The use of bar code technology in medication administration. *Clinical Nurse Specialist, 19*(2), 55–56.

Mendelson, C. (2003). Gentle hugs: Internet listservs as sources of support for women with Lupus. *Advances in Nursing Science, 26*(4), 299–306.

Middleton, B. (2005). Achieving U.S. information technology adoption: The need for a third hand. *Health Affairs, 24*(5), 1269–1272.

Moore, D., Cheng, Y., McGrath, P., & Powell, N. J. (2005). Collaborative virtual environment technology for people with autism. *Focus on Autism and Other Developmental Disabilities, 20*(4), 231–243.

Noll, J. G., Shenk, C. E., Barnes, J. E. & Putnam, F. W. (2009). Childhood abuse, avatar choices, and other risk factors associated with Internet-initiated victimization of adolescent girls. *Pediatrics, 123*(6), e1078–e1083.

Olivieri, N. F., Matsui, D., Hermann, C., & Koren, G. (1991). Compliance assessed by the medication event monitoring system, *Archives of Disease in Childhood, 66,* 1399–1402.

O'Malley, P. (2008). Think bar-code medication administration eliminates adverse drug events? Think again! *Clinical Nurse Specialist, 22*(6), 269–270.

Park, I. H., Kim, J. J., Ku, J., Jang, H. J., Park, S., Kim, C., . . . Sim, S. I. (2009). Characteristics of social anxiety from virtual interpersonal interactions in patients with schizophrenia. *Psychiatry, 72*(1), 79–93.

Parr, M. B., & Sweeney, N. M. (2006). Use of human patient simulation in an undergraduate critical care course. *Critical Care Nursing Quarterly, 29*(3), 188–198.

Perez, E. (2009). e-Health: How to make the right choice. *Nursing Forum, 44*(4), 277–282.

Pike, T., & O'Donnell, V. (2010). The impact of clinical simulation on learner self-efficacy in preregistration nursing education. *Nurse Educator Today, 30*(5), 405–410.

Preece, J. (1999). Empathic communities: Balancing emotional and factual communication. *Interacting with Computers, 12,* 63–77.

Reed, K. (2005). Telemedicine: Benefits to advanced practice nursing and the communities they serve. *Journal of the American Academy of Nurse Practitioners. 17*(5), 176–180.

Reilly, A., & Spratt, C. (2007). The perceptions of undergraduate student nurses of high-fidelity simulation-based learning: A case report from the University of Tasmania. *Nurse Educator Today, 27*(6), 542–550.

Robinson, T. N., Patrick, K., Eng, T. R., & Gustafson, D. (1998). An evidence-based approach to interactive health communication: A challenge to medicine in the information age. *JAMA, 280*(14), 1264–1269.

Sandelowski, M. (1997). Irreconcilable differences? The debate concerning nursing and technology. *Image: The Journal of Nursing Scholarship, 29*(2), 169–174.

Sandelowski, M. (1999). Troubling distinctions: A semiotics of the nursing/technology relationship. *Nursing Inquiry, 6,* 198–207.

Scheuermann, R. H. & Milgrom, H. (2010). Personalized care, comparative effectiveness research and the electronic health record. *Current Opinions In Clinical Immunology, 10,* 168–170.

Schoening, A. M., Sittner, B. J., & Todd, M. J. (2006). Simulated clinical experience: Nursing students' perceptions and the educator's role. *Nurse Educator, 31*(6), 253–258.

Schulz, J. K. (1980). Nursing and technology. *Medical Instrumentation, 14,* 211–214.

Sensmeier, J. (2010). Alliance for nursing informatics statement to the Robert Wood Johnson Foundation Initiative on the Future of Nursing: Acute care, focusing on the area of technology. *Computers, Informatics, Nursing,* 63–67.

Shreve, J., Van Den Bos, J., Gray, T., Halford, M., Rustagi, K. & Ziemkiewicz, E. (2010). *The economic measurement of medical errors.* Retrieved from http://www.soa.org/research/health/research-econ-measurement .aspx

Simpson, R. L. (2002). Issues in telemedicine: Why is policy still light-years behind technology? *Nursing Administration Quarterly, 26*(4), 81–84.

Skinner, H. A., Maley, O, & Norman, C. D. (2006). Developing internet-based e-health promotion programs: The spiral technology action research (STAR) model. *Health Promotion Practice, 7*(4), 406–417.

Snider, M. (2011, January 19). New health technology may be the best medicine. *USA Today,* p. 4D.

Taylor, R., Bower, A., Girosi, F., Bogelow, J., Fonkych, K., & Hillestad, R. (2005). Promoting health information technology: Is there a case for more aggressive government action? *Health Affairs, 24*(5), 1234–1245.

Tellez, M., Spetz, J., Seago, J., Harrington, C. & Kitchener, M. (2008). Do wages matter? A backward bend in the 2004 California RN labor supply. *Policy, Politics, & Nursing Practice, 10*(3), 195–203.

Thede, L. (2008). Summer institute on nursing informatics 2008: Building connections for patient-centered records. *Computers, Informatics, Nursing,* 307–310.

Timmermans, S. (1998). Resuscitation technology in the emergency department: Towards a dignified death. *Sociology of Health and Illness, 20,* 144–167.

U.S. Department of Health and Human Services (2000). With understanding and improving health and objectives for improving health. *Healthy People 2010.* Retrieved from http://www.healthypeople.gov

Vandenkerkhof, E. G., Hall, S., Wilson, R., Gay, A., & Duhn, L. (2009). Evaluation of an innovative communication technology in an acute care setting. *Computers, Informatics, Nursing, 27*(4), 254–262.

Vidrine, D., Arduino, R., Lazev, A., & Gritz, E. (2006). A randomized trial of proactive cellular telephone interaction for smokers living with HIV/AIDS. *AIDS, 20*(2), 253–260.

Wang, D., Kogashiwa, M., & Kris, S. (2006). Development of a new instrument for evaluating individual's dietary intakes. *Journal of the American Dietary Association, 106*(10), 1588–1593.

Wang, Z., Walther, J. B., Pingree, S., & Hawkins, R. P. (2008). Health information, credibility, homophily, and influence on the Internet: Websites versus discussion groups. *Health Communication, 23,* 358–368.

West, V. L. & Milio, N. (2004). Organizational and environmental factors affecting the utilization of telemedicine in rural home health care. *Home Health Services Quarterly, 23*(4), 49–67.

Whitehead, D. (2000). Using mass media within health-promoting practice: A nursing perspective. *Journal of Advanced Nursing, 32*(4), 807–816.

Woolhandler, S., Campbell, T., & Himmelstein, D. (2003). Costs of health care administration in the United States and Canada. *New England Journal of Medicine, 349*(8), 768–775.

Yellowlees, P., Marks, S., Hogarth, M., & Turner, S. (2008). Standards-based open-source electronic health record systems: A desirable future for the U.S. health industry. *Telemedicine and e-Health, 14*(3), 284–288.

For a full suite of assignments and additional learning activities, see the access code at the front of your book.

CHAPTER 10

Evaluation, Research, and Measurement in Health Promotion Practice

Bonnie Raingruber

OBJECTIVES

At the conclusion of this chapter, the student will be able to:

- Discuss why it is challenging to conduct research and program evaluation related to health promotion.
- Apply principles of health promotion while critiquing research and evaluation strategies.
- Distinguish between formative, process, outcome, and impact evaluation.
- Identify when to use which research design.
- Discuss challenges associated with and the reasons for pay-for-performance evaluations.
- Analyze reasons for and arguments against use of QALYs.
- Describe two advantages of using logic models to plan and evaluate health promotion programs.
- Discuss the advantages and challenges associated with electronic evaluation measures.
- Critique common outcomes used in health promotion evaluations.
- Summarize why reliability, validity, utility, appropriateness, responsiveness, precision, interpretability, acceptability, and feasibility need to be considered when selecting an evaluation instrument.
- Discuss the advantages and disadvantages of objective and self-report measures.
- Critique an assortment of health promotion measures.
- Evaluate your own approach to health promotion using the Self as Role Model in Health Promotion Scale.

INTRODUCTION

Researchers claim that the evaluation phase is one of the most neglected and critical components of health promotion practice (Whitehead, 2002). The future of the discipline has been tied to the ability to develop sound evaluation strategies (Downie, Tannahill, & Tannahill, 1996). It is vital to use appropriate methods of measuring and evaluating health promotion programs if the new discipline is to be viewed as a credible science, command adequate resources, contribute to future program development, implement interventions that work in specific communities, disseminate effective outcomes and processes, and add to the research literature (Learmonth & Mackie, 2000; Tones & Green, 2004; Whitehead, 2002).

Researchers have stressed that because health promotion is a new field, innovative evaluation approaches and indicators are needed (Lima et al., 2007). However, research and program evaluation within health promotion are both very challenging tasks because health promotion is a relatively new discipline. Although the next 10 years will yield substantial growth, at present the research base and methods of program evaluation within health promotion are not yet clearly developed. Some of the outcome measures that have been published have been inappropriate for the given health promotion program, are overly simplistic, are not tested in the population in which they are being used, are lacking in reliability/validity, or deemed irrelevant by stakeholders and community members affected by the given intervention (Lima et al.).

Health promotion is a broad concept that covers the spectrum of disease prevention; treatment; and promotion of physical, mental, social, and emotional well-being. Such a broad spectrum of intervention requires methods of evaluation and measurement that are wide-reaching, diverse, and complex. Kaplan and Anderson (1996) identified several major dimensions of health that need to be addressed: physical status, functional ability, psychological status or well-being, social functioning, economic/environmental factors, and religious/spiritual influences.

Researchers have argued that examining risk factors to the exclusion of health-promoting or salutogenic factors is misguided (Antonovsky, 1996; Bauer et al., 2006). These researchers argue for adopting a person-centered approach to evaluation, not just a disease-oriented focus. They stress the need to target health resources and positive health conditions (salutogenic factors) along with risk factors and disease (pathogenic factors). The need to measure and evaluate the effect of supportive personal relationships, a sense of purpose, resilience to stress, positive self-image, and well-developed coping abilities is emphasized.

Oftentimes the outcomes of a health promotion program are not seen for years. For example, the effectiveness of dietary education on heart disease offered in an elementary or high school would not influence the rate of coronary artery disease or heart attack for 20 to 30 years. A cancer education program might not influence young women's likelihood of receiving mammography until age 30 to 40 (Macdonald, Veen, & Tones, 1996). For that reason, both short-term and long-term outcomes must be included in health promotion program evaluations. Continuing to monitor for 6 months or longer after the end of the program is common to determine if the effects can be maintained over time (Glanz, Rimer, & Lewis, 2002).

Researchers have criticized combining measures of behaviors, affect, attitudes, and knowledge into a single measure of health promotion behavior. This argument rests on the concern that specific dimensions of health promotion have not been adequately identified and documented in the literature. Other researchers have made the opposite argument, highlighting the need to evaluate a broad spectrum of awareness, knowledge, belief, attitudes, support systems, and actions because each of these factors can influence whether a person changes their behavior (Kulbok, Baldwin, Cox, & Duffy, 1997).

Recommendations for focusing simultaneously on multiple health behavior changes and the interrelationships among them rather than single-behavior interventions make research and program evaluation quite challenging (Prochaska, Spring, & Nigg, 2008). In addition, context has a major impact on whether a health promotion program is effective. However, contextual and environmental influences, because of their subtle aspects, are difficult to measure. The World Health Organization (WHO) has argued for adopting evaluation approaches that consider the input of multiple individuals, relevant communities, and varied environments while using all relevant quantitative and qualitative methodologies (Lima et al., 2007).

Stokolos (1996) stressed that health promotion programs must be evaluated using both scientific and social validity:

> Scientific validity refers to the methodological rigor and theoretical adequacy of a research or intervention program. For example, internal validity is the extent to which program outcomes are attributable to treatment conditions rather than to extraneous variables, whereas external validity is the extent to which research findings can be generalized from one intervention site to other specified populations, environments, and time intervals. An alternative, yet complementary, criterion for evaluating research and intervention programs is social validity. Social validity refers to the societal value and practical significance of the research or intervention program . . . how economically feasible is it, how likely it is to benefit a broad segment of the population, how unlikely is it to cause adverse side effects, and how consistent is it with public priorities. (p. 294)

It is also important to select relevant exclusion and inclusion criteria and to over-recruit high-risk and diverse subgroups so that a representative sample can be obtained. Health professionals need to brainstorm about all the possible mediating or extraneous variables that could affect an outcome and design a way to measure those variables. Involving community members or those who will adopt the health promotion program in the planning stage is also crucial if it is going to be widely used and continued over time.

However, if the proposed health promotion intervention is too complex, it may be hard to implement and it may be delivered in a manner that is not consistent among all those who are involved. This is called a type III error and should be avoided (Glanz et al., 2002).

Whitehead (2003) has emphasized the importance of evaluation by stressing that it is important to design "health promotion programs around an evaluation strategy rather than the other way around" (p. 494). He has argued for careful planning about the purpose of evaluation, the setting in which the evaluation will be conducted, the resources available to support evaluation, who will conduct the evaluation, whether stakeholder perspectives are included, the selection of appropriate outcome measures, and the need for a plan for how dissemination of outcomes will occur.

HEALTH PROMOTION EVALUATION PRINCIPLES

Stakeholder involvement in identifying, gathering, evaluating, and disseminating credible evidence is a principle that is consistent with health promotion values. The Centers for Disease Control and Prevention (CDC) and the WHO have both supported stakeholder involvement in program evaluation and/or health promotion research (CDC, 1999). The Institute of Medicine (IOM) supports collecting data that is "respectful of and responsive to individual patient preferences, need, and values and ensuring that patient values guide clinical decisions" (Deutscher, Hart, Dickstein, Horn, & Gutvirtz, 2008, p. 271). A main reason for this recommendation is that client reports of functional outcomes have differed substantially from clinician ratings of health-related improvement (Deutscher et al., 2008).

In 2002, the Society of Behavioral Medicine formed a special interest group to support the principle of examining interventions that target multiple health behaviors simultaneously. This focus is similar to the concept of "bundling" of services in telecommunications companies, in which complimentary interventions are packaged together for maximum effectiveness—for example, stop-smoking campaigns can be paired with interventions designed to prevent weight gain. Evidence indicates that focusing on multiple behaviors works better than targeting single-behavior interventions (Prochaska, et al., 2008).

Thirty-three percent of adults have one risk factor for disease, 41% have two risk factors and 17% have three or more risk factors for disease (Fine et al., 2004, p. 20). These risk factors include smoking, alcohol or drug abuse, physical inactivity, poor diet, lack of regular medical screenings, risky sexual behaviors, not wearing helmets and/or seatbelts, and mental health issues. Protective interventions such as completing mammography, colonoscopy, cholesterol testing, blood pressure monitoring, glucose screening, and HIV testing are positive health behaviors that are relevant targets for intervention in multiple health behavior change efforts (Fine et al., 2004; Prochaska, et al., 2008).

Even though focusing on multiple interventions simultaneously makes sense clinically, it also poses several research and measurement-related challenges. It is never clear which intervention of the many that were packaged together was the "cause" of any behavioral change. It is difficult to decide if multiple behaviors should be targeted concurrently or if one intervention should come before the other. Is the order determined by intervening with the behavior that represents the most severe risk first or the one the participants are most willing to change first (Prochaska et al., 2008)?

Researchers have argued that environmental influences, clinical relevance, equity, and community empowerment should also be considered when designing evaluations for health promotion studies (South & Tilford, 2000). The International Union for Health Promotion and Education (IUHPE) conducted a study that was funded by the European Union to examine the quality of evaluation research within health promotion disciplines. Based on the results of that study, the IUHPE advocated for using case-control groups; pre/posttesting measures; triangulation of qualitative and quantitative evaluations; and the inclusion of formative, process, and summative measures (Macdonald et al., 1996).

TYPES OF EVALUATION

It is common to consider formative evaluation, process evaluation, outcome evaluation, and impact evaluation when designing a health promotion program. In fact, these types of evaluation are seen in both research and program evaluation. Formative evaluation occurs during the process of program planning and it examines individuals who are aware of and will access the health promotion program as well as perceptions of stakeholders about the anticipated program effectiveness. Formative evaluation can consist of surveys, baseline data, qualitative interviews, or data gathering that is needed to design a quality program (Healey & Zimmerman, 2010). Numerous federal agencies, including the Health Resources and Services Administration, require formative data be included in each grant application to document the need for the proposed health promotion program.

Process evaluation occurs during program implementation. Process evaluation is designed to evaluate how the intervention is conducted and whether the program is being implemented as planned; it is used to evaluate the effectiveness of the means used to achieve programmatic goals. Process evaluation can examine the number of program participants and the number of health promotion events held. In both formative and process evaluations, the focus is on activities and interventions, not outcomes. Both formative data and process evaluations allow for self-correction of program problems while changes are still possible (Healey & Zimmerman, 2010).

Outcome evaluation, which is also called summative evaluation, focuses on whether the goals and objectives of the health program have been achieved (Healey & Zimmerman, 2010). Examples include improved well-being, heightened quality of life, increased social capital, weight loss, or blood pressure control. The push for outcomes evaluation has been driven by the need to contain spiraling healthcare costs, improve the quality of care that is available, and establish performance measures for given conditions.

For example, evidence-based medicine has been used in mainland Europe and England to establish payment guidelines for physicians and nurses who are treating clients with congestive heart failure, diabetes, and a spectrum of chronic illnesses. Monitoring mechanisms and health outcome targets are established, which influence reimbursement (Macdonald et al., 1996). A limitation of outcomes evaluation is that it provides no insight into what occurred during implementation of the health promotion program (Tones, 2000).

Impact evaluation focuses on intermediate rather than long-term outcomes and examines the effectiveness of the intervention in changing knowledge, attitudes, beliefs, and behaviors (IOM, 2001). Structural evaluation examines the influence of organizational and human resources on health promotion. Transfer evaluation explores whether the program is replicable and transferable to other settings and populations (Whitehead, 2003). Authors have argued for inclusion of, at minimum, both process and outcomes measures in every study since results and factors that facilitate and inhibit change can be simultaneously examined (Health Education Board for Scotland [HEBS], 1999).

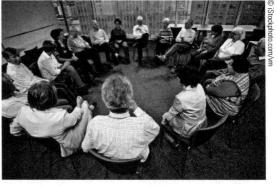

© iStockphoto.com/vm

RESEARCH AND EVALUATION DESIGNS

As you will remember from your research class, there are a variety of research designs that can be selected to evaluate health promotion interventions. Given that the discipline of health promotion is broad, a variety of research designs are needed to address the range of questions and interventions that are commonly seen in practice. In fact, a combination of both quantitative and qualitative approaches (called triangulation) is commonly used.

Evidence-Based Approaches

The Oxford Centre for Evidence-Based Medicine provided a level of evidence hierarchy for evaluating research evidence, which is presented here (ranging from highest to lowest level of evidence):

- Randomized controlled trials
- Systematic reviews of randomized controlled trials
- Systematic reviews of cohort studies
- Cohort studies
- Outcomes research
- Systematic reviews of case-control studies
- Case series research
- Expert opinions (Bauer, 2008)

However, questions have been raised about whether ethical priorities are given adequate attention in this hierarchy when health promotion research is being conducted in the community. An example was the study conducted by Johns Hopkins University in which lead paint abatement procedures were examined to determine if low-expense or high-expense methods were most effective at minimizing lead levels in blood samples from disadvantaged children. The judge ruled the quality of the research design could not take precedence over the harm to the children who were exposed to lead paint. He ruled that the children were placed at risk and being used as measurement tools in this study (Bauer, 2008). As this case illustrates, it is vital for health promotion researchers to always consider the risk and benefits to be gained from a given study before the quality of the research design.

Within the health promotion literature the use of evidence-based approaches has also been criticized as being too aligned with a positivist framework and for stressing the importance of cost-effectiveness (Whitehead, 2003). In health promotion research this evidence-based hierarchy may not be the most relevant approach to selecting an evaluation design. The advantages and disadvantages of varied research designs as they apply to health promotion programs are summarized next.

Randomized and Nonrandomized Clinical Trials

A randomized clinical trial (RCT) or true experiment is thought to provide the strongest evidence in many disciplines. When sample sizes are large this design minimizes bias and accounts for confounding variables (variables other than the primary intervention that affect outcomes) by randomizing participants into an intervention and control group. However, in most health promotion research it is difficult to randomize people into an intervention and control group. Sometimes this happens because it is not ethical to deny the control group the benefit of an intervention that is known to be effective. Sometimes a RCT is not feasible because the control and intervention groups exist within the same community, school, or institution; have contact with one another; and discuss the intervention being provided. In addition, RCTs are typically conducted in university settings, do not recruit samples that are representative of the larger population, and have large dropout rates, which undermine the generalizability of their findings.

Efficacy in a RCT is a measure of whether an intervention can work under controlled conditions. That is not a guarantee the intervention is effective and will work in actual practice settings. Some variables like culture, sociopolitical environment, and community history are things a researcher cannot control (IOM, 2001). Finally, RCTs do not lend themselves to multifaceted intervention, which is a priority in the health promotion field (Macdonald et al., 1996). The WHO (1998) has argued that RCTs can be misleading and disempowering, while also being an unnecessarily expensive way to evaluate health promotion programs.

Quasi-Experimental Designs

Quasi-experimental designs are used when randomization is not possible or practical. They are natural experiments in which a health promotion intervention is offered to an intervention and control group. Because participants are not randomly assigned to the intervention or comparison group, it is not possible to ensure that confounding variables (other than the planned intervention) did not have a substantial effect on the outcome. Quasi-experimental designs are often used to evaluate the impact of public policy changes and educational interventions. Pre- and postdesigns in which an intervention and comparison group are evaluated before and after a given health promotion program are examples of quasi-experiments.

Cohort Studies

Longitudinal cohort studies follow a specific group or cohort over a substantial period of time with the purpose of analyzing the risk a particular group has for developing a disease—the cohort is identified before anyone has developed the disease and then observed to see who develops the disease. Data is collected at regular intervals and individuals are often followed for years. A comparison group frequently is used that was not exposed to the variable that is being tracked (for example, vaccination). The group being observed and the comparison group are matched for variables such as health status, economic status, and culture. Cohort studies are expensive because they take so long to complete and often have large numbers of individuals who drop out of the study.

Case-Control Studies

Case-control studies are often used to investigate rare outcomes. A retrospective examination is done, in which people with a particular disease or health state are matched with a comparison group that does not have the disease or health state. Characteristics of both groups are compared to identify differences. Case-control studies are less expensive than cohort studies because they can be completed in a fairly short period of time. However, the actual cause of the outcome cannot be determined using a case-control study.

Cross-Sectional Surveys

Cross-sectional surveys rely on data collected at a defined time, often using survey data from large, national studies. Everyone in the population is examined at an established period in time to evaluate a particular health behavior or belief. Cross-sectional studies are used to describe the prevalence of acute and chronic health conditions. For example, the prevalence of cirrhosis among those who consume alcohol on a daily basis could be explored using a cross-sectional study.

Qualitative Research

Qualitative research is used frequently in health promotion research to examine formative and process-oriented measures as well as outcomes based on the perspective of stakeholders. Green and Tones (1999) argued for greater reliance on qualitative research in establishing the base of literature in health promotion. Focus group and interview-based data provides multiple clues as to why a health promotion program did or did not work (Macdonald et al., 1996).

Qualitative research allows the researcher to remain person-centered rather than disease-focused and to examine what stakeholders consider to be meaningful and effective. As King (1994) asserted, "Both societal and individual perceptions of health and wellness and perceived health status must be assessed" (p. 212). Qualitative research is specifically designed to obtain the perspective of individuals and communities through focus groups, individual interviews, and health diaries that include open-ended questions. Specific qualitative studies can be designed to evaluate the most relevant aspects of a given health promotion program. In addition, there are semi-structured qualitative approaches that are designed to examine individual's illness experiences.

Structured Qualitative Health Interviews

Two primary semi-structured qualitative interviews, the Explanatory Model of Illness Catalogue and the McGill Illness Narrative Interview, have been used in the health promotion literature.

The Explanatory Model of Illness Catalogue The Explanatory Model of Illness Catalogue (EMIC) is a semi-structured qualitative interview that allows people to describe their illness experience. It contains four sections and questions are organized around: patterns of distress (problems associated with the illness), perceived causes (why and how the person has been affected), help seeking and treatment behavior (ways of getting help from family, friends, and professionals), and general illness beliefs (this illness episode compared to other illness the person has experienced) (Coutu et al., 2008).

The EMIC was developed in a non-Western country and has been used effectively in 13 languages and cultures. Each section begins with a short story or metaphor to help the respondent understand that there is no right or wrong answer. It can be analyzed both qualitatively and quantitatively, although most studies have only reported qualitative results. A limitation of the EMIC is the time that the interview takes to complete (Coutu et al., 2008).

The McGill Illness Narrative Interview The McGill Illness Narrative Interview (MINI) is a semi-structured, qualitative interview designed to explore illness experiences that are medically unexplained. The interview begins with an initial narrative in which he person tells his or her story in his or her own words. The second section focuses on stereotypes or hypotheses about illness and treatment approaches that the respondent holds, while the third section examines causation. Optional sections focus on the respondent's experience with healthcare treatment and how the illness is impacting the person's life and way of coping. A limitation of the MINI is that it takes almost 2 hours to complete (Coutu et al., 2008).

Community-Based Participatory or Action Research

Community-based participatory research (CBPR) or action research is based on the belief that both researchers and participants contribute to planning, implementation, evaluation, and dissemination activities. The word *participatory* is especially important, since the research is not just conducted in the community; rather, the community is actively involved in the planning, implementation, evaluation, and dissemination of results. The focus is on empowering individuals and communities, building capacity, and identifying meaningful objectives (Whitehead, 2003).

The process begins with focus groups or surveys that help identify the health needs of the participants or community. A key task is to define the problem in such a way that stakeholders can agree on priority interventions and commit to the work required to achieve meaningful outcomes (Best et al., 2003). Community resources, strengths, and assets are listed along with needed changes. The goal is to identify community perspectives, to translate those goals into actions, and to develop ongoing partnerships between academic researchers and community members.

Intervention and evaluation methods are collaboratively selected based on input from the participants or community and the researchers. Typically, community members are employed to offer portions of the intervention and to collect agreed-upon evaluation data. Funds are returned to the community in which the evaluation is occurring. By involving community members in the research or program evaluation activity they gain skills, are empowered, and are able to continue to contribute to the community even after the research study has been completed. Finally, community members are routinely employed to disseminate the study results to other community members (Whitehead, 2000).

CBPR often "involves communities that have been marginalized on the basis of race, ethnicity, class, gender, [or] sexual orientation in examining the consequences of marginalization and attempting to reduce and eliminate it" (IOM, 2001, p. 286). Since the research is conducted in the target community, information about how context and setting influence the results can easily be obtained (IOM).

Community-based methods recognize that process is important, community-level participation and ownership is valuable, capacity development is key, and shared power/control are necessary (Best et al., 2003). This participatory approach was adopted by the National Institutes of Health and other federal agencies in order to ensure that research focuses on problems that communities are invested in changing, recognize as being relevant and significant, mesh with community values, and therefore, are more likely to result in long-term change.

Community-based participatory approaches bring together partners with "diverse skills, knowledge, expertise, and sensitivities to address complex problems" (IOM, 2001, p. 285). This type of research has the potential for overcoming the distrust of research that is an understandable reality within communities where research subjects have been poorly treated in the past (IOM). Community-based participatory approaches result in greater ownership of and commitment to the research by those who live with and understand the given health challenge on a daily basis.

The research process itself is a tool for change because an ongoing process of action and reflection result (Scott, Stern, Sanders, Reagon, & Mathews, 2008). However, as

Aronson Wallis, O'Campo, Whitehead, and Schafer (2007) commented, CBPR takes longer than traditional research and requires a great deal of time and investment from both academic and community members. It is, however, one of the major innovations being used in health promotion research today.

Triangulation

Many researchers agree that the complex nature of health promotion requires integration of quantitative and qualitative research methods within the same study (Peersman, Oakley, & Oliver, 1999). The scientific rigor and validity of the approach depends on validating data that is collected from one source (for example, qualitative) and checking it by obtaining data from another method of data collection (for example, quantitative) (Brown, Lloyd, & Murray, 2006).

Neighborhood Mapping

Neighborhood mapping is a method of research used to analyze and describe the physical condition of neighborhoods, the location of institutions and resources, the density of residential development, the availability of roads and transit, the amount of green space, and the social and demographic characteristics of residents. Community members and/or students are recruited to walk block by block to map buildings and resources. Vacant buildings, libraries, grocery stores, access to transportation, and a variety of other measures are recorded. Housing inspection data, liquor license data, crime reports, vital statistic records for births and deaths, health outcomes, and low birth weight and preterm birth data are also used.

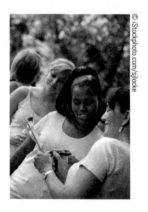

Geographic information systems are then used to map information collected from primary and secondary sources into a coherent map of the given community. The map is used to target interventions to high-need areas and to build on community strengths when planning a health promotion intervention (Aronson et al., 2007).

An important consideration in community mapping is confidentiality of community members and safeguarding residential names and addresses. Community mapping has the advantage of considering numerous contextual and community-level factors that can influence health. It does require skill and sufficient time to conduct, but also has the added advantage of involving residents and building community capacity (Aronson et al., 2007).

EVALUATION CRITERIA FOR HEALTH PROMOTION RESEARCH

Hancock and colleagues (1997) suggested four criteria for evaluating whether a health promotion evaluation strategy is effective. First, these researchers suggested examining the design, including how or whether randomization was appropriate and how the sampling was conducted to ensure that a representative sample was used. Second, these researchers stressed the importance of using outcome measures with demonstrated reliability and validity along with process measures that ensure the intervention was carried out as it was planned. Third, they emphasized the necessity of using appropriate methods of analysis. Finally, the importance of describing the intervention in sufficient detail so that another team could implement it was highlighted.

THE RE-AIM FRAMEWORK FOR EVALUATING HEALTH PROMOTION PROGRAMS

As we saw in an earlier chapter, The Reach, Effectiveness, Adoption, Implementation and Maintenance (RE-AIM) framework has been described as one comprehensive way of evaluating the five important components of health promotion programs (reach, effectiveness, adoption, implementation and maintenance). Reach focuses on whether the participants are representative of a larger population and represent a significant percentage of individuals who might be affected by the health promotion program. Effectiveness examines how well the intervention impacted planned outcomes and quality of life. Adoption targets the percentage and representation of settings and staff who will deliver the program. Implementation focuses on whether staff members are consistent and skilled at offering the intervention. Maintenance is the extent to which participants retain behavior change over time (Glasgow, Klesges, Dzewaltowski, Estabrooks, & Vogt, 2006).

The individual-level impact of a health promotion program is calculated by multiplying the reach and effectiveness scores. The number of individuals who were eligible and invited to participate is multiplied by the effect size. When the number of eligible participants is known, their health characteristics are compared to those who decline to participate. If the number of eligible participants is not known, participants are compared with characteristics of people in the area or the nation. The efficiency component of the model is determined by dividing the cost of an intervention by its individual level impact. It is also important to evaluate the setting-level impact if an intervention requires a substantial investment of time or expertise. The RE-AIM model is one way of evaluating the impact of health promotion programs (Glasgow et al., 2006).

THE EUROPEAN COMMUNITY HEALTH PROMOTION INDICATOR DEVELOPMENT MODEL

The European Community Health Promotion Indicator Development Model (EUHPID) was created to establish a common data set and group of indicators for evaluating health promotion interventions and health status. It includes both a focus on health- (salutogenic and resources) and disease-oriented indicators (risk factors). Specifically, there are three objectives of the EUHPID: "to provide a clear rationale for selecting, organizing, and interpreting health promotion indicators (a classification system); to communicate the unique health promotion approach to the larger public health community (an advocacy tool); and to develop a common frame of reference for the fields of health promotion and public health which shows their interrelationship (a dialogue tool)" (Bauer et al., 2006, p. 154).

Based on the fact that 80% of gain in life expectancy has been related to socioenvironmental changes and 20% of gain has been related to improvements in the healthcare system, there is a focus on social and economic influences in the EUHPID. The model includes: (1) environmental determinants of health (social networks, ecological, cultural, and economic); (2) individual determinants of health (lifestyle choice); and (3) health status (physical, mental, and social). The model acknowledges that current health status has a major impact on future health. It includes social factors such as social capital, a sense of community, trust, reciprocity, health capacity, health literacy, and community action, all of which contribute to health. Positive health includes a focus on "objective fitness, subjective well-being, optimal functioning, meaningful life, and a positive quality of life" (Bauer et al., 2006, p. 156).

The EUHPID model emphasizes the interdependence of all factors in creating health while recognizing that a person can experience well-being and chronic disease at the same time. Recommended indicators to be used in evaluation include those that measure environmental factors, individual determinants of health, and health status. It is designed to provide a common frame of reference and a classification system that can be used in multiple countries to monitor public health (Bauer et al., 2006).

Categories of indicators include demographic factors, mortality/morbidity, health status, health behaviors, working conditions, prevention, health protection and health promotion, healthcare resources, healthcare utilization, health expenditures, and healthcare quality measures (Bauer et al., 2003).

PERFORMANCE INDICATORS

Common performance indicators in health promotion research include effectiveness, efficiency, and equity. A program is considered to be effective if it meets its objectives, while efficiency is a measure of how successful the health promotion program was compared to the cost and resources needed to conduct it. Equity is a measure of whether participants are involved in research design, implementation, evaluation, and dissemination.

PAY-FOR-PERFORMANCE EVALUATION

Pay-for-performance evaluation in the health professions has already been implemented in a number of countries. Within the United States, the Health Resources and Services Administration has made one of their priorities the implementation of electronic medical records that will support pay-for-performance evaluation for individual providers and healthcare systems. Pay-for-performance measures are being given attention because they are one way to improve clinical outcomes and improve quality of care (Werner, Greenfield, Fung, & Turner, 2006).

One barrier to implementation of pay-for-performance is the reality that many clients have multiple clinical conditions. Methods of evaluating quality of care with these complex clients are poorly developed. For example, as of 2002, 50% of Medicare beneficiaries had "at least three chronic medical conditions and one-fifth had five or more" (Werner et al., 2007, p. 1206).

Some of these chronic conditions are concordant in that the same quality standard is an effective measure for each of the conditions—for example, coronary artery disease and diabetes are both improved by lowering hypertension. Discordant conditions, however, require different treatments based on the given medical conditions; an example of discordant conditions would be emphysema and cancer, neither of which are related to lowering hypertension. Other questions center on whether greater focus should be given to physicians and healthcare providers who attend to the most serious health risk that a client presents. Should lipid level evaluation in a diabetic client, for example, be given more attention than foot exams (Werner et al., 2006)?

COST-EFFECTIVENESS ANALYSIS

Since the need for health promotion exceeds the resources that are available to fund programs, it is necessary to examine cost effectiveness. Cost-effectiveness analysis helps identify which programs result in the greatest improvement in health status based on a given expenditure. For example, should $1 million be spent on influenza vaccinations for the elderly, which yields 7,750 additional life years, or should that same amount be spent to yield 217 additional life years from a smoking cessation program (IOM, 2001)?

Researchers have argued that the true cost of choosing a particular intervention "is not the monetary cost per se, but the health benefits that could have been achieved if the money had been spent on another service instead . . . Costs are represented by the net difference between the costs of the intervention and the total costs of the alternative to that intervention" (IOM, 2001, p. 293). The typical health measure used in cost effectiveness analysis is the quality-adjusted life year (QALY). The value of the intervention is measured by comparing the QALY produced by the intervention to the alternative intervention that could have been funded (IOM, 2001).

Quality-Adjusted Life Years

Quality-adjusted life years is a measure of life expectancy and a method of evaluation that facilitates decision making about allocation of scarce healthcare resources among competing needs or individuals. The QALY integrates mortality and morbidity in terms of equivalents of healthy life years. QALYs are used in the United Kingdom, the Netherlands, and Canada to estimate the cost effectiveness of needed interventions (McGrath, Rofail, Gargon, & Abetz, 2010). When healthcare reform in the United States is fully implemented, it will likely be driven by QALYs.

QALYs are "calculated by estimating the total life years gained from a treatment and then weighing each year with a score. This score ranges from 0 to 1 (or 100) representing the worst imaginable health and the best health respectively" (McGrath et al., 2010, p. 2). QALYs are based on the view that an extra year of good health is more valuable than a year in poor health. "The number of QALYs are then expressed as the value given to a particular health state multiplied by the period of time spent in that state to determine a composite measure of health" (McGrath et al., 2010, p. 2). A descriptor (a vignette describing a particular health state), a valuation (the value given to the health state using a visual analogue scale), and a perspective (from a healthcare provider) are required to complete a QALY calculation.

Arguments against the use of QALYs center on whether they are unethical and introduce bias in the allocation of resources that favor certain diseases over others. Instruments currently available in the literature are based on symptoms derived from the literature, not from gathering the input of clients or healthy populations. Varied agencies and authors have stressed that it is important to pay greater attention to client perspectives about health-related quality of life. Studies used to develop QALY measures to determine how much or if individuals get health care have not considered positive factors, such as coping strategies or social supports, that influence the client's perception of a given condition. Without inclusion of client perspectives and attention to factors that enhance health, there may not be an equitable way to determine how valuable a given year of life is for all populations, communities, groups, or individuals (McGrath et al., 2010).

However, decisions about whether treatment will be provided or not will be based on measures such as QALY. Moreover, healthcare providers are being asked to make decisions about provision of health care based on cost effectiveness, not client need. Concerns include the fact that QALYs discriminate against the elderly, disabled, and unemployed individuals (McGrath et al., 2010).

A CASE STUDY: WOULD QALY CALCULATION HELP OR HINDER PROVISION OF CARE FOR SARA?

Step into the experience of this graduating student nurse. Imagine telling the following story based on your work in an intensive care unit. As you read about this student's clinical experience, consider whether the use of QALYs would help or hinder him to sort out his conflicting feelings about the treatment of Sara, to whom he was assigned to provide care. The nurse shared the following story, saying:

> I took report from the day shift nurse who meticulously went over the patient's systems and outlined a few areas of concern. My eyes darted back and forth between Sara, my patient, and the reporting nurse. I made a mental note that Sara was receiving continuous doses of infusing medications that included versed, fentanyl, maintenance fluid, a blood product, and what I found out later to be an extremely expensive medication, Flolan.
>
> As the night progressed, I found Sara's care to be very challenging and complex given the ethical dilemma surrounding her case. Beginning with my initial interaction, I assessed my patient as a 43-year-old white female. Physically, she did not appear her age, but resembled someone who was closer to 60-years old. She had her eyes shut and her body was silent, head tilted to one side, anchored by an endotracheal tube that was inflating and deflating her lungs in a calculated rhythm. I looked over towards the mechanical ventilator and assessed her respirations to be near 25 breaths per minute. The sedative medications, despite her medical condition, were adequately keeping her breathing rate at a baseline. Without the current medical intervention, she would not have sustained the very rapid breathing rate that was a direct result of her disease process. As I moved on to assessing her gastrointestinal system, I noticed two quadrants that were very rigid and slightly protruding in her abdominal

area, even though she was somewhat obese. I was puzzled, but moved on to finish my assessment. After I had checked all the titratable intravenous (IV) medications, I moved back to the computer to begin gathering my thoughts and creating a plan of action for the rest of the night shift.

As I read through her electronic medical record, I pieced together a cascade of what revealed a very sick patient. Sara was on nasal cannulated 4–6 liters of oxygen at home and had a history of pulmonary hypertension secondary to methamphetamine use. About a month ago, and before her admission to this medical intensive care unit, she presented to the emergency room with shortness of breath, which quickly descended into a hypoxic respiratory failure. Within a span of 3 weeks, her declining respiratory status became exacerbated by a pneumonia, which led to intubation. During her stay at the hospital, she became septic and was placed on a triple antibiotic regiment.

The primary medical team initially tried nitrous oxide to reverse her primary pulmonary hypertension. When that failed to work, she was placed on Flolan, at an annual cost of $100,000. Administering Flolan required its own continuously infusing pump that had to function without interruption, as Sara would die within 3–5 minutes if the infusion was not restored. Flolan's primary function was to open up the pulmonary vascular beds to allow oxygen exchange to take place between the blood supply and incoming ventilated oxygen.

Heparin therapy was also initiated to thin out the blood so that microvascular clots would not develop secondary to her pulmonary hypertension. However, due to prolonged heparin use, Sara developed internal bleeding as the heparin caused her body to stop producing platelets. As it turns out, what I had earlier discovered to be two rigid areas on her abdomen were internal hematomas filled with blood.

Slightly overwhelmed, I took a step back to enumerate her current problems. Not only was Sara bleeding internally and breathing with lungs that were sustained by medications, but she had also developed an enlarged heart secondary to her almost defunct lungs. Her heart condition, paired with a blood infection, led to acute renal failure. The medical team was getting closer to reversing the acute renal failure by supporting her blood pressure with a dopamine drip and by treating the infection with antibiotics. I looked over her code status and saw that she was still a full code.

As my shift progressed a battle was forming within me as two opposing thoughts were flashing across my mind, each one overwhelming and trying to silence the other. On one side was the idealistic humanitarian in me, framing Sara's situation as a valiant conquest to save a life. In opposition, the realist side was fastidiously reminding me that it was her methamphetamine use that brought her here. Even the fact that she was also a Medicaid patient, who was supported through government sustenance, was bothersome to the realist in me. Part of me saw a woman who was using resources that could have gone to help save a life stricken down by an accident or a congenital malformation. I questioned why we continued supporting Sara even when it was known that she was on the brink of death.

I told myself that it was not up to me to make the decision whether one lives or dies: My sole duty was to provide a level of care that was unconditional and humane. As I looked up her blood work, she had 50k platelets and her hemoglobin/hematocrit came back as 9.8/28.7. Our main concern that night was monitoring her blood pressure and the amount of blood circulating in her vascular system. In the last 24 hours, we had given her a total of 10 units of blood products. On the midnight rounds, per doctor's orders, we continued this trend by starting an infusion of one unit of platelets and afterwards, two more units of whole blood.

It had become a game of watching and waiting as our primary focus was to support Sara's vascular system while the platelets would theoretically dampen her bleeding. Before any other progression could be made from a medical standpoint, it was critical that we halt her slipping platelet count and blood levels. As an hour passed, we drew blood for a complete blood count to be sent down to the lab. In the meantime, another unit of blood was hung. The lab results came back and only showed a marginal improvement with an uptick to 59k, which was insignificant as the goal of 150k was set by the attending. My preceptor and I reviewed the trending levels and saw that after the constant blood products, she managed to maintain a platelet count hovering around only 50k. It was becoming clear that her body was physically "eating up" everything we were giving her. My preceptor began suggesting that we push for either cessation of care or a milder course of treatment by approaching the family to change her status to reflect a do-not-resuscitate order.

On the one hand, I was in agreement with that decision. On the other hand, I wanted to yell in protest, "Well, why don't we just push her over the cliff and be done with it already!" I clearly understood this was an incredible ethical challenge. A decision had to be reached on whether we would begin palliative care or whether we would continue to pour finite resources into one patient. The notion of utilitarianism was flying high; surely it was appropriate to consider the facts and accept that the most good should be done for the most people. The facts were clear: She was actively bleeding internally, functioning on a pair of lungs that were supported with an extremely expensive medication, and her heart physically lacked the capacity it once had as a result of her poor pulmonary vasculature. Even if she survived, her quality of life would be less than inadequate; she would be mired in dependence on medications and confined sedentarily within the four walls of her home.

Simultaneously, I questioned whether I had forgotten what it means to help save a life. I thought about why I went to nursing school to become a patient advocate. Part of me thought it would be best to press forward until all options were completely exhausted. I asked my preceptor whether we could continue giving more blood products with the hope that the body would prevent its own demise by miraculously jump starting the platelet production again. It was futile, he responded—Sara's body was, in effect, leaking the blood into the interstitial pockets of the abdomen at a rate no amount of blood product could sustain.

A decision had been made, and the family would be allowed to begin to reconcile their and her wishes. Again, I tried to make sense of the situation, rhetorically asking myself what was the point of all these huge institutions, the brain trusts, and medical technologies.

Powerless and morally beaten down, I sat in the chair looking at Sara before I got up to check her medication drips. The last of versed, a short-acting sedative in the hanging bag, was almost empty. I asked my preceptor to pull the sedative for me. We did not have it in stock at the moment so he volunteered to go to the pharmacy a few floors down to get a replacement bag. What was only like 30 minutes felt much longer as my preceptor had not yet returned. From previous knowledge I knew that the medication had a very short half life and that it would be out of Sara's system momentarily. I had to shut off the pump as there wasn't any more medication to infuse.

Slowly, her restrained arms began to nudge and the frown on her face neatly folded the skin on her forehead along the well-worn creases. She was beginning to move her neck and was growing more restless, opening her eyes ever so slightly. As she was regaining consciousness, the movement of her arms became more vigorous and her head moved right to left in slow motion. The first alarm went off on the room monitor screen, indicating a respiratory rate that climbed into the high 30s. Understanding her predicament, Sara began bucking the vent, trying to take her own breaths over those administered by the ventilator. The ventilator alarm started screeching, a flashing a yellow light signaling that Sara was not taking in the preset amount of tidal volume of oxygen to fill her lungs.

I started fiddling with the infusing lines and looking over the bags until three other nurses came into the room. As Sara was repeatedly told to relax, another nurse was paging my preceptor over the Vocera, a communication device for all in-house staff. In addition to the lack of a calming sedative, the Flolan pump was loudly beeping with its own warning system. By virtue of making small movements, Sara had kinked the tube leading to the port hooked up to the intrajugular intravenous catheter on the right side of her neck.

Fortunately for all of us, my preceptor strode into the room as all of this was happening. I made way to allow him better access to Sara. With the new bag of versed hung and the line unkinked, he asked Sara to relax. I thought to myself, at least she is alive. But life could not have been more grotesque. The sclera in both Sara's eyes were completely red with blood encapsulated under the surface, engulfing the iris. Fear was in her eyes as she tried to mouth, "Help me" against the tube resting between her teeth. The anxious look fixed on her face was so overpowering that I couldn't help but think how in the face of death, the living strain to apply the last bit of strength in holding out against the looming depths of a lifeless abyss.

After giving report to the oncoming day shift, sad, broken, and haunted, I left the unit. Later that evening, I shared my trials and tribulations with a few friends. When asked what was going to happen to Sara, I answered that death, of course, was imminent, not knowing if that was in fact the truth or just the captive response of my mind.

Later, a few months after I had taken care of her, I had learned that Sara had pulled through. Even though her status was changed to DNR, the internal bleeding was controlled by a surgical intervention that didn't guarantee success, but eventually worked in her favor. After spending yet another month in the intensive care unit, Sara was discharged off the floor to eventually go home on the continuous Flolan medication. A lung transplant was out of the question, but the medication bought her on average another 3–5 years of life. I returned to contemplate that shift many times, puzzled, trying to gain a better understanding of myself, and why everything transpired within me as it did.

I remembered a short story credited to Loren Eiseley. It is about a boy walking the beach after a storm. He encountered thousands of starfish who were beginning to dry out and die, having been washed too far from shore. Frantically he began throwing them back into the sea. A man strolling on the beach reminded the boy that his throwing starfish back would not help because there were too many to save. The little boy, carrying another starfish in his hands, stopped and looked into the man's eye thoughtfully. Tossing the starfish into the waves he replied, "It makes a difference to that one!" and he rushed off to try and save more of the dying starfish.

The story captured the essence and meaning I had been searching for within the confines of nursing practice. It was possible that Sara was discharged to finish the last days of her life in a quality of life that was perhaps worse than when she was admitted. But in retrospect, it was never my duty to decide whether one dies or lives. It was my duty to continue providing equal and unequivocal patient care (Personal communication, Yuri Vorobets, May 15, 2010).

Discuss how consideration of QALYs showed up in this clinical scenario. Which part of providing care to Sara would have been most difficult for you?

LOGIC MODELS

Logic models are used for program evaluation, to review grant submissions and yearly progress reports, and to ensure health promotion program success. Visual flow charts or concept maps are used within logic models to specify: (1) problems the health promotion program is designed to target; (2) inputs such as staff and resources; (3) program goals; (4) interventions or activities designed to address problems; (5) short-term outcomes such as changes in attitudes, skills change, knowledge growth, or changes in regulations; and (6) long-term health-related outcomes.

As one clearly outlines the connections among each of these six components, it is possible to tack forward from the problem to the long-term outcome or to trace backward from the outcome to the intervention, input, and problem. This allows for identifying components that contribute to the success or failure of a health promotion program. It also allows for building on successful components and modifying problematic approaches. Use of a logic model ensures that each intervention included is needed, measured, and linked to planned outcomes. Logic models help to design a well-integrated health promotion program that is efficient, consistent, and effective (Healey & Zimmerman, 2010).

Figure 10-1 is one example of a logic model for a peer navigator program for individuals with substance abuse issues that was designed to minimize re-admissions to an emergency room. This model links resources, programmatic activities, objectives, and outcomes.

FIGURE 10-1

Resources (Inputs)	Program Components (Activities) 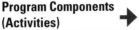	Outputs (Objectives)	Outcomes (Goals)
1. Community support as evidenced in attached letters 2. Consumer Self Help's long and successful history of providing peer-to-peer support 3. Availability of Consumer Self-Help office and meeting space near rapid transit access 4. Subcontracts with partners for program evaluation, educational, grants management, and publication expertise	**A. Peer Mentoring:** 1. Client assessment 2. 1:1 support 3. Case management services 4. Client recruitment **B. Informational Support:** 1. A list of community-based, governmental/county resources provided in English, Hmong, Vietnamese, and Spanish 2. Life-skills classes for clients, peer mentors, and family members (life management skills, anger management, assertiveness training, healthy boundaries, nutrition, budgeting, and computer literacy) **C. Instrumental Support:** 1. Bus passes 2. Access to shower facilities, washers, and dryers **D. Affiliational Support:** 1. Community Member focus groups 2. Health promotion classes for clients and family members (yoga, meditation, empowerment, art expression, poetry writing, journaling, creative writing, and self esteem) **E. Leadership Training for Peer Mentors:** 1. Eleven scheduled classes 2. Ongoing monthly supervision **F. RN Training:** 1. Cultural competency 2. Working effectively with peer mentors	Minimum number of clients with a substance abuse problem served per year: 115 Minimum number of clients who successfully complete at least 1 year of recovery program attendance: 50 **Client attendance:** 1. Clients will have at least 2 contacts per week with their peer mentor 2. Clients will attend at least 2 life skills and health promotion classes per week **Peer Mentor Program Completion:** At least 10 peer mentors per year will complete all training and supervision sessions and remain in recovery **Partnerships:** All participating agencies will remain involved throughout the 4-year grant period	1. Provide leadership training and monthly supervision to 15 peer mentors per year to develop their skills and promote their recovery 2. Provide effective support services to 115 clients with a substance abuse problem per year to prevent their relapse and promote their recovery efforts 3. Involve 60 community leaders per year (Hmong, Vietnamese, African American, and Hispanic/Latino) in designing and evaluating program success 4. Form an inpatient/outpatient partnership to strengthen linkages between treatment and recovery efforts and to involve the community in preventing relapse

Are there any components of the described logic model that you would question if you were the reviewer considering whether to fund this grant or not? What would you question and why?

ELECTRONIC METHODS OF INTERVENTION AND EVALUATION

Electronic mobile technology is being used to offer and evaluate a number of health promotion programs. Palmtop computers, mobile phones, and text messages are used to encourage smoking cessation, weight loss, anxiety management, diabetes control, substance use prevention, healthy eating education, and physical activity programs. A major advantage of these methods of delivery is providing a confidential way to offer health-related interventions and collect outcome data that does not embarrass the participant or place him or her at risk of revealing information that could affect employment, schooling, or community standing (Heron & Smyth, 2010).

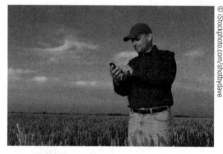

Electronic health records provide increased access to multiple ways of measuring the quality of health care that clients receive. Standardized data capture is possible using electronic health records that allow comparison of different providers, different systems of care, and regional healthcare use patterns.

A disadvantage of electronic health record use is that identifying select tracking parameters when measuring provider performance can result in practitioners focusing excessively on the assessment measures are being evaluated while ignoring other associated clinical priorities. Therefore, arguments have been made to focus on all relevant symptoms and interventions rather than a select number of tracers. RAND Corporation developed a quality assessment tool that measures 400 quality indicators for 29 conditions and preventative care measures. It tracks both under- and overuse of health care and is available online (Roth, Lim, Pevnick, Asch, & McGlynn, 2009).

Authors have cautioned that some information available in electronic health records, such as social history, medication use, and disease history, requires continual updating. It is vital, therefore, that practitioners monitor for changes in these areas on a regular basis rather than relying exclusively on the existing electronic health record data. All entries that involve a free text field in the electronic medical record, such as chief complaint or patient education, present challenges to collecting standardized responses. To evaluate patient education using electronic health records it will be important to document patient education using standardized bulleted lists or education prescriptions that clearly document what was taught (Roth et al., 2009) However, in a clinical sense the amount of standardization required for evaluation purposes may undermine individualized, patient-centered care.

SELECTING HEALTH PROMOTION MEASURES

It is important to select health promotion measures that have been tested in other studies, have good reliability and validity, are easy to administer and score, do not place excessive burden on participants, and have been normed on the population and setting in which they will be used. Most important is to select measures that will provide meaningful results given the population, setting, budget allocated to evaluation, and the type of intervention conducted (Bauman, Phongsavan, Schoeppe, & Owen, 2006).

COMMON CATEGORIES THAT ARE EXAMINED IN HEALTH PROMOTION RESEARCH

There are a number of common evaluations conducted in the literature on smoking cessation, weight loss, physical activity levels, and medication adherence that are worthwhile to discuss.

Medication Adherence

Medication adherence is one measure that has been examined as influencing the health of individuals with chronic diseases. Estimates of nonadherence to prescribed medications vary from 15% to 93%. Factors such as affordability, ease of obtaining refills, the quality of the doctor–patient relationship, and cultural beliefs affect medication adherence.

There are a variety of ways of measuring medication adherence, including "mean adherence, mean squared rate deviation, daily adherence, daily overdosing and underdosing, late dosing, and premature timing" (Balkrishnan & Jayawant, 2007, p. 1180). An accurate measure that avoids self-report bias is assaying drug concentrations in blood or urine. However, this approach is costly and burdensome for participants. In addition, rates of absorption, metabolism, and excretion differ among individuals and drug types.

Pill counts and refill records have also been used to supplement self-report measures. Pill counts and refill records rely on the premise that if a prescription is filled or an empty bottle is returned to the researcher, the medication was taken. These methods can be inaccurate because medications can be discarded by clients wishing to comply with research goals.

Electronic monitoring, in which a microchip that is placed in a pill bottle cap and transmits data each time the bottle is opened, has also been used. This method assumes that each time a bottle is opened, the medication is taken, and the participant has not inadvertently opened the wrong bottle.

A method that has shown some promise is educating family members about the importance of medication adherence so that a trusted person is reminding and supporting use of the medication. The significant other is involved in tracking and evaluating whether the client takes their medicine as prescribed. Blister pack or unit-of-use packaging and weekly pill organizers have also helped individuals recall if they have taken their daily medication and, therefore, have improved adherence rates (Balkrishnan & Jayawant, 2007).

Smoking Cessation

Smoking cessation programs have been evaluated using self-reported smoking status, cotinine (a metabolite of nicotine) levels, carbon monoxide levels, and genotyping risk factors. Usually, self-report of smoking underestimates actual amounts that individuals smoke because social desirability prompts respondents to answer surveys as they believe they should. This type of bias has become more of a factor as the social acceptability of smoking has decreased (Gorber, Schofield-Hurwitz, Hardt, Levasseur, & Tremblay, 2009).

Cotinine can be measured in the blood, urine, or saliva. Cotinine measurement is considered to be the gold standard measure in smoking cessation research. Using saliva (versus blood or urine) is both less invasive and easier for study participants, but also more sensitive. A problem is that cotinine levels are elevated in persons exposed to secondhand smoke and those who use chewing tobacco or nicotine replacement gums and patches. In addition, individual variation in metabolism, inhalation patterns, and cigarette brand influence cotinine levels. Nevertheless, cotinine levels are the most widely used measure despite costing more to analyze than other biomarkers.

One inconsistency among published studies is what level of cotinine results in a classification as a regular smoker. Ranges have "varied from 50 to 500 ng/ml of cotinine in urine, from 8 to 100 ng/ml in serum, and from 7 to 44 ng/ml in saliva" (Gorber et al.,

2009, p. 14). Other inconsistencies are seen when dilution effects within the urine based on amount of fluid intake are included in some studies but not others. Finally, some studies rely on stimulated saliva sampling of cotinine while others do not. Stimulated sampling occurs when a participant chews on cotton or some other material prior to providing a saliva sample. This procedure is not generally well accepted by participants. Unstimulated saliva samples typically result in higher cotinine levels than stimulated samples (Gorber et al., 2009). As with most measures in health-oriented research, there is a need to standardize measures so that results across studies are more understandable and comparable (Gorber et al.).

Exhaled carbon monoxide levels and thiocyanate levels have also been used, although they are influenced by diet and pollution (Gorber et al., 2009). Lung function tests, spirometry results, and ultrasonography of carotid and femoral arteries, along with photographic demonstration of atherosclerotic plaques and lung age comparisons with nonsmokers, have also been used to promote risk awareness and serve as outcome measures. Studies using these measures have demonstrated mixed results, in part because sometimes smokers conclude it is too late to quit and continue smoking when provided with the results of biomedical risk assessment (Blize, Burnand, Mueller, Walther, & Cornuz, 2009).

Obesity Measurement

Measures of body mass index (BMI), dual-energy X-ray absorptiometry (DEXA) for body fat estimation, height, weight, waist circumference, hip circumference, and waist–hip ratios have been used to evaluate programs designed to prevent and minimize obesity. Body mass index is calculated as body weight adjusted for height (weight in kg/height^{2}in m). Obesity is defined as a BMI of greater than or equal to 30 kg/m^2. Online calculators are available for women, men, and children. Although BMI is the most commonly used measure, it does not include information about fat distribution. This is important because deposits of abdominal fat are associated with diabetes and cardiovascular disease (Katz et al., 2010).

DEXA scanning offers good data about muscle and body fat percentages, fat mass (grams), lean body mass (grams), and distribution of fat and muscle in the arms, legs, and trunk. DEXA scans are typically used to measure bone density but can also be used to measure soft tissue. DEXA scanning is sensitive to small changes in body composition. However, DEXA scanning is not feasible to use in large studies due to cost and lack of wide-spread access to equipment (Katz et al., 2010).

Waist circumference requires designating where the measure was obtained. A common reference point is midway between the lower portion of the ribs and the iliac crest. Hip circumference is often taken at the widest portion of the buttocks. Typically, two measurements are taken and the average number is reported for both hip and waist circumference. A waist circumference in a woman of greater than or equal to 88 cm is classified as obese, while a waist–hip ratio of greater than or equal to 0.85 is considered obese (Katz et al., 2010).

Food Environment, Food Consumption, and Dietary Exposure Measures

Researchers concerned with the availability of healthy foods within communities have used community surveys, neighborhood mapping, and product shelf space (for milk, vegetables, and whole grains as compared to liquor, for example) to examine whether people have access to healthy dietary choices. Diet diaries, food frequency questionnaires, and 24-hour food consumption recall have also been used to examine food consumption patterns. Research has shown that variability in portion size, lack of knowledge about food categories, and failure to self-report about one's usual diet as a result of being enrolled in a study have resulted in inaccurate findings.

Food frequency questionnaires tend to overestimate intake, whereas 24-hour dietary recall tends to underestimate carbohydrate and calcium intake. Twenty-four-hour urine samples have been used to measure protein intake based on urine nitrogen levels. Fatty acid intake has been estimated by measuring blood lipid levels (Fave, Beckmann, Draper, & Mathers, 2009).

A new science, metabolomics, is also being used to examine a limited range of metabolites in biofluids. Using vibrational spectrometry, nuclear magnetic resonance (NMR), infrared spectroscopy, and capillary electrophoresis, it is possible to measure certain limited food metabolites. For example, concentrations of "chlorogenic acid, gallic acid, epicateci, naringenin and hesperetin have been used to evaluate the consumption of coffee, wine, tea, cocoa and citrus juices, respectively" (Fave et al., 2009, p. 138). However, this research method is expensive and more than 60% of metabolites from raw food have yet to be identified. In addition, factors such as adipose levels, and the microbial environment within the gut influence metabolite release. The science of metabolomics, which is in its infancy, will likely yield significant findings over the next few decades (Fave, Beckmann, Draper, & Mathers, 2009).

Physical Activity Measurement

Physical activity measurements are collected using standardized self-report measures, diaries, activity logs, and direct measures such as pedometer and accelerometer counts. Direct observation measures are also used to record activity patterns of children in playgrounds or parks. The System for Observing Fitness Instruction Time and System for Observing Play and Leisure Activity in Youth are examples of structured observation protocols. Motion sensors can also be used to count the number of people using a trail or bike path to evaluate the effectiveness of a community development program (Bauman, Phongsavan, Schoeppe, & Owen, 2006). Researchers focus on how often physical activity occurs, what duration occurs per day, how intense the activity is, where the activity is performed, how much occupational or domestic activity is accomplished, and how much sedentary activity occurs (television, computer use, reading, etc) (Bauman et al., 2006).

Some self-report measures have a "met/not met" goal for activity, while others collect hours per week spent in activity. The International Physical Activity questionnaire is one instrument that is widely used. In it, individuals are asked to recall the last 7 days and record the frequency and duration of time spent walking and engaging in vigorous and moderate-level-intensity activity, along with sedentary activity. The long form details household and yard work, occupational activity, sedentary time, and leisure time activity (Bauman et al., 2006).

The Global Physical Activity Questionnaire is used in the WHO STEPS program for cardiovascular surveillance. It consists of 14 items that focus on work and domestic activity, active transport, leisure time activity, and sitting time. The Finbalt Health Monitor is used to record daily duration and intensity of physical activity that lasts at least 30 minutes. The Behavioral Risk Factor Surveillance State Questionnaire examines similar domains of leisure time activity and occupational activity. Recall periods cover the last month and a usual week. The Canadian Physical Activity Monitory Survey measures physical activity during the last year. Hours per week of activity is multiplied by the metabolic cost of each activity, its duration in hours, and the average number of times per year the activity occurred (Bauman et al., 2006).

Physical activity instruments also measure intention to be active, perceived control over exercise, exercise enjoyment, expected benefits, social support for exercise, and self-efficacy. For example, the Perceived Behavioral Control Scale examines how much control one has over exercising while the Exercise Perceived Behavioral Control Questionnaire explores whether exercising in the next 2 weeks is beyond a person's control. The Physical Activity Enjoyment Scale asks participants to rate exercise as fun, boring, or energizing. The Intention to Exercise Scale focuses on the person's intent to participate in a physical exercise program during the next year, while the Self Efficacy for Exercise scale measures whether a person feels confident they could exercise 3 times per week for 20 minutes each. The Social Support for Exercise Habits Scale looks at whether friends and family encouraged exercise during the previous 3 months (Bauman et al., 2006).

Other instruments are designed to evaluate characteristics of homes and neighborhoods that influence physical activity levels. The Neighborhood Environmental Walkability Scale evaluates residential density, land use, walking and cycling facilities, crime, and pedestrian and automobile traffic safety issues. The Home Environment Scale looks at whether the person has access to things like exercise equipment at home, a safe neighborhood, enjoyable scenery, basketball courts, bike lanes, and public parks (Bauman et al., 2006).

Exposure to Health Messages

Billboards, text messages, Internet postings, telephone recordings, and radio or television commercials and infomercials delivered to target audiences to reinforce health promotion include active ingredients (the health message) and are offered according to a set schedule (or dosage frequency). Each person who sees the message is exposed to a certain amount of content; however, people respond to health messages based on their own values, beliefs, life experiences, and level of interest. A person who has decided to quit smoking, for example, may pay more attention to a television commercial about smoking cessation than a person who plans to continue smoking (Morris, Rooney, Wray, & Kreuter, 2009).

The exposure level for an individual is different than the reach of the program, which is the proportion of the population the health message was designed to target. Exposure is measured by self-reported recall or remembering a portion of a jingle or message. Unaided recall measures require that a person remember the health message with minimal prompting; aided recall exposes a person to increasing portions of the message to measure whether they recognize the content (Morris et al., 2009).

Measuring the effectiveness of health education programs involves examining a broad spectrum of awareness, knowledge, belief, attitudes, support systems, and actions since each of these factors can influence whether a person changes their behavior. For example, Macdonald and colleagues (1996) reported that a commercial designed to influence dietary practices could result in increasing the awareness of 30% of the audience, with only 85% of that group fully understanding the content presented, only 31% of the aware audience believing the education presented, and only 40% of the aware audience having adequate support systems to initiate a change in their eating habits. (These hypothetical percentages were based on average figures documented for cancer education.) So overall, no more than a 3% likelihood of behavioral change might reasonably result from the health promotion commercial. In such a situation, should the focus of evaluation be primarily on changes in knowledge and attitudes, social/environmental changes, or behavioral change? What outcome or group of outcomes would you evaluate?

Asset Measurement

Researchers have argued that there is a need to shift the emphasis of health measurement from a deficit-focused to an asset- or resilience-focused approach. Attention to measures that promote positive health will allow for development of interventions that mitigate disease risk while building on health promotion activities and allow us to examine all the factors that influence long-term health trajectories (Best et al., 2003).

For example, in studies with children, protective and asset measures include involvement in structured activities, bonding with parents, school connectedness, family communication, healthy peer relationships, future aspirations, and involvement in community-based and religious activities. One measure, the Youth Asset Survey (Oman et al., 2002), which is designed to measure assets that promote health, examines family communication, peer role models, future aspirations, responsible choices, non-parental role models, and community involvement. Internal consistency ranges from 0.61 to 0.78 for the individual scales.

Biomarker Measurement

Biomarkers of exposure and measures of susceptibility to disease are being used in health promotion research in addition to environmental indicators of pollution. Historically measures of toxins in soil, water, and air were evaluated, but increasingly, measures of uptake of substances are being examined in body fluids. Human biomonitoring focuses on "human exposure to an environmental chemical via the measurement of that chemical, its metabolite(s), or reaction product(s) in human blood, urine, milk, saliva, adipose or other tissue in individuals taken separately" but analyzed to establish baseline values and levels of chemicals in the general population (Bauer, 2008, p. 3). The goal of human biomonitoring is to identify geographical clusters that are at risk, to examine risk trajectories over time, to explore genetic susceptibility to environmental pollution, and to serve as data for regulatory action. Examples include investigation of benzene and lead metabolites as well as DNA adducts that indicate increased cancer risk (Bauer).

RELIABILITY, VALIDITY, UTILITY, APPROPRIATENESS, RESPONSIVENESS, PRECISION, INTERPRETABILITY, ACCEPTABILITY, AND FEASIBILITY OF STANDARDIZED INSTRUMENTS

As you will remember from your research class, reliability and validity are important considerations to examine when selecting a quantitative outcome measure. In addition, there are also other criteria, such as appropriateness, responsiveness, precision, interpretability, acceptability, and feasibility, that need to be considered (Kayes & McPherson, 2010).

Reliability is a measure of whether the instrument yields results that are reproducible and stable from one data collection point to another. Similar scores are expected from repeat administration of surveys when an instrument is reliable. Interrater reliability is a measure of whether two data collectors agree when collecting data; test–retest reliability is a measure of whether an instrument yields the same measurements over time; and item reliability measures whether specific items within a scale are correlated or related to one another (Lytle, 2009).

Validity refers to whether the instrument measures what it claims to measure (Kayes & McPherson, 2010). Face validity is the degree to which an instrument is measuring what it purports to measure. Content validity examines whether the individual items comprising an instrument cover the full breadth of content the scale claims to measure. Criterion validity is whether the instrument agrees with other instruments designed to measure similar content, while construct validity is whether the instrument responds as one would expect based on theoretical projections (Lytle, 2009).

Utility across populations is a measure of whether the tool can be used in a large range of communities, settings, and populations. Utility of health concerns is a measure of whether the tool is relevant to a variety of health- and disease-related issues (Lytle, 2009). So, if one wanted a tool to be relevant in convenience stores in inner cities as well as large, suburban grocery stores, the important characteristic to examine is utility across populations. However, if you were concerned with measuring fat content in food as it applied to heart disease, high cholesterol, and obesity, then the focus should be on utility across health concerns (Lytle, 2009).

Appropriateness relates to whether the instrument is a good fit for the given study and measures what the researcher is hoping it will measure. Whether an instrument is a good fit for the study purpose, the population being studied, and the environment in which the study is conducted are some of the most important things to consider.

Responsiveness is whether the instrument measures outcomes that are meaningful to participants; precision is a measure of how precise the scores that derive from the instrument are, and interpretability is how much work is involved in translating the numerical score from an instrument into a clinically meaningful result. Acceptability is whether participants find the instrument to be acceptable without placing a high burden on them. Feasibility is whether the instrument is easily explained and used and whether downloading data and data analysis can be easily completed (Kayes & McPherson, 2010).

EFFECT SIZE

It is important to consider effect sizes because there is a difference between statistical and clinical significance. Just because a result is statistically significant does not mean that it is clinically significant. In addition, effect sizes are used in estimating the number of participants needed in a study to see the planned outcome. Most authors report an effect size that is associated with a health promotion program within a given area, such as the odds of an employment-based smoking cessation program being success- ful. When an effect size is not presented in the literature, a change of 0.2 is considered small, 0.5 is considered moderate, and 0.8 is described as large. A change of 1.0 stan- dard deviation is typically quite significant in a clinical sense (Wu, Revicki, Jacobson, & Malitz, 1997).

OBJECTIVE MEASURES

A critique of objective measures is that although they probably accurately measure out- comes, they may lack clinical relevance—for example, what range of activity reported by an accelerometer represents a healthy level of activity (Kayes & McPherson, 2010)? Accelerometers are commonly used as an objective measure of physical activity. They are sensitive in detecting activity levels among healthy individuals even when they are not very active and they can detect movement in three dimensions, so they are able to capture a range of activity as well as intensity of movement. They are compact, lightweight, and waterproof, making them relevant in a variety of activi- ties (Kayes & McPherson). They are tamper-free, so that participants cannot modify data, and result in minimal burden for those who wear them. However, the location of placement (ankle, wrist, or hip) has been shown to influence how much activity is recorded. Also, they have primarily been tested in healthy individuals (Kayes & McPherson, 2010).

Pedometers are used as motivational tools as well as methods to measure activity levels. They count steps a person takes without capturing the intensity or pace of movement. An inexpensive, durable, and accurate pedometer can be purchased in a variety of outlets, including RadioShack.

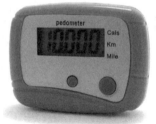

The ticking sound has been reported to serve as an auditory reminder to increase activity levels. When the pedometer is being used exclusively to report activity levels, it is important for the researcher to acknowledge that the use of the device itself may increase activity levels. It is also important to collect data on times participants were ill or forgot to wear the pedometer. They are most accurate when worn on loose clothing as they register higher step counts when worn on tight clothing, thick clothing, or belts. When collecting base- line data it is important to cover the step count register to blind the participant so that they do not decide to increase their activity level based on the measurement device reading rather than the planned health promotion program that is being evaluated (Bauman et al., 2006; Gardner & Campagna, 2009).

SELF-REPORT MEASURES

Internationally, there has been a movement toward incorporating more subjective patient-reported outcomes into health promotion program evaluations. This is being done to highlight the importance of including stakeholder perspectives. As of September 2005 all clinical trials published in a major medical or nursing journal must be registered prior to enrolling patients. The registration includes information on the trial's sponsor, an enrollment plan, the design, and the primary and secondary outcomes. This registration requirement minimizes the likelihood of bias from selective publication of outcomes and hypotheses that are different from those specified at the beginning of the trial (Scoggins & Patrick, 2009). Self-report measures include many of the scales summarized in the final section of this chapter and include outcomes such as quality of life, pain, energy levels, and perceived health.

However, when outcomes can be directly measured, such as physical activity using an accelerometer, those measures are often preferred over self-report measures. Recall bias, in which the person's memory does not match reality, and social desirability bias, in which the person reports the socially acceptable answer rather than an accurate response, continue to be problems that must be addressed if self-report measures are used.

The best self-report measures examine all dimensions of health relevant to the given study or health promotion program, are reliable and valid, are able to detect change over a long period, have a scoring mechanism that is easy to use and can be compared with normative data for the population, are easy to administer, and are adaptable to varied languages and cultures. Tools that were developed on adult populations need to be evaluated and adapted for use in pediatric and elderly populations (Winthrop, 2010).

GENERIC MEASURES VS. DISEASE-SPECIFIC MEASURES

Authors have argued for the use of generic health scales that measure the nature of health and illness across varied disease states rather than the use of disease-specific measures. Generic measures allow for comparisons across populations and disease states (Hewitt, 2007). An example of a generic measure is the SF-36, which measures quality of life across a variety of health and disease states. An example of a disease-specific measure would be the Medical Outcomes HIV survey, which measures health-related quality of life in individuals with HIV-AIDS (Wu et al., 1997).

A SUMMARY OF SELECT HEALTH PROMOTION SCALES

There are a large number of instruments that are useful in measuring outcomes of health promotion programs. Rather than being familiar with each and every one, it is important to know where and how to locate relevant scales. The *Mental Measurements Yearbook* (2007) is one resource that lists instruments, the populations they are normed on, and their reliability and validity. The *Mental Measurements Yearbook* is available in most libraries and online. Relevant instruments can be located by entering a key phrase in a search engine specific to the Mental Measurements Yearbook.

It is important to remember that once an instrument has been standardized, questions cannot be added or deleted unless the lengthy psychometric process begins again. Therefore, researchers cannot merely select a standardized instrument and only use part of the tool. They also cannot add questions to a standardized instrument.

Because there are so many instruments that are available for use, only a select few are summarized here. As you design health promotion program evaluations you will want to search the relevant literature and consult the *Mental Measurements Yearbook* to identify the instruments that are the best fit for your project. Since some instruments are free and in the public domain, while others must be purchased, it is also important to consider the amount of funding allocated to evaluation in the project budget. Selecting an instrument that has been normed on a population similar to the one you are researching is critical. Using a tool that does not place undue burden on the respondents and is easily scored and interpreted is also vital.

Quality of Life Measures

Quality of life is a common measure that is used in health promotion program evaluation. Several such instruments are summarized here.

The Short Form

The Short Form (SF-36) is a 36-item short form that is the most frequently used quality of life instrument seen in major clinical trails (Scoggins & Patrick, 1009). It consists of one multi-item scale measuring 8 health concepts including: limitations in physical activity due to physical health problems (10 items), limitations in social activities (2 items), limitations in role activity (4 items), bodily pain (2 items), psychological distress and well-being (5 items), limitations in role activities because of emotion problems (3 items), vitality (energy and fatigue—4 items), general health perception (5 items), and 1 question about health changes over the last year. A Likert scale ranging from 0 (worst possible health) to 100 (best possible health) is used. The SF-36 is for individuals age 14 and older and can be self-administered, administered by a trained interviewer, or administered via computer in 5 to 10 minutes. It has good internal consistency, reliability, and validity (Ware & Sherbourne, 1992).

A limitation of the SF-36 is that people may not be able to distinguish between health- and nonhealth-related factors that influence quality of life. Moreover, since the items on the scale were devised by researchers without being based on input from individuals in poor health, some researchers have commented that the scale cannot accurately reflect client perspectives (Hewitt, 2007).

The Quality of Life Questionnaire

The Quality of Life Questionnaire (QLQ) is a 192-item measure with 15 subscales. Both the pencil-and-paper and computer-administered scales are easy to use. Sample questions include (1) I rarely attend sports events, (2) I can usually laugh at myself, (3) I seldom lose my temper, (4) Most of the time I can depend on my relatives to help me when I need it, (5) Where I work people rarely quit their job, (6) Where I live the streets are well kept, and (7) Friends have commented on how nice my home is. Test–retest reliabilities are good, ranging from 0.77 to 0.89. However, normative data came from a homogenous group and therefore may not be generalizable (Seltzer, 1992).

The Quality of Life Enjoyment and Satisfaction Questionnaire

The Quality of Life Enjoyment and Satisfaction Questionnaire (Q-LES-Q) includes subscales for general life satisfaction, satisfaction with physical health, subjective satisfaction, satisfaction with leisure time activity, and satisfaction with social relationships. Optional subscales measure satisfaction with work, household duties, school, medication, and overall life satisfaction. The Q-LES-Q takes approximately 15 minutes to complete. Normative data is not presented and no interpretive manual exists. The main scale is reliable and has adequate convergent validity (Caruso, 2001).

Wellness and Health Promotion Measures

Numerous well-being, wellness, and health promotion scales are available. Several of those instruments are discussed here.

The Friedman Well-Being Scale

The Friedman Well-Being Scale consists of 20 adjectives used to measure an adult's well-being. Subscales include emotional stability (10 items), self esteem (3 items), joviality (3 items) sociability (3 items), and happiness (1 item). The scale takes 3 minutes to complete but is difficult to score. Reliabilities range from 0.72 to 0.96 for the subscales; however, authors have argued that the scale may actually be measuring emotional stability more so than well-being (Fleenor, 2001).

The Five Factor Wellness Inventory

The Five Factor Wellness Inventory is available in adult, teen, and elementary school versions. The adult version has 73 items, including a creative self scale, a coping self scale, a social self scale, an essential self scale, and a physical self scale. There is also a local context, an institutional context, a global context, and a chronometrical (change over time) context scale. The scale takes approximately 20 minutes to complete. It is designed for Web-based administration and scoring. The sample used for developing norms included an underrepresentation of males, an overrepresentation of African Americans, and an overrepresentation of individuals with graduate degrees. Authors have commented that there is confusion regarding reliability and validity testing, in that numerical values are presented for earlier versions of the inventory rather than the most recent version of the scale. In addition, questions have been raised about whether the instrument measures wellness-related beliefs or behaviors (Lonborg, 2007).

The Perceived Wellness Survey

The Perceived Wellness Survey (PWS) is designed to evaluate physical, spiritual, intellectual, psychological, social, and emotional dimensions of health and wellness. It has good internal consistency (alpha ranges from .88 to .93) as well as discriminant, face, and factorial validity. It has been tested with employees in diverse samples from large companies and with college students (Adams, Bezner, & Steinhardt, 1997).

The Salutogenic Wellness Promotion Scale

The Salutogenic Wellness Promotion Scale (SWPS) was designed to measure positive health including physical, social, emotional, spiritual, intellectual, vocational, and environmental aspects. It was derived from the World Health Organization's definition of health as a multidimensional state of physical, mental, and social well-being. The physical construct measures sport and lifestyle movement; the social construct measures social networks and relationships; the emotional construct measures one's ability to manage emotions; the intellectual construct measures efforts to improve verbal, reading, and thinking skills; and the vocation construct measures a respondent's perceived value of, interest in, and importance of vocation. The scale measures how often a person engages in a health-related behavior using a 6-point Likert scale (5 = Always to 0 = Never). The SWPS has a good reliability with an internal consistency of 0.89. The alphas of each subscale range from 0.70 to 0.86 (Becker et al., 2009).

The Sense of Coherence Scale

Antonovsky (1993) created the 29-item and 13-item versions of the Sense of Coherence (SOC) scale, which measures the impact of a sense of meaning or coherence in supporting health. It is in the public domain for use free of charge. The SOC scale has been translated into 15 languages and is described as clinically feasible, reliable, and valid for use with men, women, and adolescents. It has not been tested in non-Western populations.

The Social Capital Questionnaire

The Social Capital Questionnaire consists of 36 questions that measure 8 components of social capital, including participation in one's local community, social agency, feelings of trust and safety, neighborhood connections, family and friends, tolerance of diversity, value of life, and work connections. Participants rank each factor using a four-point Likert scale. This tool has been used in Mexico, Australia, Greece, and the United States. Cronbach's alpha for the scale is 0.83. Sample questions focus on whether a person volunteers, is a club member, attends community events, visits neighbors, feels safe walking outside at night, enjoys living among people with varied lifestyles, feels valued by society, knows where to find information, and feels like they are a part of the team at work (Kristsotakis, Koutis, Alegakis, & Philalithis, 2008).

The Revised Health Promoting Lifestyle Profile II

The revised Health Promoting Lifestyle Profile II (HPLPII) was designed to measure health-promoting choices rather than risk avoidance or disease prevention. After administration, one summative score is calculated. The 52-item scale includes behavioral indicators, perceptions, knowledge, and actions (Pinar, Celik, & Bahcecik, 2009).

Some authors have criticized inclusion of behaviors, perceptions, knowledge, and actions all within one summative score, suggesting rather that individual subscale scores should be developed (Kulbok et al., 1997). The profile includes subscales of nutrition, physical activity, health responsibility, stress management, interpersonal relations, and spiritual growth. A four-point Likert scale is used to measure how often participants practice the health-promoting behavior (never, sometimes, often, and routinely). It has sufficient validity and reliability and has been measured in a variety of populations. A Cronbach alpha of 0.94 for the entire scale has been reported while the 3-week test–retest reliability is 0.89. The profile has been translated into Spanish, Japanese, Arabic, and Turkish (Pinar et al., 2009).

Lifestyle Assessment Questionnaire

The Lifestyle Assessment Questionnaire is designed to evaluate an adult's habits and knowledge about health and wellness. It focuses on occupational, emotional, intellectual, physical, social, and spiritual dimensions. An assessment of a respondent's risk of death and life expectancy are provided as well as bibliographic resources focused on health. How life expectancy scores are calculated is unclear. In addition, the normative group is not described in sufficient detail. Reliability and validity data are limited (Brown, 1998).

Illness Perception Measures

Illness-related measures examine whether illness is serious, is under one's personal control, and is influenced by contextual factors. Two illness-related measures are summarized here.

The Implicit Models of Illness Questionnaire

The Implicit Models of Illness Questionnaire contains 24 items ranked on a Likert scale from strongly agree to strongly disagree. The first section addresses whether the illness is serious, contagious, caused by germs, or chronic. The second section focuses on personal responsibility and whether stress, diet, exercise, or rest influenced the illness. The third section explores whether the illness can be controlled by the individual or outside forces. The last section examines whether symptoms change over time. Internal consistency is good, ranging from 0.9 to 0.92 (Coutu et al., 2008).

The Illness Perception Questionnaire

The Illness Perception Questionnaire (IPQ) consists of 70 items divided into 3 sections. It has been used with individuals who have rheumatoid arthritis, pain, and chronic fatigue syndrome. The first section asks whether symptoms are related to the illness. The second section contains 38 items along 7 dimensions that measure whether the illness is acute or chronic, has consequences, is under one's personal control, is under control of medical providers, is understood by the person, is cyclical, and has emotional aspects. The third section consists of 18 items that focus on causes. The IPQ has been translated into 18 languages (Coutu et al., 2008).

A revised version of the IPQ, the IPQ-R, was developed to examine cognitive and emotional representations as well as the person's understanding of their illness. The test–retest reliability is acceptable at r > 0.67 and the Cronbach's alphas showed good internal consistencies (0.84 to 0.91). The IPQ-R is a widely used tool (Coutu et al., 2008).

Stress and Coping Measures

There are a multitude of standardized stress and coping measures. Only a few of the available instruments are summarized next.

Stress Audit

The Stress Audit is used to assess perception of past stress and future problems. It measures stressors and stress reactions. Normative data is available. The scale has good internal consistency, reliability, and test–retest reliability (Peterson, 1989).

Stress Indicator and Health Planner

The Stress Indicator and Health Planner (SIHP) is a self-assessment and planning tool. Subscales consist of personal distress, interpersonal stress, wellness assessment, timed-stress assessment, and occupational stress assessment. It consists of a stress indicator section (20 minutes) and a health planner section (2.5 hours). Normative data are not presented and little detail is provided about how to interpret scores (Harper, 1998).

Stress Profile

The Stress Profile is a 123-item tool (25-minute administration time) that examines circumstances that help a person withstand or remain vulnerable to stress. Subscales include stress, health habits, exercise, rest/sleep, eating, prevention, alcohol/drugs/cigarettes, social supports, Type A behavior, cognitive hardiness, coping style, positive appraisal, negative appraisal, threat minimization, problem focus, and psychological well-being. The Stress Profile is easy to administer, score, and interpret. Test–retest reliability ranges form 0.76 to 0.86. Evidence of concurrent validity is limited (Isenhart, 2003).

The Health and Daily Living Form: Second Edition

The Health and Daily Living Form (HDL) explores social resources and coping strategies that individuals use to manage stressful circumstances in both medical and psychiatric populations. There is an adult form as well as a youth form for teens from age 12 to 18. Respondents are asked to rank their health, stressful events, and perceived social support during the last year.

Subscales evaluate individual functioning, stressful life circumstances, social network resources, help seeking, health-related functioning, self-confidence, substance use, physical symptoms, medical conditions, depressive mood, alcohol consumption, smoking, and medication use. Reliability data is missing from the manual. Administration and scoring are straightforward although the manual is poorly organized (Haynes, 2003).

Exercise Measures

Numerous measures examine how frequently people exercise, how they respond to exercise, and self-efficacy related to exercise. A sampling of exercise evaluation measures are included next.

The Episode-Specific Exercise Inventory

This scale was developed to measure people's awareness of sensations, thoughts, feelings, and meanings associated with exercise. It was developed because measures of predisposition to exercise only explain a small amount of change associated with exercise behavior. A horizontal line with 10 divisions is used for individuals to indicate the direction and intensity of their exercise experience after an exercise period is over. The Episode-Specific Exercise Inventory (ESIS) includes 37 items on 6 subscales: amount of concentration required during exercise, visual observations about the exercise setting, sweat intensity, muscle and joint comfort, audible environment (what was heard during exercise), and feelings of well-being associated with exercise. Alphas range from 0.75 to 0.92 for the subscales (Kraenzle Schneider, 2009).

Sample questions include: "Today with exercise, my thinking worsened/improved; Today exercise made me feel peppy/lazy; The pumping of my heart during exercise today felt unhealthy/healthy" (Kraenzle Schneider, 2009, p. 157).

The Exercise-Induced Feeling Inventory

Developed by Gauvin and Rejeski (1993) the Exercise-Induced Feeling Inventory (EFI) asks people to use 12 descriptors to describe how they felt during exercise. Those descriptors include feeling refreshed, calm, fatigued, enthusiastic, relaxed, energetic, happy, tired, revived, peaceful, worn-out, and upbeat. A Likert scale ranging from 0 (do not feel) to 4 (feel very strongly) is used. Coefficient alphas range from 0.72 to 0.91 for the subscales. The advantage of this scale and the Episode-Specific Exercise Inventory described here is that how people interpret their exercise-related feelings will likely influence whether they continue to exercise.

The Exercise Self-Efficacy Scale

The Exercise Self-Efficacy Scale (ESES) is a 10-item scale designed to measure a person's belief in their capacity to exercise. High self-efficacy prior to beginning exercise has been associated with being more likely to adhere to and complete an exercise program. Respondents rank items on a four-point scale (1 = not at all true, 2 = rarely true, 3 = moderately true, and 4 = always true) based on how confident they are about carrying out regular exercise. The instrument is reliable with high internal consistency, with a Chronbach alpha of 0.92. Respondents rank if they are confident that: "I can overcome barriers and challenges to exercise, I can exercise even when I am tired, I can be physically active even if I had no access to a gym," and a variety of other questions (Kroll, Kehn, Ho, & Groah, 2007, Table 1).

Food Consumption and Eating Behavior Scales

A variety of scales are available to track eating behaviors, food choices, and emotionally-driven eating. A sampling of these scales is summarized next.

The Eating Inventory

The Eating Inventory is a two-part questionnaire that looks at cognitive restraint of eating, disinhibition, and hunger. It can be used with adolescents or adults. The first 36 items are rated as true or false. The second portion of the questionnaire consists of 15 items. In this section the respondent uses a Likert scale to agree with or disagree with whether statements such as "Eat whatever you want when you want" corresponds to his or her behavior. The Eating Inventory is easy to administer and score because the answer sheet includes a built-in scoring system. A table for interpreting scores is also available, as are case studies that illustrate how to use the inventory. A major weakness is that the Eating Inventory has not been standardized on a large sample of individuals (Bloom, 1998).

The Food Choice Inventory

The Food Choice Inventory provides an estimate of the nutritional quality and diversity of a person's diet, although it is not based on dietary recall. The Food Choice Inventory lists 40 familiar foods, including culturally specific choices. Twenty-five foods are classified as high nutrient while 15 are considered low nutrient choices; this classification is based on a ratio that examines the amount of nutrients in food choices compared to the number of calories. Respondents indicate if they (1) would eat the food, (2) would like to try but did not eat the food, or (3) would not eat the food. The total number of foods an individual would eat is used to estimate how diverse their diet is. The Food Choice Inventory is easy to administer and score. However, critiques have focused on the category of "would not eat," which some authors have argued should be "do not eat." Interpreting scores is challenging because no standard scores are given. The inventory has an acceptable level of reliability (Titchenal, 1989).

The Yale Food Addiction Scale

The Yale Food Addiction Scale (YFAS) was designed to identify individuals with addiction to high-fat and high-sugar foods. Both dichotomous and frequency scoring are used to assess excess consumption, emotional eating, and dieting. Dichotomous scoring is used to evaluate whether individuals continue to eat in spite of emotional or physical problems. Respondents are asked to rate their behavior over the past 12 months. Frequency response options include never, once a month or less, two to four times per month, two to three times per week, and four or more times per week. Sample questions include "I find that when I start eating certain foods, I end up eating more than I had planned" and "I spend a lot of time feeling sluggish or lethargic from overeating" (Gearhardt, Corbin, & Brownell, 2009, p. 433).

The Emotional Eating Scale

The Emotional Eating Scale (EES) measures whether overeating is related to emotional stimuli. The scale consists of 25 items on a 5-point Likert scale. Respondents select "no desire to eat", "an overwhelming urge to eat", "a small desire to eat", "a moderate desire to eat" or "a strong desire to eat" when assessing the relationship of their mood and eating behavior (Arnow, Kenardy & Agras, 1995, p. 82). The EES has an internal reliability of 0.95 and good construct, discriminate, and criterion validity (Arnow, Kenardy, & Agras, 1995).

Role Modeling: A Scale for Nurses

The Self as a Role Model in Health Promotion Scale

This 75-item scale was developed to help nurses reflect on how they assist clients to adopt a health-promoting lifestyle. The instrument has an internal consistency of 0.91.

Sample items from the first factor, Use of professional self, include: "I am always honest with clients about the struggles involved in trying to practice a healthy lifestyle," I always take time to understand why a client's lifestyle is the way it is," "I begin with clients' own experiences in guiding them with their health promoting efforts" (Rush, Kee, & Rice, 2010, p. 12).

Factor two focuses on whether the nurse identifies himself or herself as the ideal healthy person. Sample items include: "I feel a lot of guilt when I teach about health behaviors I am not practicing" and "I practice a healthy lifestyle because I am a nurse." (Rush et al., p. 13).

Factor three on the scale explores whether being an imperfect role model has value because imperfect nurses can empathize with client struggles. Sample questions include: "I have had clients identify with me because, like them, I have had similar struggles with changing my health practices" and "I convey to clients that I am a human being with weaknesses" (Rush et al., 2010, p. 13).

Factor four of the scale looks at valuing oneself. Sample questions include: "I practice healthy behaviors exclusively for my own personal well-being and I do something when I fall short in my personal health practices" (Rush et al., 2010, p. 13).

The last factor, factor five, focuses on the nurse as a health promoter. A sample question is "I think of myself more as a health promoter than a role model because promoting health is what I do" (Rush et al., 2010, p. 13).

You may want to look up the entire scale and see how you score; scores range from 57 to 342. Nurses who score low view themselves as ideal role models but also tend to be authoritarian in teaching clients about health promotion practices. Nurses who score high approach interactions as if their clients were partners, recognize their own imperfections, and use those imperfections when teaching others (Rush et al., 2010). Which sort of nurse do you aspire to be?

DISCUSSION QUESTIONS

1. What are the advantages of using logic models when planning and evaluating health promotion programs?

2. Why is it important to evaluate both salutogenic and pathogenic factors that influence health?

3. Why is it necessary to evaluate both short- and long-term outcomes when evaluating a health promotion program?

4. Discuss social validity and why it matters in health promotion program evaluation.

5. Should one design a health promotion around an evaluation strategy or design an evaluation strategy around that program? Explain your answer.

6. Why is stakeholder involvement in health promotion program evaluation critical?

7. How could patient and clinician ratings of health improvement differ?

8. Why is it challenging to evaluate multiple "bundled" interventions simultaneously?

9. What does the abbreviation RE-AIM stand for?

10. What are the advantages and disadvantages of using QALYs?

11. Why have researchers argued for asset measurement?

12. Should generic or disease-specific outcome measures be used to evaluate health promotion programs? Explain your answer.

13. Which method of monitoring medication adherence is most effective? Which is most practical?

14. Which measure of smoking cessation is most accurate? When is this method ineffective?

15. What is the most common measure of obesity? How does that measure compare with DEXA scanning?

16. What are the advantages and disadvantages of metabolomics?

CHECK YOUR UNDERSTANDING: EXERCISE ONE

Search the research literature for examples of community-based participatory research or action research related to a health promotion topic that is of interest to you. Describe how those approaches are consistent with principles of health promotion practice advocated by the World Health Organization.

CHECK YOUR UNDERSTANDING: EXERCISE TWO

Match the following types of evaluations with their definitions.

Evaluations

1. Formative evaluation
2. Impact evaluation
3. Process evaluation
4. Outcome evaluation
5. Transfer evaluation
6. Structural evaluation

Definitions

A. Examines the influence of human resources.
B. Includes perceptions of stakeholders about anticipated program effectiveness.
C. Focuses on whether goals have been achieved.
D. Tracks the number of program participants.
E. Tracks the number of health promotion events held.
F. Is also called summative evaluation.
G. Focuses on the effectiveness of the program on changing knowledge.
H. Assesses whether the program is replicable in other settings.
I. Focuses on the effectiveness of the program on changing beliefs.

CHECK YOUR UNDERSTANDING: EXERCISE THREE

Match the following terms with their definitions.

Terms

1. Appropriateness
2. Reliability
3. Feasibility
4. Face validity
5. Utility
6. Content validity
7. Responsiveness
8. Criterion validity
9. Interpretability
10. Construct validity
11. Acceptability

Definitions

A. Whether the tool can be used in multiple settings.
B. Whether the instrument scores agrees with similar instruments.
C. Whether the instrument yields stable data.
D. Whether the items cover the breadth of content that the scale purports to measure.
E. Whether the instrument measures what it claims to measure.
F. Whether the instrument measures outcomes that are meaningful to participants.
G. Whether a lot of work is required to translate a numerical score into a clinically relevant meaning.
H. Whether the subject burden is reasonable to participants.
I. Whether data analysis is reasonably easy.
J. Whether the instrument is a good fit for the study.
K. Whether the instrument results are consistent with theory.

WHAT DO YOU THINK?

1. If you were designing a health promotion program with multiple interventions, would you begin targeting the highest risk behavior or the one people were the most willing to change? Explain your answer.

2. If you were completing a neighborhood mapping exercise of the area where you live and the area where you go to school, what would the most notable differences and similarities be?

3. Do you agree a person can experience well-being and chronic disease at the same time? Explain your answer and describe a scenario that illustrates your view.

4. How might nursing practice change if a pay-for-performance system were universally adopted?

5. Should the "perspective" component of a QALY calculation be based on provider or patient perspectives? Explain your answer. Which is it based on?

6. Would a text message-based health promotion program work to motivate you to exercise more? Why or why not?

7. How often do you take time to understand why patients' lifestyles are the way they are? Why is that important?

8. Is your waist midway between your lowest rib and the top of your iliac crest? Why do researchers establish set guidelines for obtaining measurements?

9. Can an imperfect nurse role model still be an effective health educator? Why or why not?

10. Which exercise scale described in this chapter would work best to evaluate your physical activity level?

11. What health-related commercial do you remember well enough to repeat? Would you need aided or unaided recall to remember all of it?

12. Which of the components of social capital are most important in helping you to maintain your health?

REFERENCES

Adams, T., Benzer, J., & Steinhardt, M. (1997). The conceptualization and measurement of perceived wellness: Integrating balance across and within dimensions. *American Journal of Health Promotion, 11*(3), 208–218.

Antonovsky, A. (1993). The structure and properties of the sense of coherence scale. *Social Science and Medicine, 36*(6), 725–733.

Antonovsky, A. (1996). The salutogenic model as a theory to guide health promotion. *Health Promotion International, 11*(1), 11–18.

Arnow, B., Kenardy, J. & Agras, W. S. (1995). The emotional eating scale: The development of a measure to assess coping with a negative affect by eating. *International Journal of Eating Disorders, 18*, 79–90.

Aronson, R. E., Wallis, A. B., O'Campo, P. J., Whitehead, T. L, & Schafer, P. (2007). Ethnographically informed community evaluation: A framework and approach for evaluating community-based initiatives. *Maternal Child Health Journal, 11*, 97–109.

Balkrishnan, R., & Jayawant, S. S. (2007). Medication adherence research in populations: Measurement issues and other challenges. *Clinical Therapeutics, 29*(6), 1180–1183.

Bauer, S. (2008). Societal and ethical issues in human biomonitoring—A view from science studies. *Environmental Health, 7*(Suppl 1), 11–13.

Bauer, G., Davies, J. K., & Pelikan, J. (2006). The EUHPID health development model for the classification of public health indicators. *Health Promotion International, 21*(2), 153–159.

Bauer, G., Davies, J. K., Pelikan, J., Noack, H., Broesskamp, U., & Hill, C. (2003). Advancing a theoretical model for public health and health promotion indicator development: Proposal from the EUHPID consortium, *European Journal of Public Health, 13*(3), 107–113.

Bauman, A., Phongsavan, P., Schoeppe, S., & Owen, N. (2006). Physical activity measurement: A primer for health promotion. *Promotion and Education, 13*, 92. Retrieved from http://ped.sagepub.com/content/13/2/92

Becker, C. M., Moore, J. B., Whetstone, L., Glascoff, M., Chaney, E., Felts, M., & Anderson, L. (2009). Validity evidence for the Salutogenic Wellness Promotion Scale (SWPS). *American Journal of Health Behavior, 33*(4), 455–465.

Best, A., Stokols, D., Green, L. W., Leischow, S., Holmes, B., & Buchholz, K. (2003). Achieving a new vision: An integrative framework for community partnering to translate theory into effective health promotion strategy. *American Journal of Health Promotion, 18*(2), 168–176.

Blize, R., Burnand, B., Mueller, Y., Walther, M. R., & Cornuz, J. (2009). Biomedical risk assessment as an aid for smoking cessation. *The Cochrane Library, 2*, CD004705.

Bloom, L.A. (1998). Test review of the eating inventory. In J. C. Impara & B. S. Plake (Eds.), *The thirteenth mental measurements yearbook.* Retrieved from the Burros Institute's Mental Measurements Yearbook online database.

Brown, C. S., Lloyd, S., & Murray, S. A. (2006). Using consecutive rapid participatory appraisal studies to assess, facilitate and evaluate health and social change in community settings. *BMC Public Health, 6*, 68.

Brown, M.B. (1998). Test review of the lifestyle assessment questionnaire. In J. C. Impara & B. S. Plake (Eds.), *The thirteenth mental measurements yearbook.* Retrieved from the Burros Institute's Mental Measurements Yearbook online database.

Caruso, J. C. (2001). Test review of the quality of life enjoyment and satisfaction questionnaire. In B. S. Plake, & J. C. Impara (Eds.), *The fourteenth mental measurements yearbook.* Retrieved from the Burros Institute's Mental Measurements Yearbook online database.

Centers for Disease Control and Prevention (1999). Framework for program evaluation in public health. *Morbidity and Mortality Weekly Report, 48*(RR–11), 1–40.

Coutu, M. F., Durand, M. J., Baril, R., Labrecque, M-E., Ngomo, S., Cote, D., & Rouleau, A. (2008). A review of assessment tools of illness representations: Are these adapted for a work disability prevention context? *Journal of Occupational Rehabilitation, 18*, 347–361.

Deutscher, D., Hart, D. L., Dickstein, R., Horn, S. D., & Gutvirtz, M. (2008). Implementing an integrated electronic outcomes and electronic health record process to create a foundation for clinical practice improvement. *Physical Therapy, 88*(2), 270–285.

Downie, R. S., Tannahill, C., & Tannahill, A. (1996). *Health promotion: Models and values* (2nd ed.). Oxford, UK: Oxford University Press.

Fave, G., Beckmann, M. E., Draper, J. H., & Mathers, J. C. (2009). Measurement of dietary exposure: A challenging problem which may be overcome thanks to metabolomics? *Genes and Nutrition, 4*, 135–141.

Fleenor, J. W. (2001). Test review of the Friedman well-being scale. In B. S. Plake & J. C. Impara (Eds.), *The fourteenth mental measurements yearbook*. Retrieved from the Burros Institute's Mental Measurements Yearbook online database.

Gardner, P. J. & Campagna, P. D. (2009). Pedometers as measurement tools and motivational devices: New insights for researchers and practitioners. *Health Promotion Practice*. Accessed at http://hpp.sagepub.com/content/early/2009/06/10/1524839909334623.

Gauvin, L., and Rejeski, W. J. (1993). The exercise-induced feeling inventory: Development and initial validation. *Journal of Sport and Exercise Psychology, 15*, 403–423.

Gearhardt, A. N., Corbin, W. R. & Brownell, K. D. (2009). Preliminary validation of the Yale Food Addiction Scale. *Appetite, 52*, 430–436.

Geisinger, K. F., Spies, R. A., Carlson, J. F. & Plake, B. S. (Eds.). (2007). *The seventeenth mental measurements yearbook*. Retrieved from the Burros Institute's Mental Measurements Yearbook online database.

Glanz, K., Rimer, B. K., & Lewis, F. M. (2002). *Health behavior and health education: Theory, research and practice* (3rd ed.). San Francisco, CA: Jossey-Bass.

Glasgow, R. E., Klesges, L. M., Dzewaltowski, D. A., Estabrooks, P. A., & Vogt, T. M. (2006). Evaluating the impact of health promotion programs: Using the RE-AIM framework to form summary measures for decision making involving complex issues. *Health Education Research, 21*(5), 688–694.

Gorber, S. C., Schofield-Hurwitz, S., Hardt, J., Levasseur, G., & Tremblay, M. (2009). The accuracy of self-reported smoking: A systematic review of the relationship between self-reported and cotinine-assessed smoking status. *Nicotine & Tobacco Research, 11*(1), 12–24.

Green, J. & Tones, K. (1999). Toward a secure evidence base for health promotion. *Journal of Public Health Medicine, 21*, 133–139.

Hancock. L., Sanson-Fisher, R. W., Redman, S., Buton, R., Burton, L., Butler, J., . . . Walsh, R. (1997). Community action for health promotion: A review of methods and outcomes 1990–1995. *American Journal of Preventive Medicine, 13*, 229–239.

Harper, D. C. (1998). Test review of the stress indicator and health planner. In J. C. Impara & B. S. Plake (Eds.), *The thirteenth mental measurements yearbook*. Retrieved from the Burros Institute's Mental Measurements Yearbook online database.

Haynes, S. D. (2003). Test review of the health and daily living form: Second edition. In B. S. Plake, J. C. Impara, & R.A. Spies. *The fifteenth mental measurements yearbook*. Retrieved from the Burros Institute's Mental Measurements Yearbook online database.

Healey, B. J., & Zimmerman, R. S. (2010). Program Evaluation. In B. J. Healey & R. S. Zimmerman (Eds.) *The new world of health promotion: New program development, implementation, and evaluation* (pp. 89–104). Sudbury, MA: Jones and Bartlett.

Health Education Board for Scotland [HEBS]. (1999). *Research for a healthier Scotland: The research strategy for the Health Education Board for Scotland*. Edinburgh, UK: Author.

Heron, K. E. & Smyth, J. M. (2010). Ecological momentary interventions: Incorporating mobile technology into psychosocial and health behavior treatments. *British Journal of Health Psychology, 15*(1), 1–39.

Hewitt, J. (2007). Critical evaluation of the use of research tools in evaluating quality of life for people with schizophrenia. *International Journal of Mental Health Nursing, 16,* 2–14.

Institute of Medicine [IOM], Committee on Health and Behavior: Research, Practice and Policy Board on Neuroscience and Behavioral Health (2001). Evaluating and disseminating intervention research. In *Health and behavior: The interplay of biological, behavioral, and societal influences* (pp. 274–328). Washington, DC: National Academies Press.

Isenhart, C. (2003). Test review of the stress profile. In B. S. Plake, J. C. Impara, & R.A. Spies (Eds.). *The fifteenth mental measurements yearbook.* Retrieved from the Burros Institute's Mental Measurements Yearbook online database.

Kaplan, R. M. & Anderson, J. P. (1996). The general policy model: An integrated approach. In B. Spilker (Ed.). *Quality of life and pharmacoeconomics in clinical trials* (pp. 309-322). Philadelphia, PA; Lippincott-Raven.

Katz, P., Gregorich, S., Yazdany, J., Trupin, L., Julian, L., Yelin, E., & Crisweil, L. A. (2011). Obesity and its measurement in a community based sample of women with systemic lupus erythematosus. *Arthritis Care and Research, 63*(2), 261–268. PMID 20824801.

Kayes, N. M., & McPherson, K. M. (2010). Measuring what matters: Does objectivity mean good science? *Disability and Rehabilitation, 32*(12) 1011–1019.

King, P. M. (1194). Health promotion: The emerging frontier in nursing. *Journal of Advanced Nursing, 20,* 209–218.

Kroll, T., Kehn, M., Ho, P. S., & Groah, S. (2007). The SCI exercise self-efficacy scale (ESES): Development and psychometric properties. *International Journal of Behavioral Nutrition and Physical Activity, 4.* Retrieved from http://www.ijbnapa.org/content/4/1/34

Kulbok, P. A., Baldwin, J. H., Cox, C. L., & Duffy, R. (1997). Advancing discourse on health promotion: Beyond mainstream thinking. *Advances in Nursing Science, 20*(1), 12–20.

Kraenzle Schneider, J. (2009). Refinement and validation of the episode-specific interpretation of exercise inventory. *Journal of Nursing Measurement, 17*(2), 148–163.

Kritsotakis, G., Koutis, A. D., Alegakis, A. K. & Philalithis, A. E. (2008). Development of the social capital questionnaire in Greece. *Research in Nursing and Health, 31,* 217–225.

Lanza, A. (2010). Continuous quality improvement in health promotion programs. In B. J. Healey & R. S. Zimmerman (Eds.), *The new world of health promotion: New program development, implementation, and evaluation* (pp. 257–272). Sudbury, MA: Jones and Bartlett.

Learmonth, A., & Mackie, P. (2000). Evaluating effectiveness in health promotion: A case of re-inventing the millstone: *Health Education Journal, 59,* 267–280.

Lima, V. L., Arruda, J. M., Barroso, M. A., Tavares. M., Campos, N. Z., Zandonadi, R. C., . . . Serrano, M. M. (2007). Analyzing the outcomes of health promotion practices. *Promotion & Education, 14,* 21–26.

Lonborg, S. (2007). Test review of the five factor wellness inventory. In K. F. Geisinger, R.A. Spies, J. F. Carlson, & B. S. Plake (Eds.). *The seventeenth mental measurement yearbook.* Retrieved from the Burros Institute's Mental Measurements Yearbook online data base.

Lytle, L. A. (2009). Measuring the food environment: State of the science. *American Journal of Preventative Medicine, 36*(4S), S134–S136.

Macdonald, G., Veen, C., & Tones, K. (1996). Evidence for success in health promotion: Suggestions for improvement, *Health Education Research, Theory, and Practice, 11*(3), 367–376.

McGrath, C., Rofail, D., Gargon, E., & Abetz, L. (2010). Using quality methods to inform the trade-off between content validity and consistency in utility assessment: The example of type 2 diabetes and Alzheimer's disease. *Health and Quality of Life Outcomes, 8*(23), 2–13.

Morris, D. S., Rooney, M. P., Wray, R. J., & Kreuter, M. W. (2009). Measuring exposure to health messages in community-based intervention studies: a systematic review of current practices. *Health Education and Behavior, 36*(6), 979–998.

Oman, R. F., Vesley, S. K., McLeroy, K. R., Harris-Wyatt, V., Aspy, C. B., Rodine, S., & Marshall, L. (2002). Reliability and validity of the Youth Asset Survey (YAS). *Journal of Adolescent Health, 31,* 247–255.

Peersman, G. V., Oakley, A. R., & Oliver, S. (1999). Evidence based health promotion? Some methodological challenges. *International Journal of Health Promotion and Education, 37,* 59–64.

Peterson, R.A. (1989). Test review of the stress audit. In J. C. Conoley & J. Kramer (Eds.), *The tenth mental measurements yearbook.* Retrieved from the Burros Institute's Mental Measurements Yearbook online database.

Pinar, R., Celik, R., & Bahcecik, N. (2009). Reliability and construct validity of the health-promoting lifestyle profile II in an adult Turkish population. *Nursing Research, 58*(3), 184–193.

Prochaska, J. J., Spring, B. & Nigg, C. R. (2008). Multiple health behavior change research: An introduction and overview. *Preventive Medicine, 46,* 181–188.

Roth, C. P., Lim, Y., Pevnick, J. M., Asch, S. M., & McGlynn, E. A. (2009). The challenge of measuring quality of care from the electronic health record. *American Journal of Medical Quality, 24*(5), 385–394.

Rush, K. L., Kee, C. C., & Rice, M. (2010). The self as role model in health promotion scale: Development and testing. *Western Journal of Nursing Research Online, 32*(6), 814–832. doi: 10.1177/0193945910361595

Scoggins, J. F., & Patrick, D. L. (2009). The use of patient-reported outcomes instruments in registered clinical trials: Evidence from ClinicalTrials.gov. *Contemporary Clinical Trials, 30*(4), 289–292.

Scott, V., Stern, R., Sanders, D., Reagon, G., & Mathews, V. (2008). Research to action to address inequities: The experience of the Cape Town Equity Gauge. *International Journal for Equity in Health, 7*(6). Retrieved from http://www.equityhealthj.com/content/7/1/6

Seltzer, G.B. (1992). Test review of the quality of life questionnaire. In. J. J. Kramer, & J. C. Conoley. *The eleventh mental measurements yearbook.* Retrieved from the Burros Institute's Mental Measurements Yearbook online database.

South, J. & Tilford, S. (2000). Perceptions of research and evaluation in health promotion practice and influences on activity. *Health Education Research Theory and Practice, 15*(6), 729–741.

Stokols, D. (1996). Translating social ecological theory into guidelines for community health promotion. *American Journal of Health Promotion. 10*(4), 282–298.

Titchenal, C. A. (1989). Test review of the food choice inventory. In J. C. Conoley & J. Kramer (Eds.), *The tenth mental measurements yearbook.* Retrieved from the Burros Institute's Mental Measurements Yearbook online database.

Tones, K. (2000). Evaluating health promotion: A tale of three errors. *Patient Education and Counseling, 39,* 227–236.

Tones, K., & Green, J. (2004). *Health promotion: Planning and strategies.* London, UK: Sage.

Ware, J. E. & Sherbourne, C. D. (1992). The MOS 36-item short-form health survey (SF-36). *Medical Care, 30*(6), 473–483.

Werner, R. M., Greenfield, S., Fung, C., & Turner, B. J. (2007). Measuring quality of care in patients with multiple clinical conditions: Summary of a conference conducted by the Society of General Internal Medicine. *Society of General Internal Medicine, 22,* 1206–1211.

Whitehead, D. (2000). A stage planning programme model for health education/health promotion practice. *Journal of Advanced Nursing, 36*(2), 311–320.

Whitehead, D. (2003). Evaluating health promotion: A model for nursing practice. *Journal of Advanced Nursing, 41,* 490–498.

Winthrop, A. L. (2010). Health-related quality of life after pediatric trauma. *Current Opinions in Pediatrics, 22,* 346–351.

World Health Organization [WHO]. (1998). *Health promotion evaluation: Recommendations to policymakers. Report of the WHO European Working Group on Health Promotion.* Copenhagen, Denmark: Author.

Wu, A. W., Revicki, D. A., Jacobson, D., & Malitz, F. E. (1997). Evidence for reliability, validity and usefulness of the medical outcomes study HIV health survey (MOS-HIV). *Quality of Life Research, 6,* 481–493.

For a full suite of assignments and additional learning activities, see the access code at the front of your book.

CHAPTER 11

Entrepreneurship and Health Promotion

Bonnie Raingruber

OBJECTIVES

At the conclusion of this chapter, the student will be able to:

- Define entrepreneurship.
- Distinguish entrepreneurship from social entrepreneurship and intrapreneurship.
- Describe the advantages and challenges associated with running a health promotion business.
- Discuss the characteristics of a successful entrepreneur.
- List the types of health promotion business ventures that nurses have created.
- Distinguish between the different types of business structures.
- Outline the components of a business plan.
- Describe effective marketing strategies.
- Discuss methods and challenges associated with billing for services and hiring staff.
- Articulate why having adequate malpractice insurance is a must.
- List agencies that provide help to small business owners.
- Determine whether being a nurse entrepreneur is one of his/her long-term career goals.

DEFINITIONS OF ENTREPRENEURSHIP

Richard Cantillon, an Irish banker working in Paris, coined the term "entrepreneur" somewhere between 1680 and 1734. He classified doctors, lawyers, and beggars, among other professions, as entrepreneurs. Cantillon defined an entrepreneur as the bearer of an uninsurable business risk (Martin, 1984). Many definitions of entrepreneurship have been proposed since that time. Entrepreneurs variously have been defined as: (1) one who conceptualizes, implements, and operates services to influence social change (Leong, 2005); (2) someone who perceives an opportunity and creates an organization to pursue it (Orga, 1996); (3) a person with the skill of turning ideas into action; (4) a person who "sets up a business, taking on financial risks in the hope of profit" (Boore & Porter, 2011, p. 184); (5) an individual who assumes total responsibility and risk for discovering or creating unique opportunities to use personal talents, skills, and energy, and who employs a strategic planning process to transfer that opportunity into a marketable service or product" (Hewison & Badger, 2006, box 2); (6) a person who develops, organizes, manages, and assumes the risk of a business that offers nursing services of a "direct care, educational, research, administrative, or consultative nature" (Wilson, Averis, & Walsh, 2003, p. 237); and (7) a nurse who recognizes trends and identifies nursing skills that can be marketed to meet consumer needs (Powell, 1984). Because of the nature of health promotion, a multitude of educational and service-oriented businesses are possible. Entrepreneurship has been described as "sui generis, an irreducible form of freedom" (Kauffman Foundation, 2007, p. 6).

As a nurse entrepreneur, it is important to provide a specific service rather than developing a mission statement for the business that is too broad (Muscari, 2004). When considering starting an entrepreneurial venture, Dawes (2009) suggested that nurses ask themselves the following:

1. What do I excel at?
2. Which people would benefit from what I do best?
3. Who would pay for the services I plan on providing?
4. How much one might pay for those services (Dawes, 2009)?

It has been estimated that as of 2004, 1% of nurses worked in entrepreneurial roles (International Council of Nurses [ICN], 2004). Nurses, who function as entrepreneurs, according to the ICN, need to be passionate about their area of interest, be willing to take risks and make commitments, believe in their dreams, have plenty of self-confidence, have a drive to achieve, and possess a strong customer orientation.

Because of the independent nature of entrepreneurship, it has been described as being "foreign to nurses' educational, social, and professional experience" (Martin, 1984, p. 408). Even though entrepreneurship requires nurses to step out of their comfort zone, it brings an opportunity to address the many challenges confronting today's healthcare system (Martin, 1984).

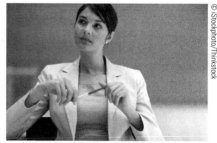

As Banham and Connelly (2002) commented: "Drawing on the core concept of professionalism, that defines its own tasks . . . nurses entrepreneurs advocate for a wider role for nursing, to be achieved by extending the types of services available to patients" (p. 1541). Entrepreneurship allows for "diversification of nursing practice beyond traditional boundaries" (Austin, Luker, & Martin, 2006, p. 1542). Entrepreneurs build their business on best practice models and a clinically based understanding of client needs (Austin et al., 2006).

SOCIAL ENTREPRENEURSHIP
AND INTRAPRENEURSHIP

Entrepreneurship "relates to the ways in which people, in all kinds of organizations, behave in order to cope with and take advantage of uncertainty and complexity and how in turn this becomes embodied in ways of doing things, ways of seeing things, . . . ways of communicating things, and ways of learning things" (Gibb, 2000, p. 16). The term "intrapreneur" has been used to describe a salaried person who behaves in an entrepreneurial way within the organization where they typically work (Drennan et al., 2007), such as someone who creates an innovative healthcare program for their employer (Hewison & Badger, 2006). Often, intrapreneurs make suggestions for program revision, develop a radically new procedure that transforms how care is provided within an institution, or devise a money-saving strategy that benefits the agency where they work. Intrapreneurship "is when an organization encourages and develops the entrepreneurial talents of staff in order to establish an innovative and effective organization" (Boore & Porter, 2011, p. 185). An example of an intrapreneur is a nurse who created a storybook to prepare children in her hospital for tonsillectomy surgery (Boore & Porter, 2011). Another example is the Heartcheck program, which included an individualized cardiovascular risk evaluation, blood work, and a care plan to decrease alterable risks. The program was developed by a staff nurse and used to generate outpatient revenue at her hospital while providing needed services (Wolfson & Neidlinger, 1991).

The term social entrepreneurship means that one "uses entrepreneurial skills to accomplish social needs or lead social change from within private, public, and not-for-profit organizations" (Boore & Porter, 2011, p. 184). Social entrepreneurs are change agents who create a mission to sustain social values (Boore & Porter, 2011). Florence Nightingale, for example, has been described as a notable social entrepreneur (Center for Advancement of Social Entrepreneurship [CASE], 2008).

A classic perception is that "nursing is about caring while business is about making money" (Elango, Phil, Hunter, & Winchell, 2007, p. 203). Some have argued that nursing and business are therefore incompatible. As Elango and colleagues commented, while the view that entrepreneurship is incompatible with the service mentality is "understandable, nurses seeking to become entrepreneurs should also recognize the societal role of entrepreneurship, wherein specific needs of society are fulfilled and new wealth is generated. Nurses having such conflicts should ask themselves, 'Would the world be a better place if there were no entrepreneurs?'" (p. 203).

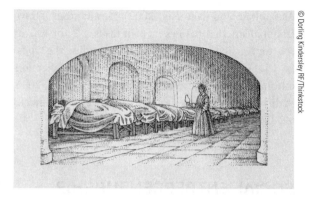

© Dorling Kindersley RF/Thinkstock

An advantage for nurse entrepreneurs is that many health promotion–related businesses have a relatively low overhead and can be used to supplement or provide care to underserved populations (Elango et al., 2007). Entrepreneurship, intrapreneurship, and social entrepreneurs are needed in today's healthcare climate. Demographic changes and economic constraints necessitate offering innovative healthcare options in what has been described as an "era of chaos and complexity" (White & Begu, 1998, p. 40). Entrepreneurs expand the range of health services that are available (Wilson et al., 2003).

THE ADVANTAGES AND CHALLENGES ASSOCIATED WITH RUNNING A SMALL BUSINESS

There are numerous advantages associated with creating and running a health promotion business. Advantages discussed in the literature include: (1) flexible time management, (2) control over the quality of the practice (Leong, 2005), (3) autonomy and creative license, (4) the diversity of the job (Sankelo & Akerblad, 2009), (5) the ability to generate income in ways that mesh with family responsibilities (Drennan et al., 2007), and (6) the fact that you can't be fired (Orga, 1996).

Many nurses are motivated to start a small business because of challenges with their existing work environment. Positions may have been downsized; high workload or time pressure can be a factor; shift work, including holidays and weekends, is often required of nurses, and nurses may not have sufficient influence over their job responsibilities. All of these are reasons nurses have cited for deciding to develop a small business (Sankelo & Akerblad, 2008). Dawes (2009) discussed the push and pull motivations that prompt a nurse to become an entrepreneur. Push factors include unemployment and job dissatisfaction, whereas pull factors are clinical opportunity and excitement about providing a needed service. Some nurses move gradually toward self-employment; this helps ensure that a steady income stream is available until the business can provide a secure income and insurance coverage (Muscari, 2004). However, other nurses have commented that part-time regular employment diverted their attention from developing their business (Wilson et al., 2003). It is also the case that some nurses work in positions that require them to sign a no-competition clause that prohibits them from offering any service such as starting a clinic in the area where they practice, receiving reimbursement from a grant that their institution might have applied for, or working simultaneously for another health-related agency (Elango et al., 2007).

Overall, nurse entrepreneurs report being pleased with their role and experiencing a sense of well-being at work that encompasses physical, mental, financial, and social needs. Among those entrepreneurs who are most stressed are nurses who have started a business within the last year, which is the case because many small businesses fail within the first year and that period is filled with challenges (Sankelo & Akerblad, 2009).

There are a variety of ongoing challenges associated with running a health promotion business. Among the challenges are the pressure associated with maintaining the bottom line; the 24/7 responsibility for running the company and always feeling tied to the job; limited vacation scheduling; feeling responsible for the income of one's employees (Sankelo & Akerblad, 2009); working long hours and having to do whatever is necessary to make the business a success; variable income based on market trends (Orga, 1996); inadequate reimbursement from public and private insurance (Wilson et al., 2003); lack of healthcare insurance and retirement benefits (Caffrey, 2005); and working in relative isolation (Drennan et al., 2007). It is always a radical change to move from being a salaried worker to a small business owner (Caffrey, 2005).

It is possible to create a home-based business. This approach saves the overhead involved in renting, leasing, or purchasing office space. However, one can become easily distracted by childcare challenges and other priorities associated with running a home. To be successful, Schulmeister (1999a), who runs a home-based oncology nursing consultation practice, suggests having a designated work area that is only used for the business, allowing the message machine to pick up calls and only returning calls four times per day, turning the television off, not reading the mail when it arrives, and setting established goals to be completed each day. For example, one could decide to work 6 hours on business-related activities each day and use a clock to monitor that this amount of time had been devoted to the business. She also suggested paying for a toll-free number so that customers and other businesses in outlying areas can easily contact you. Having a toll-free number gives the impression the business is well-established.

When the business is growing during the start-up years, it is vital to accept each patient who makes contact with the practice and to schedule visits around patient's work schedules (Muscari, 2004).

THE CHARACTERISTICS OF A SUCCESSFUL ENTREPRENEUR

Entrepreneurs have been described as being risk-takers (Schulmeister, 1999a) and having a higher internal locus of control than other nurses (Orga, 1996). While entrepreneurs must take risks, they are typically described as moderate risk-takers who spend time evaluating and calculating risk as compared to high-risk seekers (Martin, 1984). Shirey (2008) suggested that emotional endurance is a requirement for nurses who wish to start a business, which is necessary in order to "persist despite personal fears or perceived obstacles" (p. 9). She comments that nurses who are considering starting a business should ask themselves "What would I like to do even if I were not paid to do it?" (p. 10). Shirey also stresses that a would-be business owner should write down goals five or more times because being clear about a goal and committed to it is likely to result in success.

Entrepreneurship requires "creativity, innovation, and risk taking, as well as the ability to plan and manage projects in order to achieve objectives" (Boore & Porter, 2011, p. 184). The major tool of an entrepreneur is innovation, the mechanism through which they exploit change and translate it into an opportunity for different businesses or services (Drucker, 1985). Entrepreneurs need to be able to be goal-oriented, to recognize trends, and to act on opportunities that arise.

Entrepreneurs need the ability to deal with failure, ambiguity, and uncertainty. They must have integrity, reliability, patience, accountability, perseverance, determination, flexibility, courage, resourcefulness, initiative, independence, optimism, enthusiasm, confidence, self-discipline, perceptiveness, a need to achieve, and the ability to be proactive (Hewison & Badger, 2006; Martin, 1984; Wilson et al., 2003). Entrepreneurs must possess assertiveness, expertise in negotiation, time management skills, a strong customer service focus, skill in networking, and a visionary mindset (Wilson et al., 2003). They must be able to toot their own horn. Entrepreneurs are driven by "a sense of excitement and innovation that gives one the feeling energetic change is about to happen" (Kowal, 1998, p. 278). They seek challenge and realize that because they are learning on a daily basis, they will feel like a novice when they encounter new situations even though they have had years of experience in the clinical arena (Blaich, 2004). Mackey (2005) stressed that entrepreneurs habitually act on potential opportunities, keep inventories of credible options, and "seize the day" whenever possible (p. 501). However, they only pursue the best opportunities so they can remain focused and successful given their current goals.

Some nurses have managed family responsibilities, latex allergies, and back injuries by going into business. However, studies have shown entrepreneurs are not in business because they are unemployable or unable to find work; rather, they enjoy being self-employed. Nurses comment that the advantages of being self-employed outweigh the disadvantages (Wilson et al., 2008).

Many entrepreneurs are experienced nurses because it is necessary to have a well-grounded clinical understanding before one can develop a realistic practice (Wilson et al., 2003). Often, entrepreneurs have a master's or doctoral degree and years of experience, although those are not requirements. To charge private insurance or Medicare for a number of nursing services, licensure as a nurse practitioner or a clinical nurse specialist is needed. All registered nurses, however, can charge cash for activities within their scope of practice.

EXAMPLES OF HEALTH PROMOTION PRACTICES THAT NURSES HAVE CREATED

There is an abundance of opportunities related to health promotion that lend themselves to entrepreneurial activities. Numerous health promotion practices that have been created by nurses are listed in the literature:

- A lymph edema therapy practice (Leong, 2005);
- A home-based oncology consultation practice (Schulmeister, 1999a);
- A diabetes education service (Moore & Dayhoff, 2002);
- A cosmetic practice (e.g., Botox or collagen injections offered at home or in a discreet manner);
- Per diem nurse registries (Elango et al., 2007);
- A private care home for adolescents, the elderly, or disabled;
- An expert witness practice (Boore & Porter, 2011);
- Dementia care;
- A young adult cancer service;
- A substance abuse service for mothers;
- A home-based mobile minor injury treatment team (Hewison & Badger, 2006);
- A complementary and alternative healthcare practice (Drennan et al., 2007);
- A corporate wellness practice;

- Child care education;
- A pain management practice;
- Nutrition and weight counseling;
- Stoma care;
- Midwifery and lactation services;
- Infertility counseling;
- Continuing education courses;
- Individual, group, couples, and family therapy.

Entrepreneurs also work as continence advisors, tissue viability nurses, nurse consultants, nurse authors, and coaches who offer career development advice. Other examples include "Nurses on Call," a service that contracts with pediatricians to offer after-hours phone screening and an after-school program that emphasized enjoyable exercise and health food choice education for elementary age children. Toilet training classes for children and babysitting workshops that focus on child safety and effective discipline have also been offered by nurse entrepreneurs (Schulmeister, 1999b).

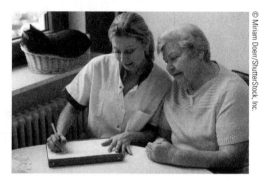

© Miriam Doerr/ShutterStock, Inc.

TYPES OF BUSINESS STRUCTURES

Three main types of businesses exist. Those include a sole proprietorship, a general partnership, and a corporation. Among the corporations there are S-Corporations, limited liability companies (LLC), and limited liability partnerships (LLP) (Leong, 2005). Sole proprietorship means the nurse and the business are one entity. Profits and losses are reported on one's individual income tax, and the individual running the sole proprietorship assumes complete financial and professional liability for the business. A sole proprietorship is the easiest type of business structure to establish because in most states no registration requirements or legal fees are required for a sole proprietorship (Moore & Dayhoff, 2002; Schulmeister, 1999b). The sole proprietorship remains in existence as long as the individual wishes to stay in business. However, individuals who operate a sole proprietorship from their home have been encouraged to take out business liability insurance to cover possible injuries as clients enter or leave the home (Lyon, 2003).

In a general partnership, several individuals jointly manage the business; an example would be two clinical nurse specialists working with a physician. In a general partnership each partner assumes professional and financial liability for all partners. An S-Corporation consists of 75 or fewer stockholders. Profit and loss is reported on an individual tax return, but the corporation assumes professional and financial liability for the business, thus placing a limit on personal liability (Moore & Dayhoff, 2002).

An LLC or limited liability partnership is separate from the individual creating the business. The business assumes professional and financial liability. LLCs and LLPs must file articles of incorporation with the state and federal government and be granted a Tax Identification Number. It is important to contact a lawyer to determine which type of organizational structure is the best fit for a business depending on associated legal and tax purposes (Mackey, 2005; Moore & Dayhoff, 2002).

A nurse who is interested in starting a business needs to decide if it is best to (1) set up a solo practice from a home office, (2) run a solo practice in leased or rented space, (3) join insurance panels to obtain third-party reimbursement, (4) partner with other nurses interested in a similar business venture, or (5) work with a physician in a collaborative practice (Barry, 2005). Which model is the best fit for a given business in the select location, along with the nurse's personality and the specific patient population, are all factors that must be considered.

CREATING A BUSINESS PLAN

Having a business plan is necessary to motivate investors or obtain a loan in order to establish a business. A business plan is also needed to make sure adequate planning has been done to ensure the business will be successful, to attract skilled employees, and to facilitate obtaining large contracts (Shirey, 2007). Business plans begin with a signed and co-signed nondisclosure statement to notify the reader that the plan is not to be shared with anyone without permission (Mackey, 2005).

Next, one develops an executive summary (approximately three pages in length) describing the company and location, products or services, date the business will begin, market potential (uniqueness of services offered compared to the existing community services, economic trends, and growth prospects), types and numbers of clients anticipated, hours of operation, space/equipment needs, start-up funds, marketing strategies, personnel, an operating budget, organizational chart, and a resume of key personnel (Mackey, 2005; Moore & Dayhoff, 2002; Shirey, 2007). To describe the services your business will provide, begin by listing your skills and knowledge and identifying which of those skills a customer would purchase. A section of the business plan focuses on customers, their location, number, and characteristics. Customers may include individual patients or insurance groups, hospitals, and other healthcare facilities or schools.

An overview of the given industry, called a market analysis, is included in the business plan along with a timeline over which the business can be expected to become profitable (Schulmeister, 1999b). Formal surveys or trends in health care or demographic data can be used to produce a market analysis (Muscari, 2004). It is also important to discuss how you will market your business; how pricing for, cost of, and quality of services provided will differ from that of competitors; and how your business is different or unique. There is a section of the business plan that includes forecasts of future success, such as when the business can expect to break even (revenues equal or exceed expenses). Typically the forecast covers a 3- to 5-year period and includes benchmarks that can be used to evaluate yearly progress (Mackey, 2005; Muscari, 2004).

The business plan includes a section on the organizational structure, the office location (access to public transportation and parking, square footage, handicap access, lease agreement terms), start-up expenses needed to begin the business, and operating expenses. Start-up expenses include things such as a fax machine, a computer, a printer, a duplicating machine, a telephone, chairs, desks, trade name license fees, business incorporation fees, lawyer fees, business cards, and stationary. Ongoing operating expenses include payroll costs, telephone and Internet fees, rent, postage, utilities, accounting fees, liability insurance, marketing costs, and supplies (Moore & Dayhoff, 2002). As Elango and colleagues (2007) commented, one should not "buy new what you can buy used, buy used what you can lease, lease what you can borrow, borrow what you can barter, barter what you can beg, beg what you can scavenge, or scavenge what you can get for free" (p. 203). Recommendations are that a new business should have enough cash on hand to cover 3 months of expenses so that delayed reimbursement does not pose problems (Schulmeister, 1999b). Letters of support from "potential patients, hospitals, or other healthcare providers in the area who will refer patients to you" are helpful to include in the business plan for lenders to review (Mackey, 2005, p. 504).

HIRING AND SUPERVISING STAFF

Another decision one has to make as a business owner is whether you can see all of the anticipated patients yourself or whether to hire staff to assist you. Whether an office manager, a billing service, or an accountant is needed are also key decisions (Mackey, 2005). Depending on the type of services provided by employees, checking their license may suffice. Or, it may be important to do drug testing, background checks, and reference checks. As an employer, one has to deduct taxes and worker's compensation from the employee's check. Depending on the size of the business, healthcare coverage and benefits such as sick leave and vacation time may also be needed (Smith, 2007).

All employees must be oriented to the company mission, policies and procedures, and expectations regarding their performance. Training costs should be included in the budget. Ways of recognizing exceptional care, such as an employee-of-the-month program, are valuable ways to enhance productivity and promote retention. Allowing employees flexibility in terms of scheduling or types of patients they prefer to work with will result in a greater commitment to company goals (Smith, 2007).

BILLING FOR SERVICES

Nurse practitioners (NPs) and many clinical nurse specialists (CNSs) are able to bill private insurances for many diagnoses and procedures. To bill insurances, one must join provider panels of health maintenance organizations (HMO). This is an important decision because sometimes HMO panels require a 6-month notification before you can resign from the panel, during which time you must continue to see patients they refer (Barry, 2005 & 2006a). Often, receiving timely payments from HMOs is a challenge requiring multiple contacts. Keeping detailed records is a necessity, as is being tenacious about asking for written justification for why a claim was denied. It is important to factor in the cost of billing time for overdue or inaccurate payments when establishing a payment schedule (Barry, 2006a; Muscari, 2004).

Muscari (2004) stressed the importance of tracking the percentage of fees that are collected from each insurance company and evaluating the history of the reimbursement from that carrier when deciding whether to accept a new client. She also recommended doing one's own billing during the first year of the business to become familiar with what insurances will pay. After that, if one selects to hire a self-employed business manager to handle billing, that person can be expected to receive 8 to 10% of the net collections (Muscari, 2004).

Experienced entrepreneurs have stressed it is important to clarify from the initial telephone contact what the patient will pay and what their insurance will cover as well as to have policies in place for what occurs if insurance does not cover the visit. Barry (2006a) suggested providing clients with a list of questions to ask of their insurance company, such as:

1. Do I have out-of-network insurance coverage?
2. What is my deductible?
3. What is the maximum allowable yearly reimbursement?
4. Is a referral necessary (p. 135)?

It is also necessary to be explicit with patients about late or missed appointment fees. After enactment of Public Law 105-33 in 1998, NPs and CNSs became eligible to bill Medicare part B if the services would have been billable by a physician and the services are within the NP's or CNS's scope of practice. Nurses who bill must have a master's degree in a defined clinical area from an accredited institution and have a collaborative practice with a physician. Collaboration with a physician involves working with a physician to "deliver healthcare services within the scope of the practitioner's professional expertise, with medical direction and appropriate supervision as provided for in jointly developed guidelines as defined by the law of the state in which the services are performed" (Schulmeister, 1999b, p. 2). A Medicare part B provider number unique to the nurse submitting the claim is required. "Reimbursement rates for NP and CNS services are 80% of the lesser of the actual charge or 85% of the fee schedule amount" allowed by Medicare (Schulmeister, 1999b, p. 6).

In select states such as Oregon, nurse practitioners and clinical nurse specialists can obtain Medicaid waivers to pay for care provided to low-income, community-dwelling seniors. A collaborative practice with a physician is not required (Caffrey, 2005). Irrespective of the payment mechanism, it is critical before charging to determine if the patient would be eligible for financial assistance through another program. "To accept clients with limited means and who are eligible for financial assistance from another program is unethical" (Caffrey, 2005, p. 15).

Businesses can also be structured on a private pay model that does not seek private insurance, Medicare, or Medicaid reimbursement. All nurses are able to accept private pay reimbursement if the services offered are within their scope of practice. Structuring a business on private pay monies is much easier and involves less paperwork and billing time. However, it is clear that one would be targeting higher income patients if private pay billing were selected (Smith, 2007).

When establishing a per-visit rate, one has to consider what other agencies who offer similar services charge, the expertise of the involved personnel, and when the services are provided. For example, a private pay nurse who visited elderly individuals in their home charged $40 for a daytime visit, but $75 if she made a home visit between 7 PM and 7 AM or on weekends or holidays (Caffrey, 2005). When establishing a rate, one has to consider the demographics of the area where one's practice is located; whether employees qualified to provide the specific services are available; what the costs associated with recruiting, hiring, and training employees are; and the costs associated with scheduling and payroll (Smith, 2007).

MARKETING AND OTHER BUSINESS-RELATED DECISIONS

The term "marketing" includes logo/brand design; creation of websites; and advertising to attract, maintain, and satisfy customers (Mackey, 2008). When beginning to advertise, Mackey suggests identifying organizational talents, outcomes you are most proud of, and qualities of your service customers need to consider. Mackey also stresses the importance of having a single, clear, compelling statement of your niche or what makes your service unique. You should be able to explain what you offer and to whom in a short statement. The statement should describe how the health problem your business targets affects individuals, how you can solve the problem, and why your service is superior.

There are low and high budget forms of marketing. Flyers describing hours of operation, business location, and services are a low budget form of marketing. Business cards and brochures can be placed on bulletin boards at grocery stores, car washes, and public areas. Bulk mailing can be used to reach large numbers of individuals (Schulmeister, 1999b). One can also offer free workshops on the health topic your business addresses at local schools, churches, and clubs. Creating a monthly newsletter is yet another option, as is establishing a toll-free phone number. Newspaper and yellow page ads and websites are reasonably affordable. Giveaways such as pens and refrigerator magnets are another approach, or one can pay for fairly expensive television ads (Mackey, 2008). An affordable form of television advertising is agreeing to be a guest on a cable show about a given health topic such as cancer or childhood obesity (Schulmeister, 1999b). Joining a professional, business, or religious organization is also a good way to network and reach out to potential clients (Smith, 2007).

Word-of-mouth advertising from previous patients and other healthcare professionals is one of the most effective forms of advertising. This form of marketing requires that you build a patient base that is satisfied with the services your business provides (Mackey, 2008). Being an insider and knowing key individuals in the community such as school nurses, case managers, physicians, and other referral sources is critical (Caffrey, 2005). Following up with other healthcare providers who make referrals is also important. Muscari (2004) suggests sending a detailed letter to professionals who sent you a referral outlining symptom improvements and thanking them for the referral.

MALPRACTICE AND MALPRACTICE INSURANCE

Although all nurses benefit from having malpractice insurance, it is critical for nurse entrepreneurs to carry adequate amounts of malpractice insurance and to select a practice model consistent with the amount of personal liability they are willing to assume. "Malpractice occurs when a practitioner does not exercise the level of learning or skill normally applied by a reputable practitioner in the field" (Barry, 2006b, p. 201). Having a malpractice suit filed against you is a time-consuming event that "puts your license, livelihood, business, and personal assets at risk" (Barry, 2006b, p. 201). It is important to select a reputable malpractice insurance agency and to pay for adequate amounts of coverage.

If an entrepreneur is notified of a lawsuit, it is critical to notify the insurance carrier immediately. Often, insurance companies will settle cases rather than going to trial, so it is important to not only practice in a safe manner but to keep detailed records. If one is reported to the nursing board of examiners it is a serious event. Barry (2006b) suggests only answering simple questions such as how long you have been in practice and where you are located. Beyond that, having the advice of an attorney and offering to provide a written answer to the question is a good idea.

AGENCIES THAT PROVIDE HELP TO INDIVIDUALS SETTING UP A BUSINESS

The Internal Revenue Service maintains a website that offers detailed information on tax laws affecting small businesses (http://www.irs.gov). The Business Hotline Online is a resource that is available free of charge for advice on topics such as accounting and finance, legal issues, direct mailing, public speaking, and marketing, and it also offers a mentoring program (http://view.fdu.edu/default.aspx?id=1249). Network solutions (http://www.internic.net) is a company that registers and authorizes Internet domain names for a fee (Schulmeister, 1999a). The Service Corps of Retired Executives (SCORE) (http://www.score.org), an association of retired business executives, provides free help to small businesses regarding start-up questions and day-to-day challenges encountered in running a practice (Elango et al., 2007).

The Small Business Association is located in every state and offers support through its small business development centers (http://www.business.gov). An alphabetical listing is provided of all small businesses along with direct links to their websites. Online workshops are available 24 hours a day, covering topics such as developing a business plan, targeting your market, managing cash flow, creating a profit and loss statement, attracting and retaining clients, creating a website, and advertising (Barry, 2005). The Medical Group Management Association (MGMA) offers information about the average number of support persons and space required per healthcare provider/physician based on the geographic area and size of the practice (Mackey, 2005).

Creating a health promotion business is an adventure. Networking with others who have been successful in establishing a business and taking advantage of existing resources is vitally important.

DISCUSSION QUESTIONS

1. Does entrepreneurship allow for pushing the boundaries of nursing practice? Explain your answer.
2. Is entrepreneurship incompatible with a service mentality? Why or why not?
3. Why don't more nurses start their own business?
4. What constitutes malpractice and how can a nurse entrepreneur protect against a malpractice claim?
5. Should an entrepreneur do their own books or hire an accountant right away? Explain your answer.
6. What sort of marketing approaches are most affordable and most effective?
7. When should an entrepreneur hire employees?
8. Why do more doctors than nurses start businesses?

CHECK YOUR UNDERSTANDING: EXERCISE ONE

If you were living in a middle-class, rural neighborhood with large numbers of retired individuals and households headed by a single parent, what sort of business might be profitable to consider developing? Assume you are going to proceed with starting this business. Answer the following questions as you plan for your venture.

1. Which type of business structure would be easiest to develop? Which type of business structure would be safest to use?
2. Who might provide referrals?
3. What type of payment would you seek (Medicare, private insurance, private pay)?
4. What sort of experience should the nurses setting up and providing care in the business have?
5. How could/should the business be marketed?
6. Would a loan be needed to set up the proposed business? What expenses would the loan cover if it were needed?
7. What factors might motivate a nurse entrepreneur to consider establishing this business?
8. What challenges could be expected during the first year of the business?
9. Who would you seek assistance from if you were going to set up this venture?

CHECK YOUR UNDERSTANDING: EXERCISE TWO

Place a True or False beside each of the following characteristics of a successful entrepreneur.

Successful entrepreneurs are:

____ Good at networking

____ Risk averse

____ Able to identify healthcare trends

____ Have an external locus of control

____ Have low self-efficacy

____ Value working autonomously

____ Are good communicators

____ Lack emotional endurance

____ Prefer having a set schedule

____ Dislike challenge

____ Need a consistent income

____ Need group coverage for insurance and retirement

CHECK YOUR UNDERSTANDING: EXERCISE THREE

Identify each of the following statements about creating a business plan or starting a business as being primarily True or primarily False.

_____ It is easy to get a business loan without a business plan.

_____ Having an accountant is a necessity.

_____ A good business plan analyzes market trends.

_____ It is not required that employers deduct for employee's worker's compensation.

_____ You can create an operating budget anytime within the first 12 months of starting your business.

_____ HMO reimbursement should be a primary source of income for nurse entrepreneurs.

_____ A business plan should include a forecast of future success.

_____ It is sufficient to outline benchmarks for each 5-year period.

_____ Only master's and doctoral-prepared nurses can bill for services.

_____ Word of mouth advertising is not as effective as other methods.

_____ Operating expenses are more important than start-up expenses.

_____ Billing rates depend on the demographics of the area.

_____ You need at least enough cash to cover 6 months of business expenses.

CHECK YOUR UNDERSTANDING: EXERCISE FOUR

Match the following types of businesses with the best description of that type of business.

1. A general partnership
2. A sole proprietorship
3. A limited liability company
4. An S-corporation

Descriptions

A. Consists of 75 or fewer stock holders
B. The nurse and the business are one entity.
C. Requires having a Tax Identification Number.
D. Must involve several business owners.

WHAT DO YOU THINK?

1. Would you make a good entrepreneur? Why or why not?
2. What part of being an entrepreneur would you enjoy? What part of being an entrepreneur would be challenging for you?
3. Read over the types of practices nurses have developed. What sort of business would you focus on if your long-term goal was to be an entrepreneur?
4. At what point in your career would you consider setting up a health promotion business? Provide a rationale for your answer.
5. What would "trigger you to move from a job with a predictable paycheck and benefits to an uncertain income and personal responsibility for a business" (Moore & Dayhoff, 2002, p. 548)?
6. What type of business structure would you select for your business?
7. Which business created by a nurse that was discussed in this chapter do you think was most innovative? Which was the most needed?

REFERENCES

Austin, L., Luker, K., & Martin, R. (2006). Clinical nurse specialists as entrepreneurs: Constrained or liberated. *Journal of Clinical Nursing, 15*, 1540–1549.

Banham, L., & Connelly, J. (2002). Skill mix, doctors and nurses: Substitution or diversification? *Journal of Management in Medicine, 16*, 259–270.

Barry, P. (2005). Questions and answers for the nurse psychotherapist in private practice. *Perspectives in Psychiatric Care, 41*(1), 42–44.

Barry, P. (2006a). Handling the finances: HMO versus private pay. *Perspectives in Psychiatric Care, 42*(2), 133–136.

Barry, P. (2006b). Professional malpractice insurance and practicing within professional guidelines. *Perspectives in Psychiatric Care, 42*(3), 201–203.

Blaich, B. S. (2004). Expert to novice: A journey from administrator to entrepreneur. *Clinical Nurse Specialist, 18*(5), 235–237.

Boore, J. & Porter, S. (2011). Education for entrepreneurship in nursing. *Nurse Education Today, 31*, 184–191.

Caffrey, R. A. (2005). Independent community care gerontological nursing. *Journal of Gerontological Nursing*, 13–17.

Center for Advancement of Social Entrepreneurship [CASE]. (2008). *Developing the field of social entrepreneurship: A report from the Center for Advancement of Social Entrepreneurship (CASE)*. Alberta, Canada: Canadian Centre for Social Entrepreneurship, Duke University: The Fuqua School of Business.

Dawes, D. (2009). A guide to setting up social enterprises. *Nursing Management, 15*(10), 18–20.

Drennan, V., Davis, K., Goodman, C., Humphrey, C., Locke, R., Mark, A., . . . Traynor, M. (2007). Entrepreneurial nurses and midwives in the United Kingdom: An integrative review. *Journal of Advanced Nursing, 60*(5), 459–469.

Drucker, P. F. (1985). *Innovation and entrepreneurship*. Oxford, UK: Butterworth Heinemann.

Elango, B., Phil, M., Hunter, G. L., & Winchell, M. (2007). Barriers to nurse entrepreneurship: A study of the process model of entrepreneurship. *Journal of the American Academy of Nurse Practitioners*, 198–204.

Gibb, A. A. (2000). SME policy, academic research and the growth of ignorance: Mythical concepts, myths, assumptions, rituals and confusions. *International Small Business Journal, 18*(3), 13–29.

Hewison, A. & Badger, F. (2006). Taking the initiative: Nurse intrapreneurs in the NHS. *Nursing Management, 13*(3), 14–19.

International Council of Nurses [ICN]. (2004). *Guidelines for the nurse entre/intrapreneur providing nursing service*. Geneva, Switzerland: Author.

Kauffman Foundation (2007). *Entrepreneurship in American higher education: A report from the Kauffman panel on entrepreneurship curriculum in higher education*. Kansas City, MO: Author.

Kowal, N. (1998). Specialty practice entrepreneur: The advanced practice nurse. *Nursing Economics, 16*(5), 277–278.

Leong, J. (2005). Clinical Nurse Specialist Entrepreneurship. *Internet Journal of Advanced Nursing Practice, 7*(1), 15236064.

Lyon, B. A. (2003). A clinical nurse specialist private practice in nursing. *Clinical Nurse Specialist, 17*(3), 131–132.

Mackey, T. A. (2005). Planning your nursing business. *Journal of the American Academy of Nurse Practitioners, 17*(12), 501–505.

Mackey, T. A. (2008). Marketing your nurse-managed practice: Become a marketpreneur. *Clinical Scholars Review, 1*(1), 13–17.

Martin, S. S. (1984). Exploring the concept of enterprise. *Nursing Economics, 2*, 406–408.

Moore, P. S. & Dayhoff, N. E. (2002). The diabetes educator as an entrepreneur: Starting your business. *The Diabetes Educator, 28*(4), 547–552.

Muscari, E. (2004). Establishing a small business in nursing. *Oncology Nursing Forum, 31*(2), 177–179.

Orga, J. (1996). Becoming a nurse entrepreneur. *Tennessee Nurse, 59*(2), 10553134.

Powell, D. J. (1984). Nurses: High touch entrepreneurs. *Nursing Economics, 2*(1), 33–36.

Sankelo, M., & Akerblad, L. (2008). Nurse entrepreneurs' attitudes to management, their adoption of the manager's role and managerial assertiveness. *Journal of Nursing Management, 16*, 829–836.

Sankelo, M., & Akerblad, L. (2009). Nurse entrepreneurs' well-being at work and associated factors. *Journal of Clinical Nursing, 18*, 3190–3199.

Schulmeister, L. (1999a). The challenges of a home-based nursing consultation business. *Clinical Nurse Specialist, 13*(2), 101–103.

Schulmeister, L. (1999b). Starting a nurse consultation practice. *Clinical Nurse Specialist, 13*(2), 94–100.

Shirey, M. R. (2007). The entrepreneur and the business plan. *Clinical Nurse Specialist, 21*(3), 142–144.

Shirey, M. R. (2008). Endurance and inspiration for the entrepreneur. *Clinical Nurse Specialist, 22*(1), 9–11.

Smith, C. (2007). Turning caring into business: The nuts and bolts of starting a private-duty home care business. *Home Healthcare Nurse, 25*(9), 560–565.

White, K. R. & Begu, J. W. (1998). Nursing entrepreneurship in an era of chaos and complexity. *Nursing Administration Quarterly, 22*(2), 40–47.

Wilson, A., Averis, A., & Walsh, K. (2003). The influences on and experiences of becoming nurse entrepreneurs: A Delphi study. *International Journal of Nursing Practice, 9*, 236–245.

Wolfson, B., & Neidlinger, S. H. (1991). Nurse entrepreneurship: Opportunities in acute care hospitals. *Nursing Economics, 9*(1), 40–43.

For a full suite of assignments and additional learning activities, see the access code at the front of your book.

CHAPTER 12

Health Promotion Policy

Bonnie Raingruber

OBJECTIVES:

At the conclusion of this chapter, the student will be able to:

- Discuss examples of successful health policy reform, as well as factors motivating current policy reform efforts.
- Describe the relationship between development of health policy and health promotion policy.
- Identify components of the Patient Protection and Affordable Care Act, along with timeframes for implementing components of that law.
- Describe why electronic health records are a critical component of health policy reform.
- Evaluate the impact that medical homes will have on health policy and reimbursement.
- Discuss the role of the Patient-Centered Outcomes Research Institute.
- Evaluate proposed methods of allocating health care to vulnerable groups.
- Describe the role of patients/consumers in health policy formation, implementation, and evaluation.
- Discuss the role of nursing in health policy formation.

INTRODUCTION

Tones and Tilford (1994), early pioneers in health promotion, suggested that health promotion consists primarily of two components: health education and health policy. The World Health Organization (WHO) defined health policy as "a consensus on the health issues, goals, and objectives to be addressed, the priorities among those objectives, and the main directions for achieving them" (Vogel, Burt, & Church, 2010, p. 85). In 2000, the WHO emphasized that nurses should be actively involved in the planning and implementation of health policy at all levels (WHO, 2001). Health policy is not just about content; it is also about process and power and "who influences whom . . . and how that happens" (Walt, 1994, p. 1). As we will learn in this chapter, the necessity of achieving a community-level and political-level consensus is critical when developing health promotion policies. Health policy at the county, state, and national levels is designed to influence social structures, environmental conditions, and laws that relate to both health and illness (Whitehead, 2003a).

HEALTH POLICY AND HEALTH PROMOTION POLICY

Health is influenced by genetics, gestational conditions, social circumstances (education, employment, income, housing, crime, social support), environmental conditions (toxic agents, microbes, structural hazards, infectious diseases), behavioral choices (diet, physical activity, substance abuse, coping strategies), and medical care (access to care, medical errors). The breakdown of causative factors of early deaths in the United States has been estimated as follows: 30% to genetic predispositions, 15% to social circumstances, 5% to environmental exposures, 40% to behavioral patterns, and 10% to issues related to medical care (McGinnis, Williams-Russo, & Knickman, 2002). Yet only 5% of health expenditures are devoted to health promotion policies, even though social and behavioral issues constitute the largest percentage of causes of mortality. Development of prevention policies requires compiling and analyzing large databases capable of identifying multiple causes of disease, such as dietary and physical activity, tobacco and alcohol use, and past health history (McGinnis et al., 2002). It may be that introduction of the electronic health record (EHR) will allow for collection of such data and contribute to the future development of prevention-oriented health policy.

Health policy is a complicated subject that requires consideration of multiple perspectives, establishment of a social consensus based on shared values and norms, attention to ethical guidelines, and political/legislative action. In addition, prevention policies require intervention outside the arena of traditional health policy. For example, excise taxes on tobacco and alcohol, implementation of safety standards for workers and products, zoning mandates that limit environmental hazards, laws regulating community water supplies and fluoridation, and truth in marketing are all within the domain of health promotion policy. Economic incentives and disincentives, health education, and regulation are necessary aspects of developing health promotion policy. A hefty commitment of resources is required to craft and implement health prevention policies, and economic, social, and political support is necessary to provide these resources (Boddington & Raisanen, 2009).

Several caveats should be mentioned here: (1) Health prevention policy also requires legislators to begin "thinking in terms of a health agenda rather than a health-care agenda" (McGinnis et al., 2002, p. 89); (2) It is difficult to do justice to the topic of health prevention policy in only one chapter; and (3) Health policy is especially complicated given the massive number of changes recently enacted as part of the Patient Protection and Affordable Care Act (PPACA) of 2010.

HISTORICAL ACCOMPLISHMENTS

We benefit today from a multitude of health policies that have revolutionized our daily lives, including seat belt laws, car seat regulations, speed limit laws, drunk driver initiatives, immunization/vaccination policies, nutrition labeling of food in grocery stores and restaurants, mental health parity mandates, laws related to safety in the workplace, regulation/removal of lead and asbestos from buildings and building materials, and regulation of cigarette sales and advertising as well as creation of nonsmoking areas. Most of these health policy changes have become so widely accepted and taken for granted that the majority of individuals adhere to them without requiring legal punishments for nonadherence. But each of these policies was controversial at some point in time, requiring a widespread media campaign and creation of a social and legislative consensus prior to their implementation (Ruger, 2007).

Today, we face a variety of current health policy challenges that are somewhat controversial. Embryonic stem cell research is one such topic, with some individuals supporting this approach as a way to find a cure for a spectrum of chronic diseases while others oppose it because of the impact on human embryos and the right to life (Sage, 2010). Passage of the Patient Protection and Affordable Care Act in 2010 was supported by numerous individuals and groups, as well as opposed by other individuals and groups. In the future a multitude of other health policy initiatives will be proposed, debated, and implemented, which in turn will shape the nature of nursing practice and the healthcare delivery system.

BARRIERS TO INVOLVEMENT OF NURSING IN HEALTH POLICY

Numerous authors have discussed the reality that most nurses are not educated about how to become involved in political and policy issues. Typically, nurses do not know how to lobby for health policy changes, and they are not educated to engage in health policy research or to work with the media. As Clay (1987) commented, "nursing, power, and politics are not usually words that go together" (p. 1). Typically the public and nurses themselves see nursing "as being outside politics and political power struggles" (Clay, 1987, p. 1). In addition, "the nature of intimacy and privacy in the patient–nurse relationship" has been cited as a reason nurses are not active in health policy work (Fyffe, 2009, p. 699).

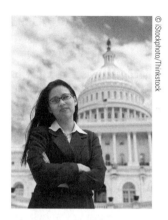

Professional organizations that lobby for specific health policy, although they do exist, are less established in nursing than in medicine, dentistry, pharmacy, or clinical psychology. The American Nurses' Association (ANA) has endorsed political candidates since the late 1980s because problems related to delivering nursing care are often associated with public policy. One of the goals of the ANA is to ensure that "nurses are a recognized political force with a prominent seat at health policy tables" (Johnson, 2002, p. 7). Success within the health policy arena takes time, resources, and persistence. When nurses try to organize a group or community around a health policy issue without success, then feelings of rejection at the individual, organizational, and societal level are to be expected. Finally, although more and more nurses are running for elected office, completing legislative internships, and being appointed to federal taskforces, nurses still lag behind other professions in terms of serving in these health policy roles (Fyffe, 2009).

FACTORS INFLUENCING HEALTH POLICY AND HEALTHCARE REFORM

Rising costs and inconsistent healthcare quality prompted the passage of the Patient Protection and Affordable Care Act, which has been called the biggest health policy change since the introduction of Medicare and Medicaid in 1965. The PPACA was designed to improve access to care, increase quality, and control healthcare costs. Health care accounts for as much as 16% of gross national product in the United States, even though we lag behind other industrialized nations in terms of life expectancy and infant mortality (Dalton et al., 2010). The United States is the only industrialized country that does not provide universal access to health care (Ruger, 2007). "Despite spending on health care being nearly double that of the next most costly nation, the United States ranks thirty-first among nations in life expectancy and thirty-sixth in infant mortality" (Berwick, Nolan, & Whittington, 2008, p. 759).

Lack of access to primary care results in a substantial cost to the state and federal government including funds used to reimburse hospitals for uncompensated care to uninsured individuals and emergency room costs (Stream & Myers, 2010). In 2001, the Institute of Medicine (IOM) identified a need for "improvements in safety, effectiveness, patient-centeredness, timeliness, efficiency, and equity" within health care (Berwick et al., 2008, p. 760; IOM, 2001).

Ruger (2007) emphasized the importance of understanding conflicting public values when analyzing whether a health policy will or will not succeed. Ruger suggested, "American political culture is full of unresolved value conflicts, especially between freedom and equality, particularly when applied to social policy" (p. 56). When considering the fate of healthcare reform in particular, there are a number of supportive core values as well as core values that stand in opposition to healthcare reform.

The libertarian value of assuming personal responsibility and individualism, along with aversion to excessive state or governmental control, undermines support for implementation of healthcare legislation. Also, concerns about loss of freedom through increased regulation are a barrier to healthcare reform. For some, concerns that one's personal health care might diminish in quality undermine support for legislation and favor the status quo. Questions about rationing of care and lower quality of care prompted some individuals to believe they were going to lose more than they gained as a result of reforms. Distrust of government and a healthy cynicism regarding the inefficiency of bureaucracies, along with a historical commitment to capitalism, also undermined support. The perceived harmful effect on business and especially small business, from laying off workers during a period of economic downturn in order to afford the cost of health care, was yet another factor. Requiring purchase of healthcare coverage even among groups who do not believe they need insurance was controversial. Some authors have called government intrusions into individual's lives the "tyranny of health" in which difficulties related to a broad expanse of human experience are medicalized and seen as belonging to the domain of medicine. Such a view is seen as undermining self-determination, which is part of the holistic notion of health (Boddington & Raisanen, 2009, p. 55; Fitzpatrick, 2001). Higher taxes required to support health care was a concern for other groups. Finally, strong interest group opposition and powerful congressional personalities played a role in opposing healthcare reform.

Opposing values that supported healthcare reform included a belief in equal opportunity for all citizens, a commitment to fair distribution of resources, the need for increased workforce productivity, decreased absenteeism, and global competitiveness, along with norms such as altruism and compassion. With the exception of hypochondriacs and those suffering from Munchausen's disorder, most people only seek health care on an as-needed basis and for preventive care. In addition, "individuals do not always have full control over their health, people can get sick for unknown reasons, and health problems can arise even when individuals are doing everything they can to be healthy" (Ruger, 2007, p. 57). Any individual or family can be devastated by a catastrophic illness. Even though the PPACA has passed, these competing values still have an influence as can be seen in the resistance to implementation of the law and overall public opinion about the law (Ruger, 2007).

THE PATIENT PROTECTION AND AFFORDABLE CARE ACT

A number of provisions of the PPACA have gone into effect since its passage in 2010, while additional provisions will go into effect between 2011 and 2014. As of 2010, uninsured individuals with preexisting conditions can join high-risk pools and receive insurance, lifetime caps on healthcare coverage were eliminated, bans were put into effect preventing insurance companies from dropping coverage for individuals who had exceeded their benefit limits, and young adults were allowed to remain on their parent's insurance policies up to age 26 (Johnson, 2010).

Of crucial importance to the field of health promotion is the establishment of a Prevention and Public Health Fund as part of the PPACA to provide support for health promotion and prevention activities. Small employers are also being funded to establish wellness programs for employees. A state-based home visiting program for at-risk families with pregnant mothers and infants/toddlers was funded by the Health Resources and Services Administration. A task force on Clinical and Preventive Services is disseminating evidence-based health recommendations. The PPACA also requires appropriate use of language services and cultural competency training for healthcare providers. Finally, a breast health campaign is funded for 2010 to 2014 (Johnson, 2010).

In 2014, it will not be possible to consider gender when setting healthcare premiums or to deny coverage due to preexisting conditions. States will be required to offer Medicaid coverage for individuals whose income is 133% of the defined poverty level. PPACA eliminates cost-sharing for preventive care, such as requiring copays for breast cancer screening and tobacco cessation for pregnant women. PPACA allows women direct access to obstetrical and gynecological care, increases payment rates for primary care physicians seeing Medicaid and Medicare patients, supports initiatives to increase the supply of healthcare professionals, expands funding for community health centers, and provides funding for medical homes where interdisciplinary teams provide disease prevention, case management, and health education for patients. Health education programs designed to reduce teen pregnancy and prevent sexually transmitted disease will also be funded in 2014 (Johnson, 2010).

Employers with 50 or more employees will be required to provide healthcare insurance for their workers or pay a monetary penalty. Individuals will also be required to obtain coverage or pay a penalty. Supporters of PPACA claim that health care for all is an ethical mandate and a necessity if the new law is to be cost-effective (Johnson, 2010). Those who opposed the individual mandate within the PPACA believe that the federal government should not be able to require citizens to purchase insurance even though the Supreme Court ruled this was constitutional.

ELECTRONIC MEDICAL RECORDS AND PATIENT-CENTERED OUTCOMES EVALUATION

A major component of the American Recovery and Reinvestment Act (ARRA) of 2009 provides incentives for hospitals, community clinics, and primary care practices adopting electronic medical records. ARRA requires a federally-certified electronic health record (EHR) be used in a meaningful manner for activities such as order entry and medication prescribing. The EHR allows for exchange of health-related information as well as clinical quality and risk assessment measures. Incentives are provided for adoption of an EHR prior to October 2011 and reduced reimbursement penalties go into effect in 2015 if a practice or hospital has not met meaningful use goals. The goal for 2010 is establishing an EHR and using information to track key clinical conditions, the goal for 2013 is implementing care coordination and patient engagement using the EHR, and the goal for 2015 is improving performance and key health system outcomes. Electronic health records are designed to be able to track smoking patterns, substance use patterns, exposure to violence, physical inactivity, and poor nutrition through pooled databases. In addition, it will be easier to monitor waste and fraud using the EHR, including unnecessary visits or interventions that lack a solid evidence base (Berwick et al., 2008).

Some authors have argued for using EHRs to limit yearly patient service. These authors have suggested capital budget growth should be based on regional need along with budget caps on "total healthcare spending for designated populations" (Berwick et al., 2008, p. 767). Other authors (Luft, 2007) have suggested EHRs can be used to collect data and then implement bundled payment reimbursements for specific types of patients and diagnoses that require the provider to cover the cost of any needed care for a set fee. For example, a primary practice would receive a set fee for taking care of a diabetic patient and another fee for caring for a patient with congestive heart failure no matter how many hospitalizations or specialty referrals those patients needed. What do you see as the advantages, challenges, and disadvantages of bundled reimbursement for providers? How would a bundled approach to reimbursement change health care for patients, administrators, and nurses?

THE PATIENT-CENTERED OUTCOMES RESEARCH INSTITUTE

A Patient-Centered Outcomes Research Institute is planned as part of the PPACA to collect and analyze data obtained from EHRs on the clinical effectiveness of medical treatments (http://healthit.hhs.gov/). This institute will be a private nonprofit entity designed to compare the effectiveness of health treatments. It will be overseen by a board of governors, include stakeholders, and work with an expert advisory panel. The institute cannot mandate reimbursement or insurance coverage and is prohibited from using research data alone to deny coverage. In addition, a Center for Comparative Effectiveness Research within the Agency for Healthcare Research and Quality will be funded to conduct and synthesize research evidence on patient outcomes, clinical effectiveness, and quality of healthcare services (Johnson, 2010).

The stated goal of collecting demographic data, clinical data, environmental data, risk factor history, and effectiveness data via EHRs is that predictive, preventative, and participatory care involving patients as an active members of the healthcare team will become a reality. Collection of large amounts of data and pooled clinical trial results will allow researchers to identify which treatments are effective with a given subpopulation. "By creating information networks of databases that follow patients longitudinally over time, and identifying patients who share both clinical characteristics and molecular biomarkers . . . clinicians may be able to predict clinical outcomes and determine the value of certain diagnostics or interventions for specific patient populations" (Dalton et al., 2010, p. 5988). The goal is to match the right treatment to the right patient at the right time. Costly treatments that are now simply provided as the standard of care will be replaced with evidence-based interventions. Ineffective and unnecessary diagnosis and treatment costs will be eliminated. Cost-effective treatments that have the greatest likelihood of benefit with the fewest side effects can be identified using EHRs. Decision-making tools and individual provider-level quality control methods can be embedded to improve the quality of care. These quality-of-care metrics will also be used to influence reimbursement strategies and control cost (Dalton et al., 2010). What do you see as the primary benefit of EHRs and the primary limitation in terms of health policy development?

MEDICAL HOMES: A COMPONENT OF INTEGRATED HEALTH POLICY

Patient-centered medical homes are designed to provide individualized, accessible, and coordinated care including health promotion and disease prevention activities (Blount, 2010). Appointment times are to be scheduled at a time that is convenient for patients, email communication between providers and patients is encouraged, and a case manager is assigned to minimize delays associated with obtaining specialty referrals (Sia, Tonniges, Osterhus, & Taba, 2004). Medical homes are built on a foundation of sustaining patient–clinician relationships; treating people, not the disease; adopting an interdisciplinary approach to care; implementing continuous quality improvement; using outcomes evaluation based on data from EHRs; and ensuring enhanced reimbursements for providers so that case managers can be hired within a primary care practice (Blount, 2010).

Medical home demonstration projects are being funded by the government and also by private insurers (Blue Cross, 2009). In some medical home models, case managers who work for the insurance company are embedded in a primary care practice to provide health coaching, motivational interviewing, patient education, assessments, and telephone follow-up contact for patients with chronic illness (Case Management Advisor, 2008).

Medical homes are designed to improve integration of care; reduce overuse of primary care, emergency rooms, and hospitals; and save on healthcare costs (Sia et al., 2004). This occurs in part because finely tuned coordination of care minimizes unnecessary referrals and admissions. One issue to keep in mind is that participating physicians and nurse practitioners who serve in a lead role in the medical home receive bonus reimbursements of up to $50,000 per year if healthcare costs are managed. Therefore, it will be necessary to advocate for patients to ensure that needed health care is recommended and specialty referrals are obtained. Limiting needed care in order to obtain a bonus reimbursement would not be ethical (Case Management Advisor, 2010).

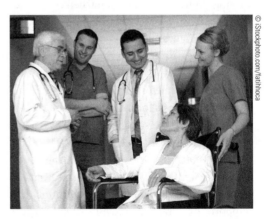
© iStockphoto.com/fatihhoca

ALLOCATING HEALTH CARE: THE QUESTION OF RATIONING, COST-UTILITY ANALYSIS, AND PRACTICE GUIDELINES AS WAYS OF CONTROLLING COST

A disproportionate amount of resources in the United States is directed toward health-care spending. This limits funding for education, housing, food, and crime prevention, all of which impact health. "Although public opinion polls tell us that Americans are unwilling to ration health care, in fact we already do." (Goold, 1996, p. 71). Until full implementation of the PPACA we "ration by restricting the availability of insurance to those who can pay for it or those who qualify for public assistance" (Goold, 1996, p. 71).

Goold (1996) suggests rationing should rely on moral reasoning that respects an individual's autonomy and their right to make decisions for themselves; this means not using age, prognosis, or cost in rationing decision making. She advocates for involvement of patients in decision making and provision of education about acceptable indications for and outcomes of proposed treatments. Goold disputes the use of cost-utility measures because intangibles such as quality of life and well-being cannot be accurately measured and because individual patients often differ markedly from statistical averages. Furthermore, Goold asserts that cost-utility analysis can be nonsensical. An example could be considering the treatment of a 50-year-old with asthma and pneumonia to be the same as that for someone in a vegetative state who has pneumonia. Cost-utility analysis relies on aggregated costs; it does not calculate the realities of widely varying clinical scenarios even when comorbid conditions and age are factored into the formula. Diverse patient values and preferences have never been used in determining cost-utility figures.

Debate exists between those who believe a physician or nurse practitioner should use his or her expertise in treating patients based on unique clinical symptoms and environmental factors and those who believe objective, universally valid knowledge should be the basis for care. The debate centers on whether medical knowledge should be based on "the personalized authority of clinical judgment or the impersonal authority of practice guidelines" (Matthews, 1999, p. 301).

The 1990s saw a resurgence in the use of practice guidelines based on universally validated knowledge. Aggregated data based on large numbers of patients and clinical outcomes were used to determine the most appropriate medical intervention. Supporters of practice guidelines herald that they will be "the means by which clinical judgment will finally be transformed from a subjective art into an objective science" (Matthews, 1999, p. 276). These individuals argue for the use of economics, statistics, probability, and decision theory in establishing practice guidelines (Matthews, 1999). Procedures are reimbursed if "the expected health benefits of a procedure exceed its expected negative consequences by a sufficiently wide margin such that the procedure is worth doing" (Chassin et al., 1987, p. 2534).

Critics counter that practice guidelines favor the use of "cookbook medicine" rather than expert tacit knowledge that is consistent with the unique cultural, socioeconomic, and environmental needs of individual patients. Furthermore, they argue that practice guidelines "filter out the particulars that are essential and . . . that statistical justice . . . replaces the individual with the average; the case at hand with a generality, and the exercise of judgment with the application of rules" (Gigerenzer et al., 1989, p. 260).

The Agency for Health Care Policy and Research, within the federal government, has the primary mission of collecting large volumes of outcome data from EHRs and other sources to develop national practice guidelines capable of containing cost and improving the quality of medical care. Data repositories are also being developed that allow for examining and publicizing health system and provider level practice parameters including cost, quality, and access. This provider level data will enable consumers to compare providers and healthcare systems. Practice guidelines are also being used in malpractice cases to protect practitioners and limit medical liability (Matthews, 1999).

Health policy is now relying on health technology assessment, comparative effectiveness studies, and cost–benefit studies to restrict access to expensive and scarce interventions. Once studies have been done showing a given treatment is superior, access will be limited and decisions will be made by administrative panels in the government or by insurance agencies about which treatments are acceptable and for whom (Reese, Caplan, Bloom, Abt, & Karlawish, 2010).

Some experts have argued that this approach is equivalent to age-based rationing and have used dramatic labels such as death panels to describe these policies. Concerns exist that administrative panels "will not allocate treatments in a way that respects the circumstances of individual patients," the elderly, the chronically ill, or the disabled (Reese et al., 2010, p. 1982). Priority scores used in allocating treatment have been based on projected years of survival after a given intervention. Such a model does not account for the health, functional abilities, or other comorbidities of a given individual.

Administrative panels that were designed to control costs conform to "the utilitarian theory of optimizing outcomes for the greatest number of individuals" (Reese et al., 2010, p. 1982). Ezekiel Emanuel, a special advisor to President Obama, argued that rationing health care and directing healthcare resources to younger individuals "maximizes the possibility that every person experiences all the different stages of life" (p. 1982). Areas such as withholding vaccinations, transplants, and intensive care unit admissions for older individuals are included in the policy advocated by Mr. Emanuel. Some have suggested the "devil is in the dataset" because not all factors that influence treatment response have been systematically captured or even identified (Reese et al.,

2010, p. 1983). Those who collect and analyze the data need to be free of conflicts of interest. Dataset reliability should be monitored on an ongoing basis (Reese et al.). Concern exists that "narrow webs of power . . . concentrated wealth and the influential elites around them" could influence health policy and determine who receives rationed care (Greider, 1992, p. 12). Even after laws have been passed, a mechanism must exist to ensure policies are fairly implemented so that lobbyist activity is minimized.

CONSUMER INVOLVEMENT

Consumer involvement is a core tenet being stressed in health policy circles. Increasing efforts are being directed toward educating consumers about health choices; health promotion activities; the benefits and limits of specific interventions; and ways of influencing, implementing, and monitoring policy decisions (Berwick et al., 2008; Whitehead, 2003a). Tritter (2009) commented that "giving the public a more direct say in shaping the organization and delivery of healthcare services is central to the current healthcare reform agenda," as it is necessary to realign "public services around those they serve based on evidence from service user's experiences" and to design systems of care "with and by the people rather than simply on their behalf" (Tritter, 2009, p. 275). Evaluation of which services should be eliminated or expanded based on consumer input has also been proposed (Forbat, Hubbard, & Kearney, 2009).

Involving patients in developing shared plans of care they can agree to implement themselves is a necessity, as is providing case managers who can help individuals navigate inpatient, specialist, and primary care settings. By creating an EHR, it will be possible to provide access to self-scheduling, results of lab work, requests for medication renewal, and connection to community resources. Given the amount of health promotion information available on the Internet, individuals can be encouraged to better manage aspects of their health care and understand treatment options (Berwick et al., 2008). Authors have suggested consumer involvement will help contain costs because patient satisfaction will increase, as will provider accountability and quality of care (Tritter, 2009).

On a macro level, Ruger (2007) commented that every health policy that is passed requires sufficient mobilization of public opinion, creation of a social consensus, and the marshaling of a collective commitment prior to political and legislative action. Ruger emphasized that major legislation, whether it be the New Deal, Civil Rights legislation, or women's rights must necessarily derive from citizens who mobilize "around a big idea" (p. 80). Support by the clergy, grassroots organizations, and the media were key components that contributed to change in previous health policy legislation. Ruger (2007) suggested a constitutional movement in which citizens mobilize is always needed to motivate major legislative change. Developing health policy requires "brokering partnerships and blending science and community action" (McGinnis et al., 2002, p. 88).

Multiple levels of patient involvement have been encouraged, including the patient as consumer, the patient as a partner in implementing health care, the patient as policy advocate, and the patient as co-researcher in community-based participatory research. Community-based participatory research (CBPR) includes both academic researchers and community members who are knowledgeable about a given health disparity, drawing on the community's knowledge of the given health challenge and what would work to eliminate it. Community members work with academic researchers to identify a priority health need, design an intervention to minimize the health problem, collect and analyze data, disseminate research findings by framing the message in a way that is accepted by the community, and advocate for policy change related to the given health challenge. Community members oftentimes already have established relationships with local policymakers and the organizational structure needed to advocate for change. Although CBPR is time consuming and complex, the outcomes are seen as being more relevant and longer lasting than traditional approaches to research and health policy (Israel et al, 2010).

As a consumer, a patient would decide which services to select given health plan coverage choices and which services to pay out of pocket for. As a partner in care, patients would decide which conditions should be treated and what lifestyle modifications they wish to make (Forbat et al., 2009). Consumer groups also function as powerful stakeholders who influence legislators and policymakers through consciousness-raising events, educational media campaigns, website development, patient and caretaker advocacy, and lobbying activities. Consumers serve on taskforces, advisory bodies, and provide oral evidence to policymaking groups so that the patient point of view can be considered. Information on the everyday reality of service delivery, the experience of coping with a given disease, and gaps in service are offered by consumers who have firsthand experience. For example, special interest consumer groups lobby for health policy that impacts conditions such as arthritis, cancer, heart and circulatory disease, child birth, and mental health services (Jones, Baggott, & Allsop, 2004). "It is no longer good enough to simply do things to people; a modern healthcare service must do things with the people it serves" (SEHD, 2001, p. 2).

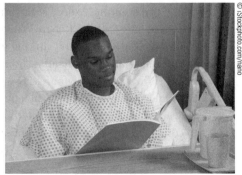

THE ROLE OF NURSING IN HEALTH POLICY WORK

Whitehead (2003a) advocated for greater participation by nurses in public health policy agenda setting, political advocacy, mass media–based health education, and lobbying efforts. Because nurses represent the largest group of highly trained healthcare providers, because nurses are patient advocates, and because the public identifies nursing as being one of the most trusted professions, nurses are well positioned to become more and more involved in health policy work. However, traditionally nurses have not been adequately trained about how to influence health policy, how to conduct the type of health policy research that will be needed, or how to implement effective lobbying strategies. To address these challenges, Whitehead (2003a) stressed the need for nurses to become more familiar with their communities and to develop a detailed understanding of how nonprofit, for-profit, and self-care organizations work in order to adopt a more activist role. As Downie and colleagues (1996) commented, "those involved in health promotion must abandon their professional isolationism and begin to work through the community rather than on it in order to do things with the community rather than to it" (p. 196).

Specifically, nurses need to take a more active role in policy development, such as increasing the numbers of nurse-run clinics, lobbying for support for nurse practitioners returning to obtain doctoral degrees, ensuring educational support for nurse educators needing to obtain a doctorate, increasing the number of nurses with a bachelor's degree, streamlining seamless educational advancement, requesting support for nursing research targeted on health outcomes, ensuring a diverse workforce, advocating for the needs of rural communities, advancing interprofessional collaboration and integrated care, and expanding laws that govern nurse–patient ratios.

The Robert Wood Johnson Foundation and the American Association of Retired Persons (AARP) are sponsoring a Campaign for Action, in which nurses play a critical role in transforming the healthcare system and ensuring that integrated, equitable, and cost-effective services are provided. This campaign is based on *The Future of Nursing: Leading Change, Advancing Health Report* (http://thefutureofnursing.org) issued by the Institute of Medicine and the Robert Wood Johnson Foundation in 2010. Regional action coalitions in the states are working with key partners to begin implementing the recommended changes. Each nurse should commit to an action step to make these goals a reality. When adopting a more active role, nurses need to adopt a unified stance and "define and own our voice" (Kennedy, 2011, p. 14). As Beverly Malone of the National League for Nursing commented, "we need to develop and communicate a clear and consistent message, aiming not to be mini-doctors but rather maxi-nurses" (Kennedy, 2011, p. 15). Developing a voice is not the same as speaking with one voice because the skills, knowledge, and expertise within varied nursing specialties are diverse and not always consistent (Buresh & Gordon, 2006).

Whitehead (2003b) quoted Plato, who commented that "one of the penalties for refusing to participate in politics is that you end up being governed by your inferiors" (p. 585). Whitehead could have made a similar comment about nurses declining to take a more active role in health policy development and implementation. Whitehead did say that changing political landscapes are offering nurses unparalleled opportunities to influence health policy. He also cautioned nurses should not end up as policy victims as a result of their reluctance to become involved in shaping and implementing health policy reforms. He recommended that nurses take an active role in consciousness rising within their communities about health policy and that they also become involved in lobbying activities. Whitehead (2003b) suggested that the relationship "between health policy reform and political activity is inseparable" (p. 586). Whitehead argued that nurses need to court and infiltrate radio stations, newspapers, and television stations in their local area to advocate for health policy change and implementation. He added that "health policy activity is the single largest influence in determining the nature of nursing and healthcare provision" (p. 590).

DISCUSSION QUESTIONS

1. What is one thing nursing students could do prior to graduation to help shape health policy reform?
2. How do practicing nurses find time to become involved in health promotion policy work?
3. Talk about the advantages of states maintaining a database of nurses willing to serve on taskforces and boards (in order to encourage nursing involvement in health policy development).
4. Why should nurses educate their patients about their own educational background and how that prepared them for practice? How would such information help the public develop a greater understanding of the varied educational levels of nurses? Why is it important that the public understand the different levels of nursing education?
5. What are the advantages and disadvantages of requiring that states collect and publicize a list of the current demand for and supply of nurses?
6. What strategies would help foster a more active role for nurses in health policy development and implementation?
7. Discuss two factors that motivated the Obama administration to pursue healthcare reform and two barriers that interfered with that effort.

CHECK YOUR UNDERSTANDING: EXERCISE ONE

Identify which of the following statements about electronic health records (EHRs) are true and which are false.

1. EHRs allow for collection and interpretation of factors that contribute to disease.
2. EHRs are not large enough to build in safety and quality of care rubrics.
3. EHRs are available and accessible 100% of the time.
4. EHRs require employers to establish wellness programs for employees.
5. EHRs facilitate creation of evidence-based recommendations.
6. EHRs mandate appropriate use of interpretative services.
7. EHRs provide for higher reimbursements for hospitals caring for Medicaid patients.
8. EHRs can be designed to promote patient engagement in their care.
9. EHRs make it easier to monitor fraud and waste.
10. EHRs make it possible to collect data on all the factors that shape treatment response.
11. EHRs undermine bundled payment policies.
12. EHRs enhance patient access to appointment scheduling.
13. EHRs can include individual provider-level quality control metrics.
14. EHR outcome data is collected by the Agency for Health Care Policy and Research.

CHECK YOUR UNDERSTANDING: EXERCISE TWO

Comment on whether the following statements about medical homes are true or false.

1. Medical homes rely on shared patient–provider responsibility.
2. Medical homes encourage e-mail communication between patients and providers.
3. Medical homes exclusively rely on physician providers.
4. Medical homes are designed to facilitate specialty referrals.
5. Medical homes encourage a higher volume of emergency room care.
6. Medical homes are based on the utilitarian theory of optimizing outcomes for the largest number of people.

CHECK YOUR UNDERSTANDING: EXERCISE THREE

Identify which of the following statements about cost-utility analysis (CUA) are true and which are false.

1. Quality of life has been accurately measured and is an important part of CUA.
2. CUA relies on aggregated cost estimates.
3. CUA factors in individual traits that impact health.
4. Patient preferences are an integral component of CUA.
5. CUA relies heavily on practitioner judgment.
6. Decision theory is an integral part of CUA.
7. Negative consequences of a procedure have no impact on CUA.
8. Consumer involvement is a core tenet of CUA.

WHAT DO YOU THINK?

1. Should advanced practice nurses be able to do the following? Why or why not?
   a. Prescribe controlled substances
   b. Perform admission assessments and certifications for patients needing home health care, admission to hospice, and skilled nursing care
   c. Order durable medical equipment
   d. Have hospital admission privileges

2. Should registered nurses be able to do the following? Why or why not?
   a. Play a key role in designing electronic medical record systems
   b. Participate in leadership training offered via telehealth
   c. Make recommendations on implementation of patient-centered medical homes
   d. Play a role in identifying healthcare delivery system improvements and recommendations about health insurance affordability
   e. Provide telephone-based care for patients with chronic health conditions (Robert Wood Johnson Foundation, 2011)

3. Are you going to sign up for e-mail alerts from the Campaign for Action Coalition? Why or why not?
4. Are you going to sign up to become a part of the American Red Cross nurse-led disaster team within your community? Explain your rationale.

5. Would you support bundled team-based reimbursements for medical home care to ease professional tensions and support the role of nurses within a medical home? (Fairman, Rowe, Hassmiller, & Shalala, 2010). Why or why not?

6. Should nurses receive continuing education hours if they develop a newspaper article that is published about a current healthcare topic? How could that process be managed, or is it unrealistic?

7. Would you vote to standardize what nurse practitioners and clinical nurse specialists across the nation are able to do within their scope of practice? Do you think prescribing privileges, maximum collaboration ratios, and physician supervision requirements should or should not be standardized across states? Explain your answer.

8. Do you agree or disagree that health policy activity is the single largest influence in determining the nature of nursing practice? Explain your answer.

9. Should advanced practice nurses be able to bill Medicaid? Should advanced practice nurses be able to bill independently of a supervising physician at a lower rate? Explain your answer.

10. Do you agree with the use of administrative panels to ration health care? If not, how would you control spiraling medical costs?

11. Imagine you are a Senator. Describe one bill you would introduce to minimize the 40% of early deaths in the United States that can be attributed to behavioral patterns. Which groups would support your bill? Which groups would oppose it?

REFERENCES

Berwick, D. M. Nolan, T. W. & Whittington, J. (2008). The triple aim: Care, health, and cost. *Health Affairs*, *27*(3), 759–769.

Blount, A. (2010). A special issue on the patient-centered medical home. *Families, Systems & Health*, *28*(4), 297–321.

Blue Cross/Blue Shield Association (2009). Blue Cross and Blue Shield Companies join primary care physician groups, national employer, and consumer groups to explore a new approach to patient care. *BCBSA News*. Retrieved from www.bcbs.com/news/bcbsa/blue-cross-and-blue-shield-14.html?templateName=tem

Boddington, P. & Raisanen, U. (2009). Theoretical and practical issues in the definition of health: Insights from Aboriginal Australia. *Journal of Medicine and Philosophy*, *34*, 49–67.

Buresh, B. & Gordon, S. (2006). *From silence to vice: What nurses must know and must communicate to the public* (2nd ed.), Ithaca, NY: Cornell University Press.

Case Management Advisor (2008). Health plan, medical practice team up on patient-centered medical home pilot. *Case Management Advisor*, *19*(9), 97–108.

Case Management Advisor (2010). Medical home model takes case management to the next level. *Case Management Advisor*, *21*(10), 108–119.

Chassin, M. R., Koesecoff, J., Park, R. E., Winslow, C. M., Kahn, K. L., Merrick, N .J., . . . Brook, R. H. (1987). Does inappropriate use explain geographic variations in the use of healthcare services? A study of three procedures. *Journal of the American Medical Association*, *258*(18), 2533–2537.

Clay, T. (1987). *Nurses: Power and politics*. Oxford, UK: Heinemann Nursing.

Dalton, W. S., Sullivan, D. M., Yeatman, T. J., & Fenstermacher, D. A. (2010). The 2010 Health Care Reform Act: A potential opportunity to advance cancer research by taking cancer personally. *Clinical Cancer Research, 16*(24), 5987–5996. doi: 10.1158/1078-0432.CCR-10-1216

Downie, R. S., Tannahill, C. & Tannahill, A. (1996). *Health promotion: Models and values* (2nd ed.), Oxford, UK: Oxford University Press.

Fairman, J. A., Rowe, J. W., Hassmiller, S., & Shalala, D. E. (2011). Broadening the scope of nursing practice. *The New England Journal of Medicine, 364*(3), 193–196. doi: 10.1056/NEJMP1012121

Fitzpatrick, M. (2001). *The tyranny of health: Doctors and the regulation of lifestyle*. London, UK: Routledge.

Forbat, L., Hubbard, G. & Kearney, N. (2009). Patient and public involvement: Models and muddles. *Journal of Clinical Nursing, 18*, 2547–2554.

Fyffe, T. (2009). Nursing shaping and influencing health and social care policy. *Journal of Nursing Management, 17*, 698–706.

Gigerenzer, G. S. Porter, T. M., Daston, L., Beatty, J. & Kruger, L. (1989). *The empire of chance: How probability changes science and everyday life*. Cambridge, UK: Cambridge University Press.

Goold, S.D. (1996). Allocating healthcare: Cost-utility analysis, informed democratic decision making or the veil of ignorance. *Journal of Health Politics, Policy, and Law, 21*(1), 69–98.

Greider, W. (1992). *Who will tell the people? A betrayal of American Democracy*. New York, NY: Simon and Schuster.

Institute of Medicine [IOM]. (2001). *Crossing the quality chasm: A new health system for the twenty-first century*, Washington, DC: National Academies Press.

Israel, B. A., Coombe, C. M., Cheezum, R. R., Schulz, A. J., McGranaghan, R. J., Lichtenstein, R., . . . Burris, A. (2010). Community-based participatory research: A capacity building approach for policy advocacy aimed at eliminating health disparities. *American Journal of Public Health, 100*(11), 2094–2102.

Johnson, T. (2002). President's pen. *Kansas Nurse, 77*(7), 7.

Johnson, K. A. (2010). Women's health and health reform: Implications of the Patient Protection and Affordable Care Act. *Current Opinions in Obstetrics and Gynecology, 22*, 492–497.

Jones, K., Baggott, R., & Allsop, J. (2004). Influencing the national policy process: The role of health consumer groups. *Health Expectations, 7*, 18–28.

Kennedy, M. S. (2011). The future of nursing: Making waves. *American Journal of Nursing, 111*(2), 14–15.

Luft, H. S. (2007). Universal health care coverage: A potential hybrid solution. *Journal of the American Medical Association, 297*(10), 1115–1118.

Matthews, J. R. (1999). Practice guidelines and tort reform: The legal system confronts the technocratic wish. *Journal of Health Politics, Policy, and Law, 24*(2), 275–304.

McGinnis, J. M., Williams-Russo, P., & Knickman, J. R. (2002). The case for more active policy attention to health promotion. *Health Affairs, 21*(2), 78–93.

Reese, P. P., Caplan, A. L., Bloom, R. B., Abt, P. L., & Karlawish, J. H. (2010). How should we use age to ration healthcare: Lessons from the case of kidney transplantation. *Journal of the American Geriatrics Society, 58*, 1980–1986.

Robert Wood Johnson Foundation (2011). *Future of nursing: Campaign for action: State and national updates by recommendation area*. Center to Champion Nursing in America. Retrieved from http://www.champion nursing.org

Stream, C. & Myers, N. (2010). Risky business: effectiveness of state market-based health programs. *Journal of Health Politics, Policy, and Law, 35*(1), 29–48.

Tones, K., & Tilford, S. (1994). *Health education: Effectiveness, efficiency, and equity* (2nd ed.), London, UK: Chapman & Hall.

Ruger, J. P. (2007). Health, healthcare, and incompletely theorized agreements: A normative theory of health policy decision making. *Journal of Health Politics, Policy, and Law, 32*(1), 51–87.

Sage, W. M. (2010). Will embryonic stem cells change health policy? *Journal of Law, Medicine, and Ethics*, 342–351.

Scottish Executive Health Department [SEHD]. (2001). *Patient focus and public involvement.* Edinburgh, UK: Author.

Sia, C., Tonniges, T., Osterhus, E., & Taba, S. (2004). History of the medical home concept. *Pediatrics, 13,* 1473–1478.

Tritter, J. Q. (2009). Revolution or evolution: The challenges of conceptualizing patient and public involvement in a consumerist world. *Health Expectations, 12,* 275–287.

Vogel, E. M., Burt, S. D., & Church, J. (2010). Case study on nutrition labeling policy-making in Canada. *Canadian Journal of Dietetic Practice and Research, 71*(2), 85–92.

Walt, G. (1994). *Health policy and introduction to process and power.* London, UK: Zed Books.

Whitehead, D. (2003a). Incorporating socio-political health promotion activities in clinical practice, *Journal of Clinical Nursing, 12,* 668–677.

Whitehead, D. (2003b). The health-promoting nurse as a health policy career expert and entrepreneur. *Nurse Education Today, 23,* 585–592.

World Health Organization [WHO]. (2001). *Strengthening nursing and midwifery.* Fifty-fourth World Health Assembly, Agenda item 13.4. WHA 54.12. Retrieved from http://ftp.who.int/gb/archive/pdf_files?WHA54/ea54r12.pdf

For a full suite of assignments and additional learning activities, see the access code at the front of your book.

Index

Figures and tables are indicated by f and t following the page number.